Table of Contents

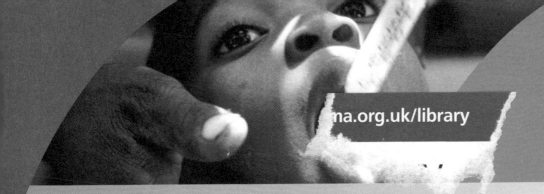

ma.org.uk/library

Essentials of Global Health

Richard Skolnik, MPA
Director of International Programs,
The Population Reference Bureau
Washington, DC

JONES AND BARTLETT PUBLISHERS
Sudbury, Massachusetts
BOSTON   TORONTO   LONDON   SINGAPORE

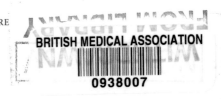

World Headquarters

Jones and Bartlett Publishers
40 Tall Pine Drive
Sudbury, MA 01776
978-443-5000
info@jbpub.com
www.jbpub.com

Jones and Bartlett Publishers
Canada
6339 Ormindale Way
Mississauga, Ontario L5V 1J2
Canada

Jones and Bartlett Publishers
International
Barb House, Barb Mews
London W6 7PA
United Kingdom

Jones and Bartlett's books and products are available through most bookstores and online booksellers. To contact Jones and Bartlett Publishers directly, call 800-832-0034, fax 978-443-8000, or visit our website www.jbpub.com.

Substantial discounts on bulk quantities of Jones and Bartlett's publications are available to corporations, professional associations, and other qualified organizations. For details and specific discount information, contact the special sales department at Jones and Bartlett via the above contact information or send an email to specialsales@jbpub.com.

Production Credits
Publisher: Michael Brown
Production Director: Amy Rose
Associate Production Editor: Rachel Rossi
Associate Editor: Katey Birtcher
Marketing Manager: Sophie H. Fleck
Manufacturing Buyer: Therese Connell
Composition: Shawn Girsberger
Cover Design: Kristin E. Ohlin
Senior Photo Researcher and Photographer: Kimberly Potvin
Associate Photo Researcher and Photographer: Christine McKeen
Illustrations: Louis Ochoa
Printing and Binding: Malloy, Inc.
Cover Printing: John P. Pow Company

Library of Congress Cataloging-in-Publication Data
Skolnik, Richard L.
  Essentials of global health / Richard Skolnik.
      p. ; cm. — (Essential public health)
  Includes bibliographical references and index.
  ISBN-13: 978-0-7637-3421-3 (alk. paper)
  ISBN-10: 0-7637-3421-7 (alk. paper)
  1. World health. 2. Public health—Developing countries. 3. Public health—International cooperation. I. Title. II. Series.
  [DNLM: 1. World Health. 2. Health Services Accessibility. 3. Public Health. WA 530.1 S628e 2008]
  RA441.S56 2008
  362.1—dc22
                    2006100605

6048

Printed in the United States of America
14 13 12 11 10 10 9 8 7 6 5

Part III.   The Burden of Disease

Part IV. Working Together to Improve Global Health

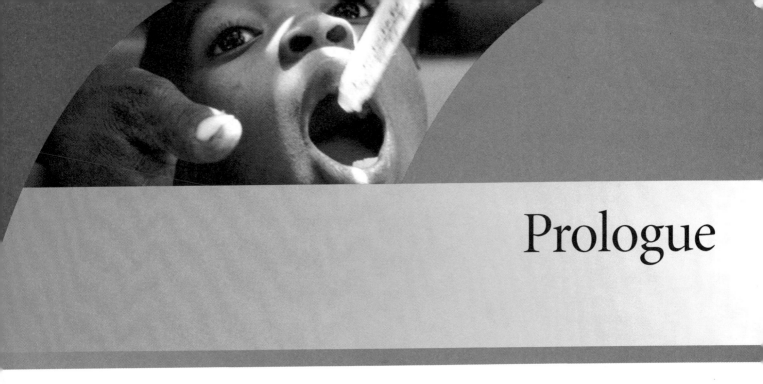

Prologue

The issues of global health have finally entered in the consciousness of the developed world through a unique union of efforts by former Presidents, software pioneers, and rock stars. It is now time that students have a textbook and accompanying casebook that systematically leads them through the issues of global health from basic principles, to the burden of disease, to examples of successful efforts to improve lives and livelihoods.

Richard Skolnik's text, *The Essentials of Global Health*, in addition to Ruth Levine's *Case Studies in Global Health: Millions Saved*, completely and artfully fulfill this need. These authors bring to their writing the clarity of thought and organization of scholars, the excitement of storytellers, and the commitment of activists to making a difference. Their book and casebook take the big picture, population health perspective, building upon classic public health principles and extending them to include the impact of the healthcare system and the relationship of health to social and economic development.

Global health belongs as an integral part of public health education as taught in Schools and Programs in Public Health. In addition, the global health curriculum needs to reach beyond public health students to the future educated citizens who will make a difference in global health such as clinicians, health administrators, lawyers, business executives, academics, and politicians—all of whom will shape the world's future from global trade to international migration to environmental sustainability. Skolnik's and Levine's book and casebook in many ways are designed to ensure that in the future the educated citizenry from Wall Street to Main Street understand public health issues and their impact on all of our lives.

I am proud that Skolnik's and Levine's efforts are part of our *Essential Public Health* series. The materials included in their books have been carefully coordinated with other books in the series to ensure that they utilize the same definitions and terminology. The content of the books has also been coordinated across the series to provide only intended overlap. You will find many of these books key to broadening and deepening your understanding of public health and global health. The full list of materials in the *Essential Public Health* series can be found at http://www.jbpub.com/essentialPublicHealth.

I am confident that you will enjoy learning from the work of Skolnik and Levine. They literally bring to you the world of global health and arrange it before you so it makes sense. The links between health and social and economic development are indisputable and fascinating. You will find an abundance of examples of ways that you can impact global health as part of your career, no matter which direction you head. They take you on an adventurous journey through the world of global health. Enjoy the ride.

Richard Riegelman, MD, MPH, PhD
Series Editor—Essential Public Health

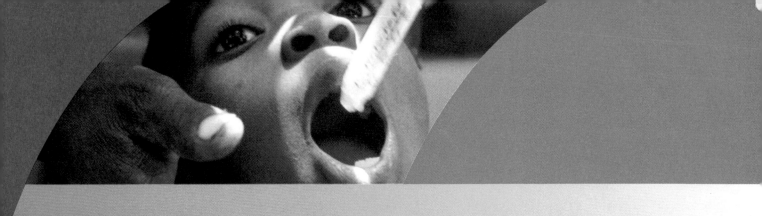

The Essential Public Health Series

Log on to *www.essentialpublichealth.com* for the most current information on availability.

CURRENT AND FORTHCOMING TITLES IN THE ESSENTIAL PUBLIC HEALTH SERIES:

Public Health 101—Healthy People–Healthy Populations—Richard Riegelman, MD, MPH, PhD

Essentials of Public Health—Bernard J. Turnock, MD, MPH

Essential Case Studies in Public Health: Putting Public Health into Practice—Katherine Hunting, PhD, MPH & Brenda L. Gleason, MA, MPH

Essentials of Evidence-Based Public Health—Richard Riegelman, MD, MPH, PhD

Epidemiology 101—Robert H. Friis, PhD

Essentials of Infectious Disease Epidemiology—Manya Magnus, PhD, MPH

Essential Readings in Infectious Disease Epidemiology—Manya Magnus, PhD, MPH

Essentials of Biostatistics in Public Health—Lisa M. Sullivan, PhD (with Workbook: Statistical Computations Using Excel)

Essentials of Public Health Biology: A Guide for the Study of Pathophysiology—Constance Urciolo Battle, MD

Essentials of Environmental Health—Robert H. Friis, PhD

Essentials of Global Health—Richard Skolnik, MPA

Case Studies in Global Health: Millions Saved—Ruth Levine, PhD & the What Works Working Group

Essentials of Health, Culture, and Diversity—Mark Edberg, PhD

Essentials of Health Behavior: Social and Behavioral Theory in Public Health—Mark Edberg, PhD

Essential Readings in Health Behavior: Theory and Practice—Mark Edberg, PhD

Essentials of Health Policy and Law—Joel B. Teitelbaum, JD, LLM & Sara E. Wilensky, JD, MPP

Essential Readings in Health Policy and Law—Joel B. Teitelbaum, JD, LLM & Sara E. Wilensky, JD, MPP

Essentials of Health Economics—Diane M. Dewar, PhD

Essentials of Community Health—Jaime Gofin, MD, MPH & Rosa Gofin, MD, MPH

Essentials of Program Planning and Evaluation—Karen McDonnell, PhD

Essentials of Public Health Communication—Claudia Parvanta, PhD; Patrick Remington, MD, MPH; Ross Brownson, PhD; & David E. Nelson, MD, MPH

Essentials of Public Health Ethics—Ruth Gaare Bernheim, JD, MPH & James F. Childress, PhD

Essentials of Management and Leadership in Public Health—Robert Burke, PhD & Leonard Friedman, PhD, MPH

Essentials of Public Health Preparedness—Rebecca Katz, PhD, MPH

ABOUT THE EDITOR:

Richard K. Riegelman, MD, MPH, PhD, is Professor of Epidemiology-Biostatistics, Medicine, and Health Policy, and founding dean of The George Washington University School of Public Health and Health Services in Washington,

DC. He has taken a lead role in developing the Educated Citizen and Public Health initiative which has brought together arts and sciences and public health education associations to implement the Institute of Medicine of the National Academies' recommendation that ". . .all undergraduates should have access to education in public health." Dr. Riegelman also led the development of George Washington's undergraduate public health major and minor and currently teaches "Public Health 101" and "Epidemiology 101" to undergraduates.

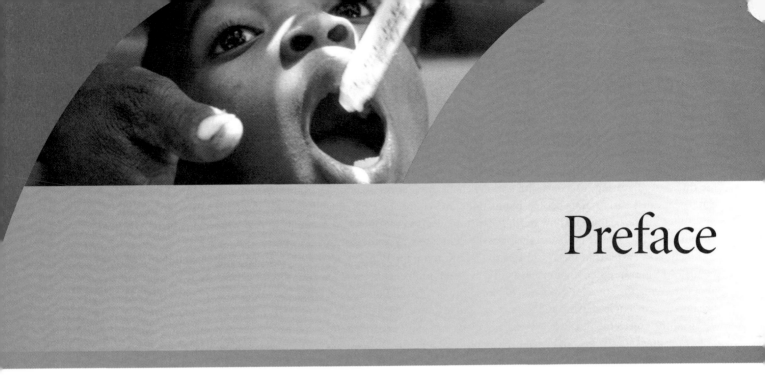

Preface

The preamble to the Constitution of the World Health Organization begins with the words, "The enjoyment of the highest attainable standard of health is one of the fundamental rights of every human being, without distinction of race, religion, political belief, economic or social conditions." In the past century, there has been enormous progress in biomedical science and public health that has truly changed the world and given life to millions of people around the world. If one takes the crudest measure of health, life expectancy at birth—that is, whether one is dead or alive at a given age—it is an astonishing fact that half of all the increase in human life expectancy over recorded time occurred in the 20th century. Can we imagine what it would have meant to have been born in 1900 in India and expected to live on average only 27 years, or in the United States to an age of 48 years? Life expectancy in India is now 61 years for men and 63 years for women, a gain of more than a whole lifetime in 1900 and, in the United States, life expectancy has similarly increased by almost 30 years over the past century.

Yet the highest attainable standard of health has not been realized by the majority of the people on the planet. Life expectancy in the 38 poorest countries of the world is about 49 years, almost the same as that in the United States in 1900. Although life expectancy in every country of the world had increased to over 40 years by 1990, it has tragically fallen since then below that level in 7 countries in Sub-Saharan Africa, largely due to HIV/AIDS. In a dramatic change, infant mortality in the industrialized countries has dropped to 6 per 1000 live births, yet it is greater than 100 per 1000 births in the least developed countries.

The huge disparities in health that exist between countries remain one of the great moral and intellectual problems of our time. This is not surprising, perhaps, when one realizes that about 3 billion people, almost half of the world's population, earn less than $2 a day and 1.2 billion earn less than $1 a day. However, there are enormous disparities in health even within countries, including the United States. A child born in 6 counties of Minnesota will live on average 13 years longer than one born in any of 7 counties in South Dakota, 12 years longer than in Baltimore, Maryland, and 9 years longer than in our nation's capital, Washington, DC. One billion of the six-plus billion people alive today enjoy a long and healthy life. The challenge of global health is to find ways to help the other five billion people live longer, healthier lives. Beyond the challenges posed by any individual disease or health problem, an overarching problem remains the disparities in health and disparities in access to knowledge and effective care and prevention, within and between countries.

From the point of view of health, there is really nowhere on the planet that is remote, and no one from whom we are disconnected. Health problems and disease do not respect national borders. This is an essential principal of global health. In a world of rapid transport, with a million people crossing our borders every day, we are all aware of the threats of a pandemic of communicable diseases and bioterrorism that can spread, as did SARS, to 38 countries in 3 months. Fewer people understand that as advances in medicine and public health increase life expectancy, hopefully in all of the countries of the world, we all increasingly share common risks of heart disease, diabetes, cancer, and mental and neurological illness.

The health problems and solutions of the third world are converging over time with health priorities in the developed world. And because modern scientific advances do translate to new vaccines and treatments, we all are faced with the threat of increasing costs of health and the challenging ethical dilemmas of how the limited resources for health can be allocated fairly among people, populations, and countries. How much is best for preventing disease, the major mission of public health, and how much for treatment of people already sick, the mission of clinical medicine? These are but a few of the huge problems that face the richest as well as the poorest countries.

Why, if the experts in the World Health Organization, the World Bank and the United Nations, and the Departments of Health in every country have not solved the problems in global health, should college students even think about studying the complex problems of global health? I would offer three arguments. The first is that it is precisely because the current leadership and technology and resources have *not* solved the major problems in global health that we need the engagement, creativity, and energy of a new generation, better schooled in science and economics and policy to enter into the field of global health. We need a new generation of idealistic leaders who believe that they can make this a better and more equitable world and who are going to learn what is needed to do so.

Second, there has never before been a single text that students could easily go to learn about what the major problems and issues in global health really are, and this book offers students a remarkable opportunity to explore global health. The final reason is simply my conviction that there is no other area of human endeavor in which the application of thought and resources can make so profound a difference in as many peoples' lives as in the world of health.

Barry R. Bloom
Dean, Harvard School of Public Health
Boston, Massachusetts

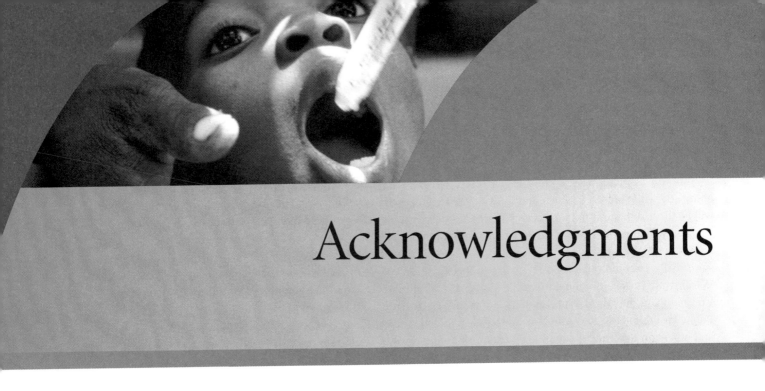

Acknowledgments

Many people graciously assisted me with the preparation of this book. Although I take full responsibility for its contents, it is clear that the book could never have been completed without their help.

Four colleagues prepared initial chapter drafts and were the co-authors of the chapters indicated: Victor Barbiero for Communicable Diseases; Michael Doney for Unintentional Injuries; Heidi Larson for Child Health; and, John Tharakan for Ethics and Human Rights. Victor also provided the Quotable Quotes at the beginning of the book.

A large number of individuals contributed case studies to the book. Florence Baingana prepared the case study on mental health in Uganda in Chapter 12. Sadia Chowdhury provided the case study on oral rehydration in Bangladesh in Chapter 5. Ambar Kulshreshtra prepared the case study of Kerala in Chapter 2. Nancy J. Haselow and Musa Obadiah, assisted by Julia Ross, prepared the case study on vitamin A and Ivermectin in Chapter 5. Peter J. Hotez, Ami Shah Brown, and Kari Stoever provided the case study on the Human Hookworm Vaccine Initiative in Chapter 16. Orin Levine prepared the case study on pneumococcal vaccine that is also in Chapter 16. Andrea Thoumi, a student at Tufts University, provided drafts of the case studies on fistula, the earthquake in Pakistan, refugees in Goma, motorcycle helmets in Taiwan, and speed bumps in Ghana. Andrea also prepared drafts of cases on cataract blindness in India and vitamin A in Nepal, based on *Case Studies in Global Health: Millions Saved*.

A large number of friends and colleagues also reviewed and commented on different book chapters, always adding great value as they did so. These people included:

Ian Anderson, Alan Berg, Florence Baingana, Stephanie Calves, Roger-Mark de Souza, Wafaie Fawzi, Charlotte Feldman-Jacobs, Adrienne Germain, Reuben Granich, Robert Hecht, Judith Justice, James Levinson, Kseniya Lvovsky, Venkatesh Mannar, William McGreevey, Anthony Measham, Tom Merrick, Elaine Murphy, Rachel Nugent, Kris Olson, Ramanan Laxminarayanan, Rudy van Puymbroeck, Richard Southby, Ron Waldman, and Abdo Yazbeck.

Several of my former students at The George Washington University, including Yvonne Orji, Sapna Patel, David Schneider, and Melanie Vant, provided background information for the book and reviewed various book chapters. Pamela Sud, a student at Stanford University, also reviewed a number of chapters.

Andrea Thoumi not only helped me to prepare cases, as noted above, but also provided background materials, help with citations, and reviewed a number of chapters.

Jessica Gottlieb, Molly Kinder, and Ruth Levine of The Center for Global Development were especially helpful to the preparation of this book. I am very grateful to them and to the Center for agreeing to make *Case Studies in Global Health: Millions Saved* the companion reader to my book. In addition, my book includes abbreviated versions of 16 of the 20 cases in *Millions Saved*, 14 of which the Center graciously prepared for me. Jessica, Molly, and Ruth, also reviewed many of the chapters of my book and Jessica Pickett from the Center also commented on a chapter.

Jessica Roeder, my former colleague at the Harvard School of Public Health, was kind enough to take on a second job at night to help me prepare tables and figures.

I am also especially grateful to my daughter, Rachel, who worked with me almost full time for months and assisted in preparing background information, tables, figures, and citations and reviewing and editing each chapter.

The staff of Jones and Bartlett were always helpful and I would especially like to thank Katey Birtcher, Mike Brown, Sophie Fleck, and Rachel Rossi.

My wife, Sophia, was exceptionally gracious in accepting the many months I worked on the book while away from home and while hidden in our home study, to the exclusion of everything else. The dogs were equally forgiving but will be thrilled that this has now been published and I can go back to playing with them a lot more.

Barry Bloom, the Dean of the Harvard School of Public Health, was kind enough to prepare the preface for this book, for which I am very appreciative.

Finally, I should offer a special thanks to Richard Riegelman. He is a Professor of Epidemiology at The George Washington University School of Public Health and Health Services, and the Founding Dean of that school. When I retired from the World Bank, he was kind enough to give me the opportunity to join the faculty of the School of Public Health at George Washington and to teach undergraduates there. He then gave me a chance to work with him and others on the Undergraduate Curriculum Committee, which was an enormously enjoyable experience for me, as we helped to build an undergraduate program in public health. He tirelessly helped me develop, prepare, and review the book.

About the Author

Richard Skolnik has worked more than 30 years in education, health, and development. At the time this book was completed, Mr. Skolnik was the director of International Programs at the Population Reference Bureau in Washington, DC.

Prior to that post, Mr. Skolnik spent almost 2 years as the executive director of the President's Emergency Plan for AIDS Relief at the Harvard School of Public Health.

From 2001 until late 2004, Mr. Skolnik was at The George Washington University, where he was the Director of the Center for Global Health, taught an undergraduate course on global health for seven semesters, and supervised Master of Public Health degree projects each semester.

From 1976 to 2001, Mr. Skolnik worked at the World Bank and for his last 15 years there he managed important components of the Bank's health and education portfolios. He has extensive experience in basic education, nutrition, reproductive health, child health, infectious disease control, and health systems development. He has been involved in country level work in these areas in Africa, East Asia, Europe, Latin America, the Caribbean, the Middle East, and South Asia.

Mr. Skolnik has also participated extensively in policy-making and program development at the international level. He was deeply involved in the establishment of the STOP TB program and served three rounds on the Technical Review Panel of the Global Fund to Fight Against AIDS, TB, and Malaria. He led independent evaluations of the International AIDS Vaccine Initiative and of the Global Alliance for the Elimination of Leprosy. He has also served on WHO working and advisory groups on DOTS expansion, TB/HIV co-infection, public and private partnerships for TB control, and follow-up to the Commission on Macroeconomics and Health.

Mr. Skolnik received a Bachelor of Arts degree from Yale University and a Master of Public Affairs degree from the Woodrow Wilson School of Princeton University. At Yale, he participated in the Five Year BA Program and spent 1 year teaching high school science in Laoag City in the Philippines, living with the same family with which he had earlier lived as a high school exchange student. Upon graduation from Yale, he was selected for a fellowship from the Yale-China Association and spent 2 years teaching at the Chinese University of Hong Kong. In between his 2 years at the Woodrow Wilson School, Mr. Skolnik was a Research Fellow at the Institute of Southeast Asian Studies in Singapore and, as part of that activity, published a monograph on education and training in Singapore.

Mr. Skolnik has studied and learned to varying degrees French, Spanish, Cantonese, Mandarin, Ilocano, and Tagalog.

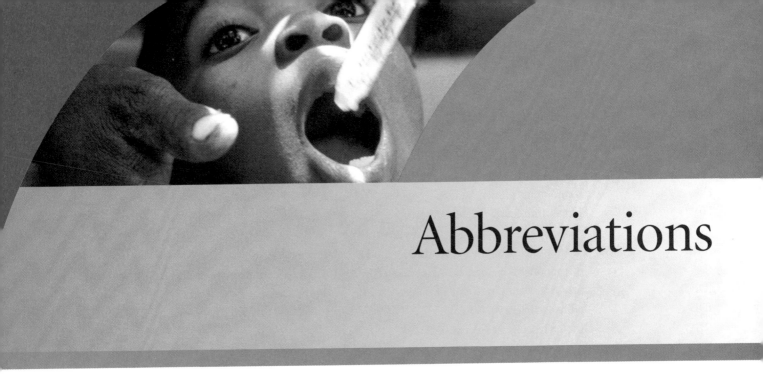

Abbreviations

TERM	DEFINITION
AIDS	Acquired Immune Deficiency Syndrome
ADB	Asian Development Bank
AfDB	African Development Bank
APOC	African Programme for Onchocerciasis Control
ARI	Acute Respiratory Infection
ART	Antiretroviral Therapy
AusAID	Australian Agency for International Development
BCG	Bacillus Calmette-Guérin (The Tuberculosis Vaccine)
BMI	Body Mass Index
BOD	Burden of Disease
CDC	The U.S. Centers for Disease Control and Prevention
CFR	Case Fatality Ratio
CHE	Complex Humanitarian Emergency
CIDA	Canadian International Development Agency
CMR	Crude Mortality Rate
CVD	Cardiovascular Disease
DALY	Disability-Adjusted Life Year
DANIDA	Danish International Development Agency
DFID	Department for International Development of the United Kingdom
DHS	Demographic and Health Survey
DPT	Diptheria, Pertussis, and Tetanus Vaccine
EPI	Expanded Program on Immunization
EU	European Union
FAO	Food and Agriculture Organization of the United Nations
FSU	Former Soviet Union
GAVI	Global Alliance for Vaccines and Immunization

GDP	Gross Domestic Product
GNP	Gross National Product
GOBI	Growth Monitoring, Oral Rehydration, Breastfeeding, and Immunization
HALE	Health Adjusted Life Expectancy
Hib	Haemophilus influenzae type b
HIV	Human Immunodeficiency Virus
IAVI	International AIDS Vaccine Initiative
IBRD	International Bank for Reconstruction and Development (World Bank)
IDA	International Development Association (the "soft" lending window of the World Bank)
IDB	Inter-American Development Bank
IDD	Iodine Deficiency Disorder
IDP	Internally Displaced Person
IEC	Information, Education, and Communication
IHD	Ischemic Heart Disease
IMCI	Integrated Management of Childhood Illness
IMF	International Monetary Fund
IMR	Infant Mortality Rate
IPV	Injectable Polio Vaccine
IQ	Intelligence Quotient
IPT	Intermittent Preventive Treatment
IRB	Institutional Review Board
ITI	International Trachoma Initiative
ITN	Insecticide-Treated Net
IUD	Intrauterine Device
LMICs	Low- and Middle-Income Countries
MCH	Maternal and Child Health
MDG	Millennium Development Goal
MDT	Multi-Drug Therapy
MI	The Micronutrient Initiative
MMR	Maternal Mortality Rate
MSF	Doctors Without Borders (Médicins Sans Frontières in French)
NCD	Non-Communicable Disease
NGO	Non-Governmental Organization
NID	National Immunization Day
NNMR	Neonatal Mortality Rate
OCP	Onchocerciasis Control Program
OPV	Oral Polio Vaccine
ORS	Oral Rehydration Solution
ORT	Oral Rehydration Therapy
PAHO	Pan American Health Organization
PDP	Product Development Partnership
PEPFAR	President's Emergency Plan for AIDS Relief
PHC	Primary Health Care
PMTCT	Prevention of Mother-to-Child-Transmission

PPP	Public-Private Partnership
RBM	Roll Back Malaria
RTI	Road Traffic Injury
SIDA	Swedish International Development Cooperation Agency
STI	Sexually Transmitted Infection
SWAp	Sector-Wide Approach
TB	Tuberculosis
TBA	Traditional Birth Attendant
TFR	Total Fertility Rate
TRIPS	Agreement on Trade-Related Aspects of Intellectual Property Rights
TT	Tetanus Toxoid
UN	United Nations
UNAIDS	United Nations Program on HIV/AIDS
UNDP	United Nations Development Program
UNFPA	United Nations Family Planning Association
UNICEF	United Nations Children's Fund
USAID	United States Agency for International Development
WFP	World Food Program
WHA	World Health Assembly of the World Health Organization
WHO	World Health Organization
WHO/TDR	WHO Special Programme for Research and Training in Tropical Diseases
WFP	World Food Program
WTO	World Trade Organization
YLD	Years Lived with Disability
YLL	Years of Life Lost

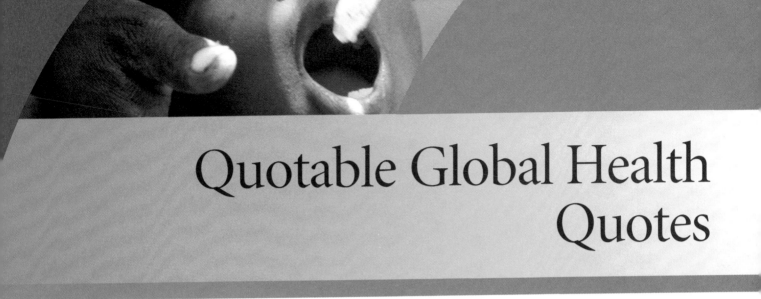

Quotable Global Health Quotes

Health is a state of complete physical, mental and social well-being and not merely the absence of disease or infirmity. The enjoyment of the highest attainable standard of health is one of the fundamental rights of every human being without distinction of race, religion, political belief, economic or social condition.

World Health Organization

Public health (. . .) represents an organised response to the protection and promotion of human health and encompasses a concern with the environment, disease control, the provision of health care, health education and health promotion.

Research Unit in Health and Behavioural Change, University of Edinburgh

Public health is the science and art of promoting health. It does so based on the understanding that health is a process engaging social, mental, spiritual and physical well-being. Public health acts on the knowledge that health is a fundamental resource to the individual, to the community and to society as a whole and must be supported by soundly investing in living conditions that create, maintain and protect health.

Ilona Kickbusch

Prevention is better than cure.

Desiderius Erasmus

Every patient carries her or his own doctor inside.

Albert Schweitzer

The doctor of the future will give no medicine, but will interest her or his patients in the care of the human frame, in a proper diet, and in the cause and prevention of disease.

Thomas A. Edison

Of all forms of inequality, injustice in health care is the most shocking and inhumane.

Martin Luther King, Jr.

It is health that is real wealth and not pieces of gold and silver.

Mohandas K. (Mahatma) Gandhi

. . . class differences in health represent a double injustice: life is short where its quality is poor.

Richard G. Wilkinson

Where once it was the physician who waged bellum contra morbum, the war against disease, now it's the whole society.

Susan Sontag

Health consists of having the same diseases as one's neighbors.

Quentin Crisp

Be careful about reading health books. You may die of a misprint.

Mark Twain

Introduction

Why should we care about the health of other people, especially that of people in other countries? Why should global health matter to those who live in Australia, France, the United States, or other developed countries? Actually, for a number of critical reasons, the health of people everywhere must be a growing concern for all of us.

First, diseases do not respect boundaries. Human Immunodeficiency Virus (HIV) has spread worldwide. A person with tuberculosis can infect 15 people a year, wherever they are. The West Nile Virus came from Egypt but occurs today in many countries. In addition, there is an important risk of a worldwide epidemic of influenza. Clearly, the health of each of us increasingly depends on the health of others.

Second, there is an ethical dimension to the health and well-being of other people. Many children in poor countries get sick and die needlessly from malnutrition or from diseases that are preventable and curable. Many adults in poor countries die because they lack access to medicines that are customarily available to people in rich countries. Is this just? Are we prepared to accept such deaths without taking steps to prevent them?

Third, health is closely linked with economic and social development in an increasingly interdependent world. Children who suffer from malnutrition may not reach their full mental potential and may not enroll in or stay in school. Sick children from developing countries are less likely than healthy children to become productive adults who can contribute to the economic standing of their family, community, or country. Adults who suffer from AIDS, tuberculosis, malaria, and other diseases lose income while they are sick and out of work, which is a major contributor to keeping their families in an endless cycle of poverty.

Finally, the health and well-being of people everywhere has important implications for global security and freedom. High rates of HIV are having a destabilizing impact on some countries, as more teachers and health workers die than are being trained, and as there are increasingly insufficient numbers of rural workers to grow and harvest crops. Outbreaks of other diseases, such as cholera, the plague, and SARS (Severe Acute Respiratory Syndrome), for example, threaten people's ability to engage freely in economic pursuits. The 1991 outbreak of cholera in Peru cost that country about $1 billion, the plague in 1994 cost India about $2 billion, and SARS in Asia in 2003 cost the economies of Asia a staggering $18 billion in lost economic activity.

Indeed, these factors have caused an increasing interest in health within universities and a growing call for all university students to study health from a global perspective. The aim of this book is to examine the most critical global health topics in a clear and engaging manner. The book will provide the reader with an overview of the importance of global health in the context of development, an examination of the most important global health issues and their economic and social consequences, and a discussion of some of the steps that are being taken to address these concerns. It will also provide numerous cases of "success stories" in dealing with important global health problems.

This book is intended to provide an introduction to global health for all students. This includes students who have never studied public health before and who will not take additional public health courses. It also includes those students, whether they have studied public health before or not, who may wish to pursue additional studies in public health later.

This book is largely based on an undergraduate course on global health that I taught for seven semesters at The George Washington University in Washington, DC. The text seeks to "speak" to the reader in a manner one would find in an exciting and motivating classroom. In addition to covering key concepts in global health and frameworks for the analysis of global health issues, this book also contains numerous examples of on-the-ground experiences in addressing key global health problems. Those students who want to explore case studies in greater depth can read the companion volume to this textbook, *Case Studies in Global Health: Millions Saved.*

Very few introductory materials on global health are available to students or their professors. Hopefully, this book will help to close that gap by providing a foundation for enhanced studies in public health, global health, and economic and social development.

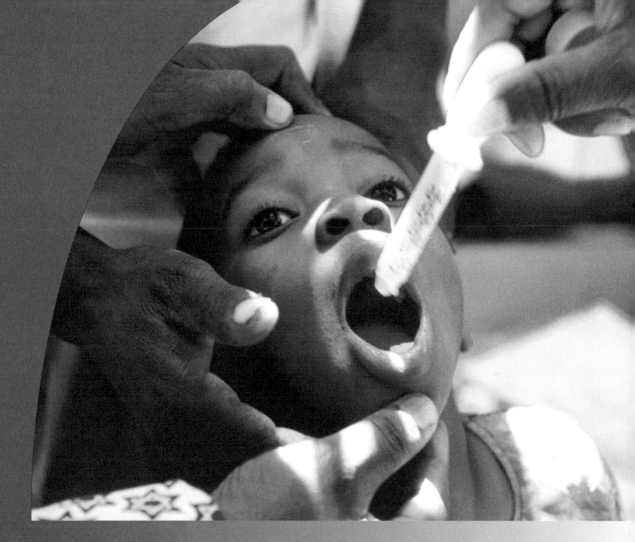

PART I

Principles, Measurements, and the Health–Development Link

CHAPTER 1

The Principles and Goals of Global Health

LEARNING OBJECTIVES

By the end of this chapter the reader will be able to:

- Define the terms *health, public health,* and *global health*
- Discuss some examples of public health efforts
- Discuss some examples of global health activities
- Describe some of the guiding principles of public health work
- Describe the Millennium Development Goals and their relation to global health
- Briefly discuss the global effort to eradicate smallpox

VIGNETTES

Laurie Smith lived in Portsmouth, Virginia, in the United States. She was fifty years old and had always been healthy. Last weekend, she woke up with a headache, a high fever, and a very stiff neck. Laurie was so sick that she went to the emergency room of the local hospital. The physicians diagnosed Laurie as having meningitis, an inflammation of the membrane around the brain and spinal cord,[1] that was caused by West Nile virus. This virus originated in Egypt in the 1930s and is transmitted by a mosquito. Over a number of decades, West Nile virus spread from Egypt to the Middle East, Africa, and Asia. In 1999, the first cases appeared in the United States, and it is now found throughout the United States, as shown in Figure 1-1.[2]

By 2005, polio was on the verge of being eradicated from every country. That year, however, rumors circulated in northern Nigeria that the polio vaccine was causing sterilization. In response to these rumors, some community leaders discouraged people from immunizing their children. Within months, polio cases began to appear in the area.

Shortly thereafter, polio cases spread from northern Nigeria to Sudan, Yemen, and Indonesia. The global campaign to eradicate polio had been dealt a major blow, stemming partly from rumors in one country about the alleged side effects of the vaccine.[3]

Getachew is a 20-year-old Ethiopian with HIV. His disease is advanced, but he receives no treatment for it. He has tuberculosis (TB) and much of his mouth is coated with a white, pasty yeast called thrush. He has lost more than 20% of his body weight. He stopped going to work some time ago, has no money, and is totally dependent on his family for care and day-to-day needs. Getachew is one of about 1.7 million people in Ethiopia with HIV.[4] In fact, in 2005 about 39 million people were living with HIV worldwide.[5] There are countries in Africa, such as Botswana and Lesotho, in which about 25% of their adults are HIV positive and Swaziland, in which almost a third of the adults are HIV positive.[6] There are communities in Africa in which more teachers are dying than are being trained. There are farms in the same areas that cannot be cared for because there are too few healthy farm workers. Some communities are collapsing socially and economically from the burden of HIV and HIV poses a threat to security throughout the world.

Jim Smith is a high school student in London, England. Early in the school year, he had a fever and cough that would not go away. He did not feel like eating. He slept badly and woke up every morning in a sweat. Jim had TB. Although many people think that TB has been eliminated from high-income countries, it has not. Rather, the spread of HIV has triggered an increase in TB worldwide. In addition, immigration is helping to spread the disease from

FIGURE 1-1 The Spread of West Nile Virus in the United States, 1999–2005

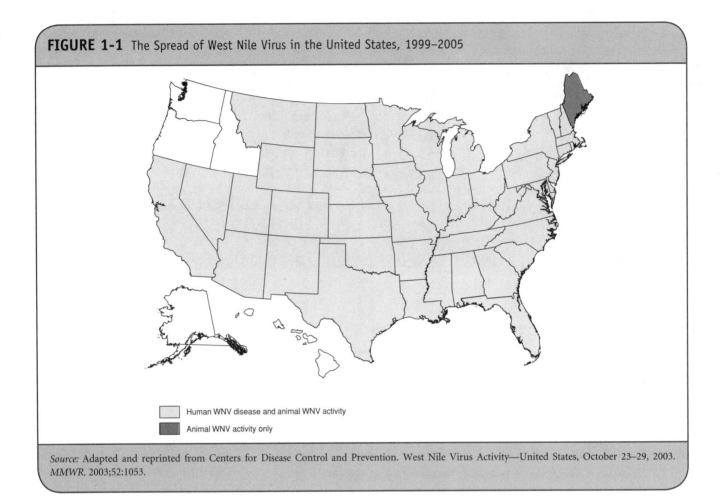

Human WNV disease and animal WNV activity

Animal WNV activity only

Source: Adapted and reprinted from Centers for Disease Control and Prevention. West Nile Virus Activity—United States, October 23–29, 2003. *MMWR.* 2003;52:1053.

lower-income to higher-income countries. In fact, there are urban areas of the United Kingdom in which the rates of TB are higher than the rates in some low- and middle-income countries.[7]

WHY STUDY GLOBAL HEALTH

Over the last fifty years, the world has made significant progress in improving human health. Since 1950, for example, the death rate of children under five years has fallen from 148 deaths per 1000 children to fewer than 60 deaths per 1000 children. During that same period, the average life expectancy in developing countries has increased from 40 years to 65 years.[8] Smallpox has been eradicated, polio has been nearly eliminated, and great progress has been made in reducing the burden of vaccine-preventable diseases in children and of parasitic infections, such as guinea worm. One reason to study global health is to gain a better understanding of the progress made so far in addressing global health problems.

Another reason to study global health, however, is to understand better the most important global health chal-

lenges that remain and what must be done to address them most effectively. Despite the important progress in improving human health:

- 10,000 babies die every day in the world before they are four weeks old[9]
- 529,000 women a year die in childbirth[9]
- More than 750,000 children die every year of measles[10]
- 1.6 million people die in the world every year of TB[10]

In addition, the world is shrinking and the health of people everywhere must be of concern to all of us. This is particularly important because many diseases are not limited by national boundaries. Tuberculosis, HIV, and polio, for example, can spread from one country to the next. Dengue fever used to be concentrated in Southeast Asia but cases are now seen in many more countries as shown in Figure 1-2.[11] The "avian flu" first appeared in East Asia but it, too, is spreading to other regions. Ten years ago, no one in the neighborhood of Laurie, mentioned in the vignette, ever thought of getting West Nile virus.

Besides the central global health challenges noted above, there are also exceptional disparities in the health of some groups compared to the health of others. Life expectancy in Japan, for example, is about 82 years but it is only 52 years in Haiti.[12] In addition, there are a number of life saving technologies that have been used in high-income countries for many years that are not yet in use in low-income countries, such as the hepatitis B vaccine. In fact, the previous points raise important ethical and humanitarian questions about the extent to which people everywhere should be concerned about disparities in access to health services and in health status.

The important link between health and development is another reason to pay particular attention to global health. Poor health of mothers is linked to poor health of babies and the failure of children to reach their full mental and physical potential. In addition, ill health of children can delay their entry into school and can affect their attendance at school, their performance in school, and, therefore, their future economic prospects. Countries with major health problems, such as high rates of malaria or HIV, have difficulty attracting the investments needed to develop their economy. Moreover, having large numbers of badly nourished, unhealthy, and ill-educated people in any country is destabilizing and a health, economic, and security threat to all countries.

The nature of many global health concerns and the need for different actors to work together to address them are more reasons why we should be concerned with global health. Although locally relevant solutions are needed to address most health problems, some health issues can only be solved using a global approach. In addition, some problems, such as ensuring access to drugs to treat HIV, require more financial resources than any individual country can provide. Still other global health issues require technical cooperation across countries because few countries themselves have the technical capacity to deal with them. Global cooperation might be needed, for example, to establish standards for drug safety, to set protocols for the treatment of certain health problems, such as malaria, or to develop an AIDS vaccine that could serve the needs of low-income countries.

The concepts and concerns of global health are also becoming increasingly prominent worldwide. The spread of

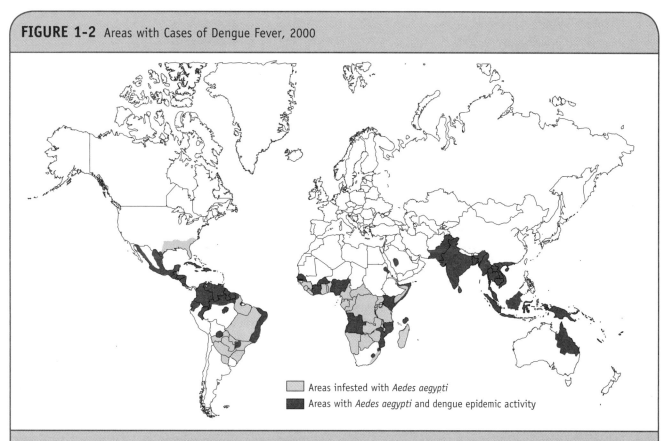

FIGURE 1-2 Areas with Cases of Dengue Fever, 2000

Areas infested with *Aedes aegypti*
Areas with *Aedes aegypti* and dengue epidemic activity

Source: Adapted and reprinted from Centers for Disease Control and Prevention. Dengue Fever. Available at: http://www.cdc.gov/ncidod/dvbid/dengue/map-distribution-2000.htm. Accessed June 11, 2005.

HIV, the SARS scare, and the fear of the avian flu have all brought attention to global health. As you will read about later in the book, the advocacy efforts of Doctors Without Borders and the rock star Bono, the establishment of the Millennium Development Goals, and the philanthropy of the Bill & Melinda Gates Foundation have also dramatically raised attention to global health. The topic has become so important that there is a push in many universities throughout the world to ensure that all students have a basic understanding of key global health issues.

HEALTH, PUBLIC HEALTH, AND GLOBAL HEALTH

Health

Before starting our review of global health in greater detail, it will be helpful to establish a set of definitions for *health*, *public health*, and *global health* that can be used throughout this book. Most of us think of "health" from our individual perspective as "not being sick." The World Health Organization, however, set out a broader definition of health in 1948 that is still widely used:

> "Health is a state of complete physical, mental and social well-being and not merely the absence of disease or infirmity."[13]

This is the definition of "health" used in this book.

Public Health

While the WHO concept of "health" refers first to individuals, this book is mostly about "public health" and the health of populations. C.E.A Winslow, considered to be the founder of modern public health in the United States, formulated a definition of public health in 1923 that is still commonly used today. In his definition, public health is:

TABLE 1-1 Selected Examples of Public Health Activities

- The promotion of hand washing
- The promotion of bicycle and motorcycle helmets
- The promotion of knowledge about HIV/AIDS
- Large scale screening for diabetes and hypertension
- Large scale screening for the eyesight of school children
- Mass dosing of children against worms
- The operation of a supplementary feeding program for poorly nourished young children

Source: The Author.

. . . the science and the art of preventing disease, prolonging life, and promoting physical health and mental health and efficiency through organized community efforts toward a sanitary environment; the control of community infections; the education of the individual in principles of personal hygiene; the organization of medical and nursing service for the early diagnosis and treatment of disease; and the development of the social machinery to ensure to every individual in the community a standard of living adequate for the maintenance of health.[14]

According to Winslow's definition, some examples of public health activities would include the development of a campaign to promote child immunization in a particular country, an effort to get people in a city to use seat belts when they drive, and actions to get people in a specific setting to eat healthier foods and to stop smoking. In addition, most levels of government also carry out certain public health functions. These include the management of a public health clinic, the operation of a public health laboratory, and the maintenance of a disease surveillance system. Other examples are shown in Table 1-1.

There are a number of guiding principles to the practice of public health that have been articulated, for example, by the American Public Health Association in its "Public Health Code of Ethics."[15] These principles focus on prevention of disease, respect for the rights of individuals, and a commitment to developing public health efforts in conjunction with communities. They also highlight the need to pay particular attention to disenfranchised people and communities and to working in public health on the basis of data and evidence. In addition, they note the importance of taking account of a wide range of disciplines and appreciation for the values, beliefs, and cultures of diverse groups. Finally, they put considerable emphasis on engaging in public health practice in a way that "enhances the physical and social environment" and that builds on collaborations across public health actors. These themes are at the foundation of this book and will recur throughout it.

Many people confuse "public health" and "medicine," although they have quite different approaches. Table 1-2 outlines these differences.[16] To a large extent, the biggest difference between the medical approach and the public health approach is the focus in public health on the health of populations rather than on the health of individuals. Exaggerating somewhat for effect, we could say, for example, that a physician cares for an individual patient whom he immunizes

TABLE 1-2 Approaches of Public Health and Medicine

Differentiating factors	Public Health	Medicine
Focus	Population	Individual
Ethical Basis	Public service	Personal service
Emphasis	Disease prevention and health promotion for communities	Disease diagnosis, treatment, and care for individuals
Interventions	Broad spectrum that may target the environment, human behavior, lifestyle, and medical care	Emphasis on medical care

Source: Modified with permission from Harvard School of Public Health. About HSPH: Distinctions Between Public Health and Medicine. Available at: www.hsph.harvard.edu/about.html#publichealth. Accessed May 27, 2006.

against a particular disease, while a public health specialist is likely to focus on how one ensures that the whole community gets vaccinated. A physician will counsel an individual patient on the need to exercise and avoid obesity; a public health specialist will work with a program meant to help a community stay sufficiently active to avoid obesity. In addition, there are branches of public health, such as epidemiology, that focus specifically on studying patterns and causes of disease in specific populations and the application of this information to controlling health problems.[17] Finally, we should note the exceptional attention which public health approaches pay to prevention of health problems.

Global Health

What exactly is *global health*? The United States Institute of Medicine defined global health as "health problems, issues, and concerns that transcend national boundaries and may best be addressed by cooperative actions . . ."[18]

Another group defined what we would now call global health as "the application of the principles of public health to health problems and challenges that transcend national boundaries and to the complex array of global and local forces that affect them."[19]

An important point concerning the study of global health is that it implies that one considers health problems from a global perspective, rather than from the point of view of any individual country. In addition, the phrase "global health" implies that countries work together not only to understand critical health issues but also to solve them. To a large extent, the expression "global health" has replaced the term "international health."[14]

Some examples of important global health concerns would include: the factors that contribute to women dying of pregnancy-related causes in so many countries; the exceptional amount of malnutrition among young children, especially in South Asia and Africa; the burden of different infectious and non-communicable diseases worldwide and what can be done to control those diseases. The impact of the environment on health globally and the effects of natural disasters and conflicts are also important to global health. Other significant global health issues include how countries can organize and manage their health systems to enable the healthiest population they can attain with the resources avail-

TABLE 1-3 Selected Examples of Global Health Issues

- The number of low birthweight babies being born
- The high rates of death of babies in the first month of life
- Measles in young children
- Diarrhea and pneumonia in young children
- The health of HIV/AIDS orphans
- Sexually-transmitted infections in young women
- Violence against women
- TB
- Malaria
- HIV/AIDS
- Parasitic infections, such as hookworm
- The rapid increase in diabetes and heart disease

Source: The Author.

able to them; the search for new technologies to improve important global health problems; and, how different actors can work together to solve health problems that are too significant for any country or actor to solve on their own. Another global health matter of importance would be the relationship between globalization and the health of different communities. Some additional global health issues of importance are shown in Table 1-3.

CRITICAL GLOBAL HEALTH CONCEPTS

In order to understand and to help address key global health issues like those noted previously, there are a number of concepts concerning global health with which one must be familiar. Some of the most important include:

- The determinants of health
- The measurement of health status
- The importance of culture to health
- The global burden of disease
- The key risk factors for different health conditions
- The demographic and epidemiologic transitions
- The organization and functions of health systems

It is also essential to understand the links between health and education and health, equity, poverty, and development.

Building on the previous concepts, those interested in global health also need to have an understanding of how key health issues affect different parts of the world and the world as a whole. These include:

- Environmental health
- Nutrition
- Reproductive health
- Child health
- Infectious diseases
- Non-communicable diseases
- Injuries

Finally, it is important to understand global health issues that are generally addressed through cooperation. Some of these concern conflicts, natural disasters, and humanitarian emergencies. Others relate to the mechanisms by which different actors in global health activities work together to solve global health problems. Harnessing the power of science and technology to serve global health needs also requires cooperation.

THE OBJECTIVES OF THE BOOK

This book aims to introduce readers, in a clear and simple manner, to the most important issues and concepts related to global health, as outlined previously. It provides an introduction to global health for people who have little or no previous exposure to this field. At the same time, it is intended to set a foundation for those who may pursue additional course work and professional activities in public health, global health, medicine, or development.

THE ORGANIZATION OF THE BOOK

This book is organized in several parts that closely follow the topics mentioned previously. Part I introduces the reader to the basic principles of global health, key measures of health, and the concepts of the health and the development link. Chapter 1 introduces readers to some key principles, themes, and goals of global health. Chapter 2 examines the determinants of health, how health is measured, and how health conditions change over time and as countries develop economically. Chapter 3 looks at the links between health and development, touching upon the connections between health and education, equity, and poverty.

Part II reviews cross-cutting themes in global health. Chapter 4 examines human rights and ethical issues in global health. Chapter 5 covers health systems. This chapter reviews the purpose and goals of health systems and how different countries have organized their health systems. The chapter also reviews the key challenges that health systems face, the costs and consequences of those challenges, and how some countries have addressed health system challenges. Culture plays an extremely important part in health, and Chapter 6 examines the links between culture and health. This chapter reviews the importance of culture to health, how health is perceived in different groups, the manner in which different culture groups seek health care and engage in health practices, and how one can promote change in health behavior.

Part III reviews the most important causes of illness, disability, and death, particularly in low- and middle-income countries. The chapters in this part of the book will examine environmental issues, nutrition, reproductive health, and child health. The book then looks at infectious diseases, non-communicable diseases, and unintentional injuries.

Part IV examines how cooperative action can address global health issues. Chapter 14 reviews the impact on health of conflicts, natural disasters, and other health emergencies. Chapter 15 examines how different actors in the global health field work both individually and cooperatively to address key global health problems. Finally, Chapter 16 reviews how science and technology have helped to improve public health and how further advances in science and technology could help to address some of the most important global health challenges that remain.

Each chapter follows a similar outline. The chapters begin with vignettes that relate to the topic to be covered and which are intended to make the topic "real" for the reader. Some of these vignettes are not true in the literal sense. However, each of them is based on real events that occur regularly in the countries discussed in this book. Most chapters then explain key concepts, terms, and definitions. The chapters that deal with cross-cutting issues in the second and fourth parts of the book then examine the importance of the topic to enhancing global health, some key challenges in further improving global health, and what can be done to address those challenges.

The chapters that focus on health conditions look at the importance of the topic to the burden of disease, key issues related to this cause of illness, disability, and death, and the costs and consequences of these issues for individuals, communities, and the world. These chapters then examine what has been learned about how to deal with these health burdens in the most cost-effective ways, the future challenges in each of these areas, and some specific cases of successful efforts at addressing such challenges.

Most chapters contain several case studies. Some of these deal with well-known cases that have already proven to be models for global health efforts. Others, however, are based on experiences that show good promise, both for success and for providing lessons, but which have not yet proven themselves.

Each chapter concludes with a summary of the main messages in the chapter and a set of study questions that can assist the reader in reviewing the materials included in the chapter. Each chapter also contains endnotes with citations for the data that is used in the book. The book does not contain any additional lists of reference materials. Those wishing to explore topics in greater depth will find ample suggestions for additional reading in the endnotes.

The reader should note that the chapters are not in order of importance. Nutrition, for example, is fundamental to all health concerns. However, it only makes sense to cover nutrition in this book after establishing the context for studying global health and after covering some cross-cutting global health issues. In addition, you will note that there is no chapter called "globalization and health." Rather, you will find that the relationships between globalization and health are integrated into all of the chapters.

THE PERSPECTIVE OF THE BOOK

The book will take a global perspective to all that it covers. Although the book includes many country case studies, topics will be examined from the perspective of the world as a whole. The book also pays particular attention to the links between poverty and health and the relationship between health and equity. Special attention will also be given to gender and to ethnicity and their relation to health. Another theme that runs through the book is the connection between health and development.

The book follows the point of view that health is a human right. The book is written with the presumption that governments have an obligation to try to ensure that all of their people have access to an affordable package of healthcare services and that all people are protected from the costs of ill health. The book is also based on the premise, however, that the development of a health system by any country, as discussed further in Chapter 5, is inextricably linked to the value system and the political structure of that country.[20]

The book covers key global health topics, including those that affect developed and developing countries; however, the book pays particular attention to developing countries and to poor people within them. The rationale for this is that improving health status indicators within and across countries can only be accomplished if the health of the poor and other disadvantaged groups is improved. In addition, the idea of social justice is at the core of public health. The basic tenet of social justice in relation to health "is that the knowledge obtained on how to ensure a healthy population must be extended equally to all groups in any society . . ."[14]

SOME KEY TERMS

The book will often speak of "developed countries" and "developing countries." These terms are not precise. "Developed countries" are those, such as the United States, France, Australia, and the United Kingdom, that have relatively high income per capita and that are often thought of as "industrialized." "Developing countries" are those, such as Haiti, Liberia, Laos, and Papua New Guinea, that have relatively low per capita incomes and that are not heavily industrialized.

Although the book will use the terms "developed" and "developing countries," it will also use the terms "low-income," "middle-income," and "high-income" to refer to countries. These terms will follow the definitions used by the World Bank, which divides countries into four income groups, based on their gross national income per person (see Table 1-4):[21]

- $825 or less—low-income
- $826 to $3255—lower middle-income
- $3256 to $10,065—upper middle-income
- $10,066 or above—high-income

Much of the data discussed in this book will be broken down by the geographic regions used by the World Bank.

- East Asia and the Pacific
- Europe and Central Asia
- Latin America and the Caribbean
- Middle East and North Africa
- South Asia
- Sub-Saharan Africa

Occasionally, however, data will be discussed according to the regions that are used by the World Health Organization. For comparative purposes, data is sometimes also shown for high-income countries that belong to the Organization for Economic Cooperation and Development (OECD).

THE MILLENNIUM DEVELOPMENT GOALS

This book will make continuous references to the Millennium Development Goals (MDGs). The MDGs were formulated in 2000 at the United Nations Millennium Summit and were articulated in the Millennium Declaration.[22] There are 8 MDGs and 15 core targets that relate to them. The countries that signed the declaration pledged to meet the MDGs by 2015. Keeping the MDGs in mind as you read this book is important because the MDGs are an explicit statement of the goals that many countries have set for an important part of their development efforts and, therefore, are an important part of the context for understanding global health issues. The MDGs and their related targets are noted in Table 1-5.

As you can see, all eight of the MDGs relate to health. The goals of reducing child mortality, improving maternal heath, and combating HIV/AIDS, malaria, and other diseases directly concern health. However, each of the other goals also relates to health. Hunger and poverty, referred to in goal 1, are intimately linked with health status, both as causes of ill

health and as consequences of ill health. The goal of universal primary education can only be met if children are well enough nourished and healthy enough to enroll in school, attend school, and have a good capacity to learn while they are there. As you will read throughout the book, the gender disparities referred to in goal 3 are central to the health issues that affect women globally, many of which relate to their lack of empowerment. Goal 7 is meant to address the need for safe water and sanitation, the lack of which is a major cause of ill health and death. The last chapter of the book discusses how different actors in global health can work together to help countries improve health status, as indicated in goal 8 on partnerships for development.

ADDITIONAL COMMENTS ON THE CASE STUDIES

Many of the case studies in this book were provided by the Center for Global Development and are elaborated upon further in a companion piece to this book entitled *Case Studies in Global Health: Millions Saved*.[8] That book provides detailed case studies of 20 successful interventions in global health. The cases were carefully selected on the basis of five selection criteria: scale, importance, impact, duration, and cost-effectiveness. When considered together, the cases suggest a number of important lessons that will be reflected throughout this book:

- Success in addressing important health problems *is* possible, even in the poorest countries
- Governments in poor countries *can* manage major public health successes and often can fund them as well
- Technology does enable progress in health; however, many successes stem from basic changes in

TABLE 1-4 Examples of Low-, Middle- and High-income Countries, Following World Bank Classification

Low-income	Lower middle-income	Upper middle-income	High-income
Bangladesh	Angola	Barbados	Aruba
Cambodia	Bolivia	Botswana	Belgium
Ethiopia	Brazil	Costa Rica	Canada
Haiti	Egypt	Czech Republic	Denmark
Mozambique	Iraq	Hungary	Portugal
Nigeria	Morocco	Panama	Italy
Senegal	Philippines	South Africa	Netherlands
Vietnam	Swaziland	Turkey	Singapore
Zimbabwe	Tunisia	Venezuela	Switzerland

Source: Data from the World Bank. Data and Statistics: Country Groups. Available at: http://web.worldbank.org/WBSITE/EXTERNAL/DATASTATISTICS/0,,contentMDK:20421402~pagePK:64133150~piPK:64133175~theSitePK:239419,00.html#lincome. Accessed May 22, 2006.

TABLE 1-5 The Millennium Development Goals and Their Related Targets

Goal	Targets
Goal 1: Eradicate Extreme Hunger and Poverty	**Target 1.** Halve, between 1990 and 2015, the proportion of people whose income is less than $1 a day **Target 2.** Halve, between 1990 and 2015, the proportion of people who suffer from hunger
Goal 2: Achieve Universal Primary Education	**Target 3.** Ensure that, by 2015, children everywhere, boys and girls alike, will be able to complete a full course of primary schooling
Goal 3: Promote Gender Equality and Empower Women	**Target 4.** Eliminate gender disparity in primary and secondary education, preferably by 2005, and in all levels of education no later than 2015
Goal 4: Reduce Child Mortality	**Target 5.** Reduce by two thirds, between 1990 and 2015, the under-five mortality rate
Goal 5: Improve Maternal Health	**Target 6.** Reduce by three quarters, between 1990 and 2015, the maternal mortality ratio
Goal 6: Combat HIV/AIDS, Malaria, and other diseases	**Target 7.** Have halted by 2015 and begun to reverse the spread of HIV/AIDS **Target 8.** Have halted by 2015 and begun to reverse the incidence of malaria and other major diseases
Goal 7: Ensure Environmental Sustainability	**Target 9.** Integrate the principles of sustainable development into country policies and programs and reverse the loss of environmental resources **Target 10.** Halve, by 2015, the proportion of people without sustainable access to safe drinking water and basic sanitation **Target 11.** Have achieved by 2020 a significant improvement in the lives of at least 100 million slum dwellers
Goal 8: Develop a Global Partnership for Development	**Target 12.** Develop further an open, rule-based, predictable, nondiscriminatory trading and financial system **Target 13.** Address the special needs of the Least Developed Countries **Target 14.** Address the special needs of landlocked developing countries and small island developing states **Target 15.** Deal comprehensively with the debt problems of developing countries through national and international measures in order to make debt sustainable in the long term

Source: Data from Millennium Project: Goals and Targets. Available at http://www.unmillenniumproject.org/goals/goals02.htm. Accessed June 6, 2006.

people's behavior, such as filtering water, giving infants oral rehydration for diarrhea, and cessation of smoking

- Cooperation among global health actors can make a major difference to the achievement of health aims
- It is possible to find evidence of what works and does not work in global health efforts
- Success comes in all shapes—different types of programs in different types of settings have been and can be successful

SMALLPOX ERADICATION—THE MOST FAMOUS SUCCESS STORY

It is fitting to end this introductory chapter with a summary of the most famous public health success story of all, the case of smallpox eradication. This effort was not only a great triumph of public health, but was also a great accomplishment for mankind. In addition, the history of smallpox eradication is well known to everyone who works in public health, and it provides many lessons that can be applied to other public health efforts.

The history of smallpox eradication and the lessons learned from dealing with it also remain very important because of the new threat of smallpox being used as a biological weapon.

Background

In 1966, smallpox ravaged over 50 countries, affecting 10 million to 15 million people, of whom almost 2 million died each year.[23] At the time, smallpox killed as many as 30% of those infected. Those who survived might suffer deep pitted scars and blindness as a result of their illness.[24]

The Intervention

Although a vaccine against smallpox was created by Edward Jenner in 1798, eradication of smallpox became a practical goal only in the 1950s when the vaccine could be mass produced and stored without refrigeration. A later breakthrough came in the form of the bifurcated needle, a marvel of simple technology that dramatically reduced costs by allowing endless reuse after sterilization, and by requiring a far smaller amount of vaccine per patient. The needle also made vaccination easy, thereby reducing the time and effort required to train villagers in its use.

In 1959, the Word Health Organization (WHO) adopted a proposal to eradicate smallpox through compulsory vaccination, but the program languished until 1965, when the United States stepped in with technical and financial support. A Smallpox Eradication Unit was established at the WHO, headed by Dr. D.A. Henderson of the Centers for Disease Control and Prevention (CDC) in the United States. As part of the smallpox eradication program, all WHO member countries were required to manage program funds effectively, report smallpox cases, encourage research on smallpox, and maintain flexibility in the implementation of the smallpox program to suit local conditions.

The Smallpox Eradication Unit proved to be a small but committed team, supplying vaccines and specimen kits to those countries that still had smallpox. Although wars and civil unrest caused disruptions in the program's progress, momentum was always regained with new methods and extra resources that focused on containing outbreaks by speeding with motorized teams to seek out new cases, isolate new cases, and vaccinate everyone in the vicinity of the new cases.

This military-style approach proved effective even in the most difficult circumstances. It also took practical account of the facts that: (1) it would have been extraordinarily difficult to immunize the whole world against smallpox, and (2) the transmission of the smallpox virus could be stopped by focusing vaccination efforts around new cases.

The Impact

In 1977, the last endemic case of smallpox in the world was recorded in Somalia. In 1980, after two years of surveillance and searching, the WHO declared smallpox the first disease in history to have been eradicated. Smallpox had previously been eradicated in Latin America in 1971 and in Asia in 1975.[25]

Costs and Benefits

The annual cost of the eradication campaign between 1967 and 1979 was $23 million. For the whole campaign, international donors provided $98 million, while $200 million came from the endemic countries.[26] The United States saves the total of all its contributions every 26 days because it no longer needs to spend money on vaccination or treatment, making smallpox eradication one of the best values in health interventions ever achieved.[27] Estimates for economic loss due to smallpox in a developing country are available only for India. Based on these, it has been estimated that developing countries as a whole suffered economic losses related to smallpox of about $1 billion each year at the start of the intensified campaign.[26]

Lessons Learned

The success of the program can be attributed to the political commitment and leadership exemplified in the partnership between WHO and the US Centers for Disease Control and Prevention. Success in individual countries hinged on having someone who was responsible, preferably solely, for the eradication effort. In addition, small WHO teams made frequent field trips to review progress, and a small number of committed people working in the program were able to motivate large numbers of staff. Moreover, in the days before the Internet and email, the program managers held a monthly meeting in which they exchanged information about the progress of the campaign and the lessons learned from working on it in different countries.

No two national campaigns were alike, which makes flexibility essential in program design. The plan for eradicating smallpox used existing healthcare systems, and it also forced many countries to improve their health services. This benefited immunization programs more generally and offset the cost of the initial smallpox campaign.

Monitoring standards were established across the program to constantly evaluate the progress of the program against agreed benchmarks. The participation of communities provided strategic lessons for later community-based projects. The value of publicity about the program was highlighted when news about the program's progress triggered large donations in 1974 to complete eradication in five remaining countries. An important discovery made during the campaign was that immunization programs could vaccinate people with more than one vaccination at a time. This helped to pave the way for later programs of routine immunization, about which you will read later.

The eradication of smallpox continues to inspire efforts against other diseases, but it must be remembered that the particular features of smallpox made it a prime candidate for eradication. The disease was passed directly between people, without an intervening vector, so there were no reservoirs; the distinctive rash of smallpox made diagnosis easy; survivors gained lifetime immunity; and, the severity of symptoms, once the disease became infectious, made patients take to their beds and infect few others. Good vaccination coverage could therefore disrupt transmission entirely. Unfortunately, almost 30 years after eradication, funds are still allocated to precautionary measures against the disease because of the continuing threat of smallpox being used as an agent of bio-terrorism.

CENTRAL MESSAGES OF THE BOOK

Because this is the introductory chapter of the book, it will not end with a summary, as the other chapters do. Rather, it will be most valuable to end this chapter by highlighting some of the central messages of the book as a whole. They are presented below in outline form, without citations or recitation of the evidence behind them. That evidence will be provided and cited in the chapters that follow. It will be very important to keep these messages in mind as you go through the book.

- There are strong links between health, human development, labor productivity, and economic development.
- Health status is determined by a variety of factors, including income, education, knowledge of healthy behaviors, social status, sex, genetic makeup, and access to health services.
- There has been enormous progress in improving health status over the last 50 years in many countries. This is reflected in the substantial increases these countries have witnessed in that period, for example, in life expectancy.
- Some of this progress has come about as a result of overall economic development and improvements in income. However, much of it is due to improvements in public hygiene, better water supply and sanitation,

and better education. Increased nutritional status has also had a large impact on improvements in health status. Technical progress in some areas, such as the development of vaccines against childhood diseases and the development of antibiotics, has also improved human health.

- The progress in health status, however, has been very uneven. Hundreds of millions of people, especially poorer people in low and middle-income countries, continue to get sick, be disabled by, or die from preventable causes of disease. In many countries, nutritional status and health status of lower-income people have improved only slowly. In addition, HIV/AIDS is causing a decline in health and nutritional status and life expectancy in a number of countries in Sub-Saharan Africa.
- There are enormous disparities in health status and access to health services both within and across countries. Wealthier people in most countries have better health status and better access to health services than poorer people. In general, urban dwellers and ethnic majorities enjoy better health status than rural people and disadvantaged ethnic minorities. In addition, women face a number of unique challenges to their health.
- Countries do not need to be high-income to enjoy good health status. By contrast, there are a number of examples, such as China, Costa Rica, Cuba, Kerala state in India, and Sri Lanka, that make clear that low-income countries or low-income areas within countries can help their people to achieve good health, even in the absence of extensive financial resources to invest in health. However, this requires strong political will and a focus on public hygiene, education, and investing in low-cost but high yielding investments in nutrition and health.
- Some global health issues can only be solved through the cooperation of various actors in global health. This could include, for example, the development of an AIDS vaccine.
- However, an important part of health status is determined by an individual's and families' own knowledge of health and hygiene. People and communities have tremendous abilities to enhance their own health status.
- The world continues to shrink at a very rapid pace. For health, security, and humanitarian reasons, each of us should be concerned about the health of everyone else.

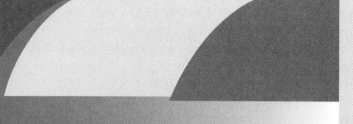

Study Questions

1. What has been some of the most important progress in health worldwide over the last fifty years?

2. What are some of the global health challenges that remain to be addressed?

3. How might one define: *health*, *public health*, and *global health*?

4. What are some examples of public health activities?

5. What are some examples of global health issues?

6. What are the key differences between the approach of medicine and the approach of public health?

7. What are some of the most important challenges to health globally?

8. Why should everyone be concerned about critical global health issues?

9. What are the Millennium Development Goals and how do they relate to health?

10. What were some of the keys to the eradication of smallpox? What lessons does the smallpox eradication program suggest for other global health programs?

REFERENCES

1. Centers for Disease Control and Prevention. Meningococcal Disease. October 12, 2005; Available at: http://www.cdc.gov/ncidod/dbmd/diseaseinfo/meningococcal_g.htm. Accessed May 27, 2006.

2. Mayo Clinic. Infectious Disease: West Nile Virus. Available at: http://www.mayoclinic.com/health/west-nile-virus/DS00438. Accessed May 28, 2006.

3. New polio cases confirmed in Guinea, Mali and the Sudan. Available at: http://www.who.int/mediacentre/news/releases/2004/pr57/en/. Accessed June 10, 2006.

4. HAPCO. Federal Democratic Republic of Ethiopia: Report on Progress Towards Implementation of the Declaration of Commitment on HIV/AIDS. Available at: http://data.unaids.org/pub/Report/2006/2006_country_progress_report_ethiopia_en.pdf?preview=true. Accessed June 14, 2006.

5. UNAIDS Wa. AIDS Epidemic Update 2006. Available at: http://data.unaids.org/pub/EpiReport/2006/2006_EpiUpdate_en.pdf. Accessed January 2, 2007.

6. UNAIDS. Countries. Available at: http://www.unaids.org/en/Regions_Countries/Countries/default.asp. Accessed May 26, 2006.

7. Health Protection Agency of the United Kingdom. Focus on Tuberculosis. Available at: http://www.hpa.org.uk/publications/2006/tb_report/pdfs/introduction.pdf. Accessed January 2, 2007.

8. Levine R., *Case Studies in Global Health: Millions Saved.* Sudbury, MA: Jones and Bartlett Publishers; 2007.

9. World Health Organization. The Executive Summary of The Lancet Neonatal Survival Series. *The Lancet Neonatal Survival Series.* Available at: http://www.who.int/child-adolescent-health/New_Publications/NEONATAL/The_Lancet/Executive_Summary.pdf. Accessed June 17, 2006.

10. Mathers CD, Lopez AD, Murray CJL. The Burden of Disease and Mortality by Condition: Data, Methods, and Results for 2001. In: Lopez AD, Mathers CD, Ezzati M, Jamison DT, Murray CJL, eds. *Global Burden of Disease and Risk Factors.* New York: Oxford University Press; 2006:126.

11. Centers for Disease Control and Prevention. World Distribution of Dengue - 2003. Available at: http://www.cdc.gov/ncidod/dvbid/dengue/map-distribution-2003.htm. Accessed June 8, 2006.

12. The World Bank. Data & Statistics: Key Development Data & Statistics. Available at: http://web.worldbank.org/WBSITE/EXTERNAL/DATASTATISTICS/0,,contentMDK:20535285~menuPK:1192694~pagePK:64133150~piPK:64133175~theSitePK:239419,00.html. Accessed June 10, 2006.

13. Preamble to the Constitution of the World Health Organization 1946, as adopted by the International Health Conference, New York, 19 June–22 July 1946.

14. Merson MH, Black RE, Mills A. *International Public Health: Diseases, Programs, Systems, and Policies.* Gaithersburg, MD: Aspen Publishers; 2001: xvii.

15. American Public Health Association. Code of Ethics. Available at: www.apha.org/codeofethics/ethics.htm. Accessed February 8, 2006.

16. Harvard School of Public Health. Distinctions Between Medicine and Public Health. Available at: http://www.hsph.harvard.edu/about.html#publichealth. Accessed February 8, 2006.

17. Last JM. *A Dictionary of Epidemiology.* 4th ed. New York: Oxford University Press; 2001.

18. Institute of Medicine. *America's Vital Interest in Global Health: Protecting our People, Enhancing our Economy, and Advancing our International Interests.* Washington, DC: National Academy Press; 1998.

19. Merson MH, Black RE, Mills A. *International Public Health: Diseases, Programs, Systems, and Policies.* Gaithersburg, MD: Aspen Publishers; 2001: xix.

20. Roberts MJ, Hsiao W, Berman P, Reich MR. *Getting Health Reform Right: A Guide to Improving Performance and Equity*: New York: Oxford University Press; 2004.

21. Data and Statistics: Country Groups. Available at: http://web.worldbank.org/WBSITE/EXTERNAL/DATASTATISTICS/0,,contentMDK:20421402~pagePK:64133150~piPK:64133175~theSitePK:239419,00.html#lincome. Accessed May 22, 2006.

22. United Nations. 55/2. United Nations Millennium Declaration. Available at: http://www.un.org/millennium/declaration/ares552e.htm. Accessed May 16, 2006.

23. World Health Organization. WHO Fact Sheet on Smallpox. Available at: http://www.who.int/mediacentre/factsheets/smallpox/en/. Accessed August 6, 2004.

24. World Health Organization. Media Centre, Smallpox: Historical Significance. Available at: http://www.who.int/mediacentre/factsheets/smallpox/en/. Accessed June 13, 2006.

25. Roberts M. How Doctors Killed Off Smallpox. July 3, 2005; Available at: http://news.bbc.co.uk/1/hi/health/4072392.stm. Accessed June 11, 2006.

26. Fenner F. *Smallpox and its Eradication*: World Health Organization; 1988.

27. Brilliant LB. *The Management of Smallpox Eradication in India.* Ann Arbor: University of Michigan Press; 1985.

Health Determinants, Measurements, and Trends

LEARNING OBJECTIVES

By the end of this chapter the reader will be able to:

- Describe the determinants of health
- Define the most important health indicators
- Discuss the differences between incidence and prevalence; morbidity, disability, and mortality; and non-communicable and communicable diseases
- Discuss the concepts of Health Adjusted Life Expectancy (HALE), Disability Adjusted Life Years (DALYs), and the burden of disease
- Describe the leading causes of death in low-, middle-, and high-income countries
- Describe the demographic and epidemiological transitions

VIGNETTES

Shawki is a 60-year-old Jordanian man who lives in Jordan's capital of Amman. Unfortunately, Shawki's health has deteriorated in the last year. His blood pressure and cholesterol are too high. He has developed diabetes. He is sometimes short of breath. What are the causes of his ill and declining health? Do these problems stem from any genetic issues? Could they come from a lack of understanding about a healthy lifestyle and diet? Could it be that Shawki lacks the income he needs to eat properly and to ensure that he gets health checkups when he needs them?

Life expectancy in Botswana prior to the spread of HIV/AIDS was about 65 years.[1] Today, it is about 40 years.[1] Life expectancy in Russia in 1985 was about 64 years for males and 74 years for females. In 2001, however, it had fallen to about 59 years for males and 72 years for females.[2] What does

life expectancy measure? What are the factors contributing to its decline in both of these countries? What has happened to trends in life expectancy in other countries? Which countries have the longest and shortest life expectancies and why?

In Cambodia today, families have, on average, four children and those children, on average, will live about 57 years.[3] Many children will die in their first month of life, and the leading causes of infant and child death will be diarrhea and pneumonia. Thirty years ago, the demographic and epidemiological profile of Thailand looked a lot like Cambodia looks today. Today, however, Thai families have on average about two children and those children on average will live 71 years.[3] Children in Thailand rarely die, and when they do, 50 percent of them die from injury.[4] What causes these shifts in fertility and mortality? Do they occur consistently as countries develop economically? How long will it take before Cambodia has the same fertility and disease burden that Thailand has today?

In Peru, the people who are poor tend to live in the mountains, be indigenous people, be less educated, and have worse health status than other people. In Eastern Europe, the same issues occur among their ethnic groups that are of lower socioeconomic status, such as the Roma people. In the United States, there are also enormous health disparities, as seen in the relative health status of African Americans and Native Americans. If one wants to understand and address differences in health status among different groups, then how do we have to measure health status? Do we measure it by age? By gender? By socioeconomic status? By level of education? By ethnicity? By location?

THE IMPORTANCE OF MEASURING HEALTH STATUS

If we want to understand the most important global health issues and what can be done to address them, then we must understand what factors have the most influence on health status, how health status is measured, and what key trends in health status have occurred historically. We must, in fact, be able to answer the questions that are posed in the narratives above.

This chapter, therefore, covers four distinct, but closely related topics. The first section concerns what are called "the determinants of health." That section examines the most important factors that relate to people's health status. The second section reviews some of the most important indicators of health status and how they are used. The third section discusses the burden of disease worldwide and how it varies across countries. The last section looks at how fertility and mortality change as countries become more developed and what this means for the types of health problems countries face.

THE DETERMINANTS OF HEALTH

Why are some people healthy and some people not healthy? When asked this question, many of us will respond that good health depends on access to health services. Yet, as you will learn, whether or not people are healthy depends on a large number of factors, many of which are interconnected, and most of which go considerably beyond access to health services.

There has been considerable writing about the "determinants of health" and one way of depicting these determinants is shown in Figure 2-1. The next section largely follows the approach to the determinants of health that is discussed in "What Determines Health" by the Public Health Agency of Canada.[5]

The first group of factors that helps to determine health relates to the personal and inborn features of individuals. These include genetic makeup, sex, and age. Our genetic makeup has much to do with what diseases we get and how healthy we live. One can inherit, for example, a genetic marker for a particular disease, such as Huntington's disease, which is a neurological disorder. One can also inherit the genetic component of a disease that has multiple causes, such as breast cancer. Sex also has an important relationship with health. Men and women are physically different, for example, and may get different diseases. Women face the risk of childbearing. They also get cervical and uterine cancers that men do not get. Women also have higher rates of certain health conditions, such as thyroid and breast cancers. For similar reasons, age is also an important determinant of

health. Young children in developing countries often die of diarrheal disease, while older people are much more likely to die of heart disease, to cite one of many examples of the relationship between health and age.

Social and cultural issues also play important roles in determining health. Social status is an important health determinant. There is good evidence that people of higher social status have more control over their lives than people of lower status, and people of higher social status also tend to have higher incomes and education, both of which are strongly correlated with better health.[6] In addition, the gender roles that are ascribed to women in many societies also have an important impact on health. In such environments, women may be less well treated than men and this, in turn, may mean that women have less income, less education, and fewer opportunities to engage in safe employment. All of these militate against their good health.

The extent to which people get social support from family, friends, and community has also been shown to have an important link with health.[6] The stronger the social networks and the stronger the support that people get from those networks, the healthier people will be. Of course, culture is also an extremely important determinant of health.[6] Culture helps to determine how one feels about health and illness, how one uses health services, and the health practices in which one engages.

The environment, both indoor and outdoor, is also a powerful determinant of health. Related to this is the safety of the environment in which people work. Although many people know about the importance of outdoor air pollution to health, few people are aware of the importance of indoor air pollution to health. In many developing countries, women cook indoors with very poor ventilation, thereby creating an indoor environment that is full of smoke and that encourages respiratory illness and asthma. The lack of safe drinking water and sanitation is a major contributor to ill health in poor countries. In addition, many people in those same countries work in environments that are very unhealthy. Because they lack skills, social status, and opportunities, they may work without sufficient protection with hazardous chemicals, in polluted air, or in circumstances that expose them to occupational accidents.

Education is a powerful determinant of health for several reasons. First, it brings with it knowledge of good health practices. Second, it provides opportunities for gaining skills, getting better employment, raising one's income, and enhancing one's social status, all of which are also related to health. Studies have shown, for example, that the single best predictor of the birth weight of a baby is the level of educational attainment of the mother.[7] Most of us already know that throughout the world, there is an extremely strong and positive correlation between the level of education and all key health indicators. People who are better educated eat better, smoke less, are less obese, have fewer children, and take better care of their children's health than do people with less education. It is not a surprise, therefore, that they and their children live longer and healthier lives than do less well educated people and their children.

Of course, people's own health practices and behaviors are also critical determinants of their health. Being able to identify when you or a family member is ill and needs health care can be critical to good health. As noted previously, however, one's health also depends on how one eats, or if one smokes, drinks too much alcohol, or drives safely. We also know that being active physically and getting exercise regularly is better for one's health than is being sedentary.

Another important determinant of future health is the way in which infants and young children are cared for and nourished and the manner in which their health is attended. Being born premature or of low birthweight can have important negative consequences on health. There is a strong correlation between the nutritional status of infants and young children and the extent to which they meet their biological potentials, enroll in school, or stay in school. In addition, poor nutritional status in infancy and young childhood may be linked with a number of chronic diseases, including diabetes and heart disease. [8]

Of course, one's health does depend on access to appropriate healthcare services. Even if one is born healthy, raised healthy, and engages in good health behaviors, there will still be times when one has to call on a health system for help. The more likely you are to access services of appropriate quality, the more likely you are to stay healthy. To address the risk of dying from a complication of pregnancy, for example, one must have access to health services that can carry out an emergency cesarean section if necessary. Even if the mother has had the suggested level of prenatal care and has prepared well in all other respects for the pregnancy, in the end, certain complications can only be addressed in a healthcare setting.

Finally, one should note that the approach that governments take to different policies and programs in the health sector and in other sectors has an important bearing on people's health. People living in a country that promotes high educational attainment, for example, will be healthier than people in a country that does not promote widespread education of appropriate quality, because better educated people engage in healthier behaviors. A country that has universal

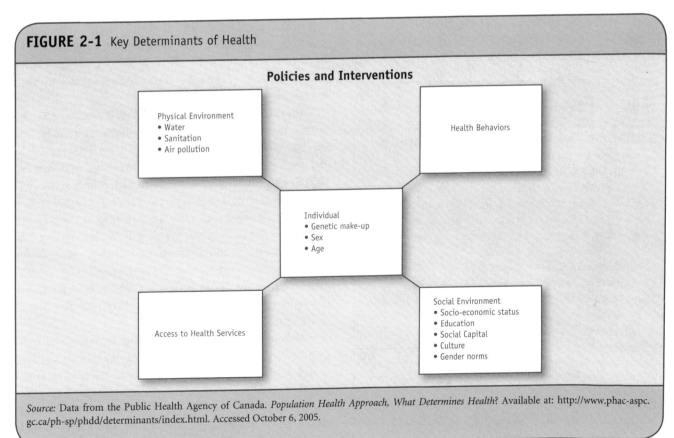

FIGURE 2-1 Key Determinants of Health

Source: Data from the Public Health Agency of Canada. *Population Health Approach, What Determines Health?* Available at: http://www.phac-aspc. gc.ca/ph-sp/phdd/determinants/index.html. Accessed October 6, 2005.

health insurance is likely to have healthier people than a country that does not insure all of its people, because the uninsured may lack needed health services. The same would be true, for example, for a country that promoted safe water supply for all of its people, compared to one that does not.

KEY HEALTH INDICATORS

It is critical that we use data and evidence to understand and address key global health issues. Some types of health data concern the health status of people and communities, such as measures of life expectancy and infant and child mortality, as discussed further hereafter. Some concern health services, such as the number of nurses and doctors per capita in a certain country or the indicators of coverage for certain health services, such as immunization. This book will discuss health service data only briefly, mostly in Chapter 5 on health systems. Other data concern the financing of health, such as the amount of public expenditure on health or the share of national income represented by health expenditure. This book also provides only a limited discussion of health financing, which is also primarily in the chapter on health systems.

There are a number of very important uses of data on health status, which we shall explore further and discuss throughout the book.[9] We need data, for example, to know what are the health conditions from which people suffer. We also need to know the extent to which these conditions cause people to be sick, to be disabled, or to die. We need to gather data to carry out disease surveillance. This helps us to understand if particular health problems such as influenza, polio, or malaria are occurring, where they are infecting people, who is getting these diseases, and what might be done to address them. Other forms of data also help us to understand the burden of different health conditions, the relative importance of them to different societies, and the importance that should be attached to dealing with them.

If we are to use data in the previously mentioned ways, then it is important that we use a consistent set of indicators to measure health status. In this way, we can make comparisons across people in the same country or across different countries. There are, in fact, a number of indicators that are used most commonly by those who work in global health and in development work, as well, as noted later. These are listed and defined in Table 2-1 and are discussed briefly below.

Among the most commonly used indicators of health status is "life expectancy at birth." Life expectancy at birth is "the average number of additional years a newborn baby can be expected to live if current mortality trends were to continue for the rest of that person's life."[10] In other words, it measures how long a person born today can expect to live, if there were no change in their lifetime in the present rate of death for people of different ages. The higher the life expectancy at birth, the better the health status of a country. In the United States, life expectancy at birth is about 77 years; in a middle-income country, such as Jordan, life expectancy is 72 years; in a very poor country, such as Mali, the life expectancy is 48 years. Figure 2-2 shows life expectancy at birth by region.[3]

Another important and widely used indicator is the "infant mortality rate." The infant mortality rate is "the number of deaths of infants under age 1 per 1000 live births in a given year."[10] This rate is usually expressed in deaths per 1000 live births. In other words, it measures how many children younger than 1 year of age will die for every 1000 who were born alive that year. Each country seeks as low a rate of infant mortality as possible, but we will see that the rate varies largely with the income status of a country. Some of the poorer countries, such as Niger, have infant mortality rates as high as 150 infant deaths for every 1000 live births, whereas in Sweden only about 3 infants die for every 1000 live births.[12] (See Figure 2-3).

Although the infant mortality rate is a powerful indicator of health status of a country, most children younger than 1 year of age who die actually die in the first month of life. Thus, the "neonatal mortality rate" is also an important health status indicator. This rate measures "the number of deaths to infants younger than 28 days of age in a given

---

TABLE 2-1 Key Health Status Indicators

Infant Mortality Rate—The number of deaths of infants under age 1 per 1000 life births in a given year

Life Expectancy at Birth—The average number of years a newborn baby could expect to live if current mortality trends were to continue for the rest of the newborn's life

Maternal Mortality Ratio—The number of women who die as a result of pregnancy and childbirth complications per 100,000 live births in a given year

Neonatal Mortality Rate—The number of deaths to infants under 28 days of age in a given year per 1000 live births in that year

Under Five Mortality Rate (Child Mortality Rate) —The probability that a newborn baby will die before reaching age five, expressed as a number per 1000 live births.

Source: Haupt A, Kane TT. Population Handbook. Washington, DC: Population Reference Bureau; 2004; World Bank. Beyond Economic Growth: Glossary. http://www.worldbank.org/depweb/english/beyond/global/glossary.html. Accessed April 15, 2007.

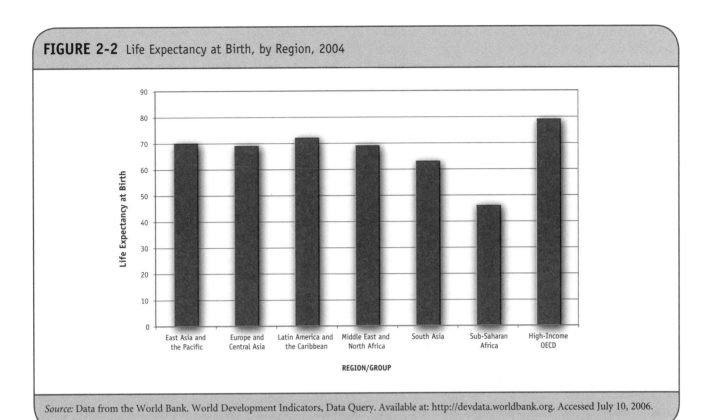

FIGURE 2-2 Life Expectancy at Birth, by Region, 2004

Source: Data from the World Bank. World Development Indicators, Data Query. Available at: http://devdata.worldbank.org. Accessed July 10, 2006.

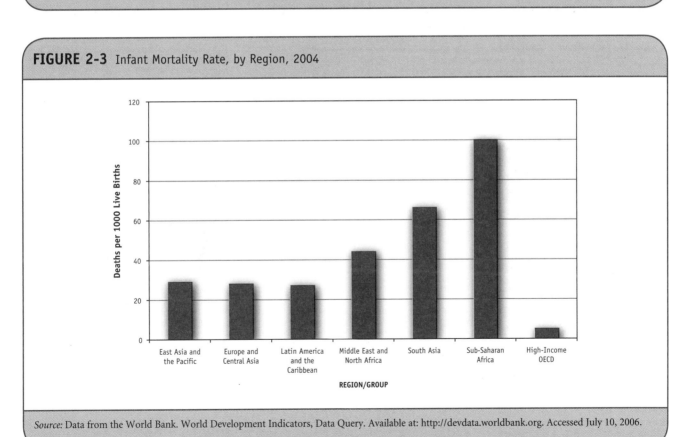

FIGURE 2-3 Infant Mortality Rate, by Region, 2004

Source: Data from the World Bank. World Development Indicators, Data Query. Available at: http://devdata.worldbank.org. Accessed July 10, 2006.

year, per 1000 live births in that year."[10] Like the infant mortality rate, this rate will generally vary directly with the level of income of different countries. Poorer countries will have a much higher neonatal mortality rate then the richer countries. The neonatal mortality rate is about 40 per 1000 live births in Sub-Saharan Africa but below 5 per 1000 live births in developed countries.[14] The neonatal mortality rate by region is portrayed in Figure 2-4.

The under-five child mortality rate is also called the "child mortality rate." This is "the probability that a newborn will die before reaching age five, expressed as a number per 1000 live births."[10] Like the infant mortality rate, this rate is also expressed per 1000 live births. Of course, this rate is very similar to the infant mortality rate, and here, too, the lower the rate the better. This rate also varies largely with the wealth of a country. In the developed countries the rate is about 20 per 1000 live births. However, in the poorest countries, the rate can be as high as 170 per 1000 live births, as in the Africa Region of the World Health Organization (WHO).[16] The under-five child mortality rate is depicted in Figure 2-5. As infant mortality declines, the under-five child mortality rate becomes a more important health indicator. The relative standing of different regions in under-five child mortality, as shown in Figure 2-5, looks very similar to that for infant mortality.

The maternal mortality ratio is a measure of the risk of death that is associated with childbirth. Because these deaths are more rare than infant and child deaths, the maternal mortality ratio is measured as 'the number of women who die as a result of pregnancy and childbirth complications per 100,000 live births in a given year.'[10] The rarity of maternal deaths and the fact that they largely occur in low-income settings also contributes to maternal mortality being quite difficult to measure. Very few women die in childbirth in rich countries and the maternal mortality rate in Sweden, for example, is 5 per 100,000 live births. On the other hand, in very poor countries, in which women have low status and there are few facilities for dealing with obstetric emergencies, the rates can be over 500 per 100,000 live births, as they are in Gabon, India, and Laos.[18] As you can see in Figure 2-6, the maternal mortality ratio is also very strongly correlated with a country's income.

There are a few other concepts and definitions that are important to understand as we think about measuring health status, and they are summarized in Table 2-3. The first is "morbidity." Essentially, this means sickness or any departure, subjective or objective, from a psychological or physiological state of well-being. Second is "mortality," which refers to death. A "death rate" is the number

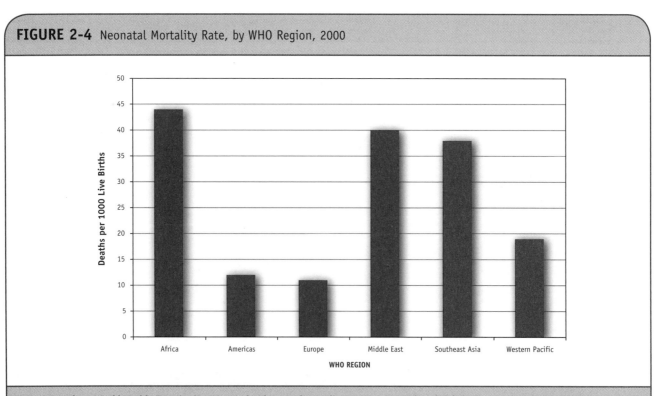

FIGURE 2-4 Neonatal Mortality Rate, by WHO Region, 2000

Source: Data from World Health Organization. Neonatal and prenatal mortality, country, regional, and global estimates. Geneva: WHO; 2006:Annex 2.

FIGURE 2-5 Under-five Child Mortality, by Region, 2006

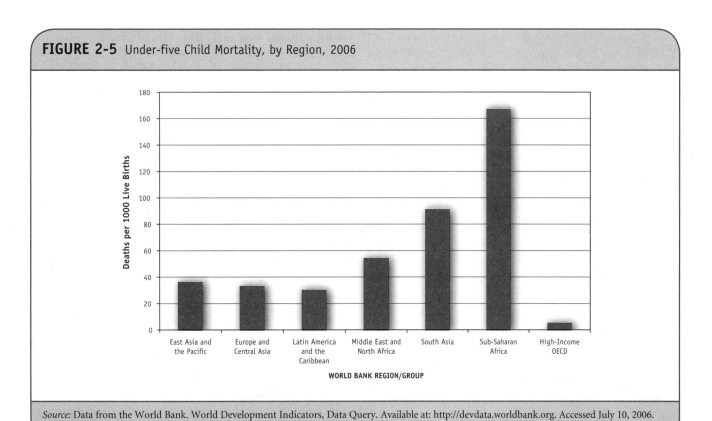

Source: Data from the World Bank. World Development Indicators, Data Query. Available at: http://devdata.worldbank.org. Accessed July 10, 2006.

FIGURE 2-6 Maternal Mortality, by Region, 2000

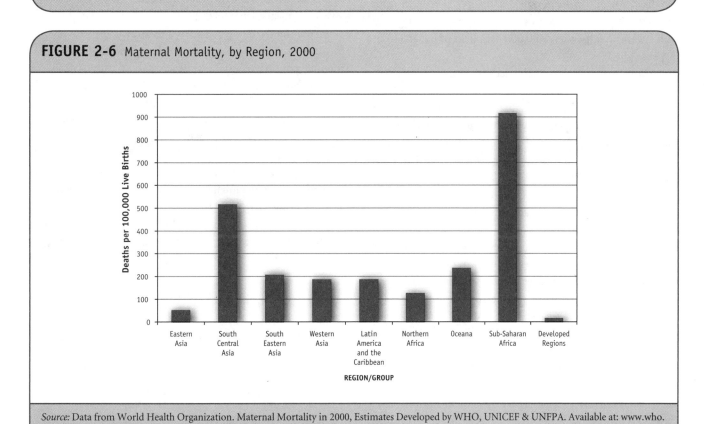

Source: Data from World Health Organization. Maternal Mortality in 2000, Estimates Developed by WHO, UNICEF & UNFPA. Available at: www.who.int/reproductive-health/publications/maternal_mortality. Accessed July 10, 2006.

of deaths per 1000 population in a given year.[10] The third is "disability." Although some conditions cause people to get sick or die, they might also cause people to suffer the "temporary or long-term reduction in a person's capacity to function."[21]

There will also be considerable discussion in this book and most readings on global health of the "prevalence" of health conditions. This refers to the number of people suffering from a certain health condition over a specific time period. It measures the chances of having a disease. For global health work, one usually refers to "point prevalence" of a condition, which is "the proportion of the population that is diseased at a single point in time."[22] The point prevalence of HIV/AIDS among adults in South Africa, for example, is estimated to be between 17% and 21%. This means that today between 17% and 21% of all adults between the ages of 15 and 49 in South Africa are HIV positive.[23]

The "incidence rate" is also a very commonly used term. This refers to the rate at which new cases of a disease occur in a population. Incidence measures the chances of getting a disease. Incidence rate is "the number of persons contracting a disease per 1000 population at risk, for a given period of time."[10] It is usually specified as the number of people getting the disease over a year, per 100,000 people at risk. In India, for example, the incidence rate for TB is 168 per 100,000.[25] This means that for every 100,000 people in India, 168 in the last year got TB.

Many people confuse incidence rate and prevalence rate. It may be convenient to think of prevalence as the pool of people with a disease at a particular time and incidence as the flow of new cases of people with that disease each year into that pool. You should note, of course, that the size of the pool will vary as new cases flow into the pool and old cases flow out, as they die or are cured.

Finally, one needs to be familiar with how diseases get classified. When you read about health, there will be discussions of communicable diseases, non-communicable diseases, and injuries. Communicable diseases are also called infectious diseases. These are illnesses that are caused by a particular infectious agent and that spread directly or indirectly from people to people, animals to people, or people to animals.[26] Examples of communicable diseases include influenza, measles, and HIV. Non-communicable diseases are illnesses that are not spread by any infectious agent, such as hypertension, coronary heart disease, and diabetes. Another category of health conditions is "injuries." These usually include, among other things, road traffic injuries, falls, self-inflicted injuries, and violence.[27]

MEASURING THE BURDEN OF DISEASE

We have already seen in Chapter 1 that the definition of health is "a state of complete physical, mental and social well-being and not merely the absence of disease or infirmity." Those who work on global health have attempted for a number of years to construct a single indicator that could be used to compare how far different countries are from the state of good health, as defined previously. Ideally, such an index would take account of morbidity, mortality, and disability; allow one to calculate the index by age, by gender, and by region; and, allow one to make comparisons of health status across regions within a country and across countries.[28] This kind of index would measure what is generally referred to as "the burden of disease."

One such indicator is "Health-Adjusted Life Expectancy," or HALE. It is a "health expectancy measure." The HALE "summarizes the expected number of years to be lived in what might be termed the equivalent of good health."[29] This can also be seen as "the equivalent number of years in full health that a newborn can expect to live, based on current rates of ill health and mortality."[30] To calculate the HALE, "the years of ill health are weighted according to severity and subtracted from the overall life expectancy."[6]

WHO calculated HALEs for most countries, using a standard methodology. Table 2-2 shows life expectancy at birth in 2000 for a number of low-, middle-, and high-income countries and how its compares with HALEs for those countries in the same year. As you can see from Table 2-2, the greater the number of years that people in any population are likely to spend in ill health or with disability, the greater the difference will be between life expectancy at birth and health-adjusted life expectancy.

The composite indicator of health status that is most commonly used in global health work is called the "Disability Adjusted Life Year," or DALY. This indicator was first used in conjunction with the 1993 World Development Report of the World Bank, and is a "health gap measure." It is now used in burden of disease studies. In the simplest terms, a DALY is:

> . . . a unit for measuring the amount of health lost because of a particular disease or injury. It is calculated as the present value of future years of disability free life that are lost as the result of the premature deaths or causes of disability occurring in a particular year.[31]

The DALY is a measure of premature deaths and losses due to illnesses and disabilities in a population. A DALY

TABLE 2-2 Life Expectancy at Birth and Health Adjusted Life Expectancy, Selected Countries, 2004

Country	Life Expectancy/Health Adjusted Life Expectancy Males	Life Expectancy/Health Adjusted Life Expectancy Females
Afghanistan	42/35.3	42/35.8
Argentina	71/62.5	78/68.1
Bangladesh	62/55.3	63/53.3
Bolivia	63/53.6	66/55.2
Brazil	67/57.2	74/62.4
Cambodia	51/45.6	58/49.5
Cameroon	50/41.1	51/41.8
Canada	78/70.1	83/74.0
Chile	74/64.9	81/69.7
China	70/63.1	74/65.2
Costa Rica	75/65.2	80/69.3
Cuba	75/67.1	80/69.5
Denmark	75/68.6	80/71.1
Ethiopia	49/40.7	51/41.7
Ghana	56/49.2	58/50.3
Haiti	53/43.5	56/44.1
India	61/53.3	63/53.6
Indonesia	65/57.4	68/58.9
Jordan	69/59.7	73/62.3
Malaysia	69/61.6	74/64.8
Nepal	61/52.5	61/51.1
Niger	42/35.8	41/35.2
Nigeria	45/41.3	46/41.8
Pakistan	62/54.2	63/52.3
Peru	69/59.6	73/62.4
Philippines	65/57.1	72/61.5
Singapore	77/68.8	82/71.3
Sri Lanka	68/59.2	75/64.0
Turkey	69/61.2	73/62.8
United States of America	75/67.2	80/71.3
Vietnam	69/59.8	74/62.9

Source: Data from WHO. Core Health Indicators. Available at: http://www3.who.int/whosis/core/core_select_process.cfm. Accessed September 24, 2006.

measures how many healthy years of life are lost between the population being measured and the "healthiest" possible population, which is used as a standard. It does this by adding together the losses of healthy years of life that occur from illness, disability, and death. The value of disability is based on values that have been established for the severity of different disabling conditions. The calculation of a DALY "discounts" losses so that losses from ill health, disability, and death in the future are worth less than losses that occur today, just as a dollar you get in the future will be worth less

than one you would get today.[9, 32–34] This is why the DALY is referred to as a "present value."

For calculating DALYs, health conditions are generally broken down into three categories:[35]

Group 1—communicable, maternal, and perinatal conditions, (meaning in the first week after birth), and nutritional disorders

Group 2—non-communicable diseases

Group 3—injuries, including, among other things, road traffic accidents, falls, self-inflicted injuries, and violence

To get a better sense of the meaning of DALYs, it will be valuable to construct a few simple examples of what goes into their calculation and how they would be used. Consider, for example, that a male can expect under the standard used to live to be 80 years old. Now let us suppose that this person dies of a heart attack at 40 years of age. That person would have lost 40 years of life. The value of this loss, discounted to the present, would be part of the calculation of DALYs.

Let us also imagine that a woman, who is 40 years of age, has diabetes that has disabled her in a number of ways. In principle, she should live to the standard used of 82.5 years of age. In practice, however, the person's disability is so severe that her quality of life is equal to only about half of what it would be if she were in a "disease free" state. Even if she were to live to be 80 years of age, therefore, she would have lost about half of the quality of her last 42.5 years due to disability. The value of this loss, discounted to the present, would also be part of the calculation of DALYs.

The DALYs for the society in which the two people are living would be a composite of the data calculated from the losses due to the premature death of the first person and the disability of the second.

In reality, of course, many health conditions produce both disability and premature death. Let us suppose that a man gets TB at 45 years of age. In the absence of treatment, let us say that he dies at 47 years of age. He suffered two years of disability and lost 33 years of life due to his illness, compared to the standard used for longevity. A person who suffers a severe road traffic injury at age 50 may live, let us say, 10 years with severe disability due to his injuries and then at age 60 die due to those injuries. He would have lost quality of life years during the period of his disability and 20 years of life from premature death, compared to the standard against which DALYs are calculated.

A society that has more premature death, illness, and disability has more DALYs than a society that is healthier and has less illness, disability, and premature death. One of the goals of health policy is to avert these DALYS in the most cost-efficient manner possible. If, for example, a society is losing many hundreds of thousands of DALYs due to malaria that is not diagnosed and treated in a timely and proper manner, what steps can be taken to avert those DALYs at the lowest cost?

An important point to remember when considering DALYs, compared to measuring deaths, is that DALYs take account of periods in which people are living in ill health or with disability. By doing this, DALYs and other composite indicators try to give a better estimate than measuring deaths alone of the true "health" of a population. This is easy to understand. Most mental health problems, for example, are not associated with deaths. However, they cause an enormous amount of disability. Several parasitic infections, such as schistosomiasis, also cause very few deaths, but enormous amounts of illness and disability. If we measured the health of a population with an important burden of schistosomiasis and mental illness only by measuring deaths, we would miss a major component of morbidity and disability and would seriously overestimate the health of that population. The next section on the global burden of disease will make the concept of DALYs clearer to you, especially as you see how DALYs compare to deaths for a number of health conditions. Other sections of the book will also make extensive use of the concept of DALYs.

Indeed, calculating DALYs requires information on disease prevalence and incidence that is not always available. In addition, the health expectancy measures are more widely used in developed countries, given the health information available to them. A number of critiques of DALYs have been written.[36] Nonetheless, this book will repeatedly refer to DALYs because this measure is so extensively used in global health work. In addition, a considerable amount of important analysis has been carried out that is based on the use of DALYs for measuring overall health status and assessing the most cost-effective approaches to dealing with various health problems. These uses of the DALY will be discussed in Chapter 3.

THE GLOBAL BURDEN OF DISEASE
Overview

As you start a review of global health, it is important to get a clear picture of the leading causes of illness, disability, and death in the world. As noted earlier, it is also very important to understand how they vary by age, sex, ethnicity, and socioeconomic status, both within and across countries. It is also essential to understand how these causes have varied over time and how they might change in the future. These topics are examined briefly below and in much greater detail throughout the book.

Table 2-3 shows the 10 leading causes of death and the 10 leading causes of DALYs lost for low- and middle-income countries and for high-income countries. Both deaths and DALYs are ranked in order of importance.

The table indicates that the leading causes of death in low- and middle-income countries are non-communicable diseases, which account for about 54% of all deaths. This is followed by communicable diseases at about 36% of all deaths and then injuries at about 10% of all deaths.[37]

In order of rank, heart attacks and strokes are the two leading causes of death in low- and middle-income countries.

TABLE 2-3 The 10 Leading Causes of Death and DALYs, 2001

Low- and middle-income countries		High-income countries	
Cause	Percentage of total deaths	Cause	Percentage of total deaths
1. Ischemic heart disease	11.8	1. Ischemic heart disease	17.3
2. Cerebrovascular disease	9.5	2. Cerebrovascular disease	9.9
3. Lower respiratory infections	7.0	3. Trachea, bronchus, and lung cancers	5.8
4. HIV/AIDS	5.3	4. Lower respiratory infections	4.4
5. Perinatal conditions	5.1	5. Chronic obstructive pulmonary disease	3.8
6. Chronic obstructive pulmonary disease	4.9	6. Colon and rectal cancers	3.3
7. Diarrheal diseases	3.7	7. Alzheimer's and other dementias	2.6
8. Tuberculosis	3.3	8. Diabetes mellitus	2.6
9. Malaria	2.5	9. Breast cancer	2.0
10. Road traffic accidents	2.2	10. Stomach cancer	1.9
Cause	Percentage of total DALYs	Cause	Percentage of total DALYs
1. Perinatal conditions	6.4	1. Ischemic heart disease	8.3
2. Lower respiratory infections	6.0	2. Cerebrovascular disease	6.3
3. Ischemic heart disease	5.2	3. Unipolar depressive disorders	5.6
4. HIV/AIDS	5.1	4. Alzheimer's and other dementias	5.0
5. Cerebrovascular disease	4.5	5. Trachea, bronchus, and lung cancers	3.6
6. Diarrheal Diseases	4.2	6. Hearing loss, adult onset	3.6
7. Unipolar depressive disorders	3.1	7. Chronic obstructive pulmonary disease	3.5
8. Malaria	2.9	8. Diabetes mellitus	2.8
9. Tuberculosis	2.6	9. Alcohol use disorders	2.8
10. Chronic obstructive pulmonary disease	2.4	10. Osteoarthritis	2.5

Source: Adapted with permission from The World Bank, Lopez AD, Mathers CD, Murray CJL. The burden of disease and mortality by condition: data, methods, and results for 2001. In: Lopez AD, Mathers CD, Ezzati M, Jamison DT, Murray CJL, eds. *Global Burden of Disease and Risk Factors.* New York: Oxford University Press; 2006.

However, all but one of the next leading causes of death in these countries is communicable. The third leading cause of death is lower respiratory conditions, related to pneumonia, often in children. The fourth leading cause is HIV/AIDS. The next are perinatal conditions, linked with the death of newborns. TB, diarrheal disease, and malaria are also major killers. Road traffic accidents are the 10th leading cause of death in low- and middle-income countries.[35]

Non-communicable diseases are also the leading causes of deaths in high-income countries. However, in other respects, the picture of deaths that emerges in high-income countries is quite different from that in low- and middle-income countries. In high-income countries almost 87% of the deaths are from non-communicable causes, 7.5% are from injuries, and only 5.7% are from communicable causes. In high-income countries, the first three leading causes of

death are heart disease, stroke, and lung cancers. The fourth, and the only communicable cause among the leading causes of death, is lower respiratory infections, which is associated in high-income countries mostly with death from pneumonia of older people. Colon and rectal cancers are the fifth leading cause of death and diabetes is the sixth.[35]

If we look at DALYs, rather than deaths, for low- and middle-income countries, communicable diseases and injuries become slightly more important and non-communicable diseases somewhat less important in percentage terms than they were for deaths. In terms of individual conditions, diarrheal disease, malaria, and perinatal conditions become more important percentages than they were for deaths. However, the most significant difference is for unipolar depressive disorders (depression), which were not in the 10 leading causes of death, but which are in the 10 leading causes of

DALYs. This stems from the fact that this mental illness, which is discussed more in Chapter 12, is not associated with many deaths but is associated with an exceptional amount of disability in almost all countries. In fact, when we look at DALYs compared to deaths for high-income countries, the relative shares of DALYs by cause group is generally not very different than it is for deaths. However, for high-income countries, as well as low- and middle-income countries, unipolar depressive disorders become very important, as do Alzheimer's disease and other dementias.

Causes of Death by Region

As you would expect, the burden of disease varies by region, as shown in Table 2-4. In general, the higher the level of

TABLE 2-4 The Ten Leading Causes of the Burden of Disease in Low- and Middle-Income Countries by Region, 2001

East Asia and Pacific	Percentage of total DALYs	Europe and Central Asia	Percentage of total DALYs
1. Cerebrovascular disease	7.5	1. Ischemic heart disease	15.9
2. Perinatal conditions	5.4	2. Cerebrovascular disease	10.8
3. Chronic obstructive pulmonary disease	5.0	3. Unipolar depressive disorders	3.7
4. Ischemic heart disease	4.1	4. Self-inflicted injuries	2.3
5. Unipolar depressive disorders	4.1	5. Hearing loss, adult onset	2.2
6. Tuberculosis	3.1	6. Chronic obstructive pulmonary disease	2.0
7. Lower respiratory infections	3.1	7. Trachea, bronchus, and lung cancers	2.0
8. Road traffic accidents	3.0	8. Osteoarthritis	2.0
9. Cataracts	2.8	9. Road traffic accidents	1.9
10. Diarrheal diseases	2.5	10. Poisonings	1.9

Latin America and the Caribbean	Percentage of total DALYs	Middle East and North Africa	Percentage of total DALYs
1. Perinatal conditions	6.0	1. Ischemic heart disease	6.6
2. Unipolar depressive disorders	5.0	2. Perinatal conditions	6.3
3. Violence	4.9	3. Road traffic accidents	4.6
4. Ischemic heart disease	4.2	4. Lower respiratory infections	4.5
5. Cerebrovascular disease	3.8	5. Diarrheal diseases	3.9
6. Endocrine disorders	3.0	6. Unipolar depressive disorders	3.1
7. Lower respiratory infections	2.9	7. Congenital anomalies	3.1
8. Alcohol use disorders	2.8	8. Cerebrovascular disease	3.0
9. Diabetes mellitus	2.7	9. Vision disorders, age-related	2.7
10. Road traffic accidents	2.6	10. Cataracts	2.3

South Asia	Percentage of total DALYs	Sub-Saharan Africa	Percentage of total DALYs
1. Perinatal conditions	9.2	1. HIV/AIDS	16.5
2. Lower respiratory infections	8.4	2. Malaria	10.3
3. Ischemic heart disease	6.3	3. Lower respiratory infections	8.8
4. Diarrheal diseases	5.4	4. Diarrheal diseases	6.4
5. Unipolar depressive disorders	3.6	5. Perinatal conditions	5.8
6. Tuberculosis	3.4	6. Measles	3.9
7. Cerebrovascular disease	3.2	7. Tuberculosis	2.3
8. Cataracts	2.3	8. Road Traffic Accidents	1.8
9. Chronic obstructive pulmonary disease	2.3	9. Pertussis	1.8
10. Hearing loss, adult onset	2.0	10. Protein-energy malnutrition	1.5

Source: Adapted with permission from The World Bank, Lopez AD, Mathers CD, Murray CJL. The Burden of Disease and Mortality by Condition: Data, Methods, and Results for 2001. In: Lopez AD, Mathers CD, Ezzati M, Jamison DT, Murray CJL, eds. *Global Burden of Disease and Risk Factors.* New York: Oxford University Press 2006:91.

income within the region, the more likely it is that the leading causes of the burden of disease will be non-communicable. The lower the level of income, the more likely it is that the leading causes of the burden of disease will be communicable. What is most important to note is the remarkable extent to which the burden of disease in the Africa region remains dominated by communicable diseases. The relative importance of communicable diseases in the South Asia Region also sets that region apart. Throughout the book, in fact, the relatively high burden of communicable diseases in South Asia and Sub-Saharan Africa will be highlighted. [38]

Causes of Death by Age

Tables 2-5 and 2-6 show the leading causes of death by age group for both low- and middle-income countries and high-income countries.

TABLE 2-5 [1]The Ten Leading Causes of Death in Children Ages 0–14, by Broad Income Group, 2001

Low- and middle-income countries		High-income countries	
Cause	Percentage of total deaths	Cause	Percentage of total deaths
Perinatal conditions	20.7	Perinatal conditions	33.9
Lower respiratory infections	17.0	Congenital anomalies	20.0
Diarrheal diseases	13.4	Road traffic accidents	5.9
Malaria	9.2	Lower respiratory infections	2.5
Measles	6.2	Endocrine disorders	2.4
HIV/AIDS	3.7	Drownings	2.4
Congenital anomalies	3.7	Leukemia	1.9
Whooping cough	2.5	Violence	1.8
Tettanus	1.9	Fires	1.2
Road traffic accidents	1.5	Meningitis	1.2

Source: Adapted with permission from The World Bank, Lopez A, Begg S, Bos E. Demographic and Epidemiological Characteristics of Major Regions, 1990–2001. In: Lopez A, Mathers C, Ezzati M, Jamison D, Murray C, eds. *Global Burden of Disease and Risk Factors.* New York: Oxford University Press; 2006:70.

TABLE 2-6 The Ten Leading Causes of Death in Adults 15–59, by Broad Income Group, 2001

Low- and middle-income countries		High-income countries	
Cause	Percentage of total deaths	Cause	Percentage of total deaths
HIV/AIDS	14.1	Ischemic heart disease	10.8
Ischemic heart disease	8.1	Self-inflicted injuries	7.2
Tuberculosis	7.1	Road traffic accidents	6.9
Road traffic accidents	5.0	Trachea, bronchus, and lung cancers	6.8
Cerebrovascular disease	4.9	Cerebrovascular disease	4.4
Self-inflicted injuries	4.0	Cirhossis of the liver	4.4
Violence	3.1	Breast cancer	4.0
Lower respiratory infections	2.3	Colon and rectal cancers	3.1
Cirhossis of the liver	2.2	Diabetes mellitus	2.1
Chronic obstructive pulmonary disease	2.2	Stomach cancer	2.0

Source: Adapted with permission from The World Bank, Lopez A, Begg S, Bos E. Demographic and Epidemiological Characteristics of Major Regions, 1990–2001. In: Lopez A, Mathers C, Ezzati M, Jamison D, Murray C, eds. *Global Burden of Disease and Risk Factors.* New York: Oxford University Press; 2006:70.

It is clear from Table 2-5 that children in low- and middle-income countries die overwhelmingly of communicable diseases that are no longer problems in the more developed countries. You can also see that HIV/AIDS and TB are among the leading causes of death in low- and middle-income countries among adults, while no communicable disease is among the 10 leading causes of death in the high-income countries.

Causes of Death by Gender

It is also important to examine deaths by gender. Table 2-7 shows deaths by gender for low- and middle-income countries.

For this group of countries, the causes of death among men and women are largely alike. However, it is important to note that, even in these countries, heart disease and stroke are the leading causes of death among both genders, that men die much more than women of road traffic accidents, and that diabetes has become the 10th leading cause of death among women.

Trends

Between 1960 and 2002, life expectancy at birth for the world as a whole increased from 50 to 67. In addition, as shown in Table 2-8 below, life expectancy at birth declined in

TABLE 2-7 The Ten Leading Causes of Death Ordered by Sex, in Low- and Middle-Income Countries, 2001

Males		Females	
Cause	Percentage of total deaths	Cause	Percentage of total deaths
Ischemic heart disease	11.8	Ischemic heart disease	10.8
Cerebrovascular disease	8.5	Cerebrovascular disease	7.2
Lower respiratory Infections	6.7	Lower respiratory Infections	6.9
Perinatal conditions	5.4	HIV/AIDS	6.8
HIV/AIDS	5.4	Chronic obstructive pulmonary disease	4.4
Chronic obstructive pulmonary disease	4.7	Perinatal conditions	4.4
Tuberculosis	4.1	Diarrheal diseases	4.0
Diarrheal diseases	3.6	Malaria	3.1
Road traffic accidents	3.1	Tuberculosis	2.1
Malaria	2.3	Diabetes mellitus	2.0

Source: Adapted with permission from The World Bank, Lopez A, Begg S, Bos E. Demographic and Epidemiological Characteristics of Major Regions, 1990–2001. In: Lopez A, Mathers C, Ezzati M, Jamison D, Murray C, eds. *Global Burden of Disease and Risk Factors.* New York: Oxford University Press; 2006:70.

TABLE 2-8 Life Expectancy, 1960–2002, by World Bank Region

World Bank Region	Life expectancy (years)		
	1960	1990	2002
East Asia and the Pacific	39	67	70
Europe and Central Asia		69	69
Latin America and the Caribbean	56	68	71
Middle East and North Africa	47	64	69
South Asia	44	58	63
Sub-Saharan Africa	40	50	46
High-income countries	69	76	78

Source: Data with permission from The World Bank, Jamison DT. Investing in Health. In: Jamison Dt, Breman JG, Measham AR, et al., eds. *Disease Control Priorities in Developing Countries.* New York: Oxford University Press 2006:3–36.

No data for Europe and Central Asia for 1960

Sub-Saharan Africa and stayed the same in Europe and Central Asia. The rise in life expectancy in most regions has been associated with overall economic development and some important improvements in the health of children, partly as a result of better coverage of health interventions for children under five years. The decline in life expectancy at birth in Sub-Saharan Africa from 1990 to 2002 is attributable to the spread of HIV/AIDS. The lack of improvement in life expectancy at birth in Europe and Central Asia is largely attributed to the social issues that arose in the former Soviet Union, including alcoholism, which has led to an increase in adult mortality, especially among men. These points are discussed in greater detail later.[38]

As we look forward, we can forecast that communicable diseases will continue to be very important to the burden of disease in South Asia and Sub-Saharan Africa. However, barring the advent of a new or emerging infectious disease, the exceptional worsening of the HIV/AIDS pandemic, or a continuing long-run failure of Sub-Saharan Africa to grow economically, the non-communicable diseases will become increasingly important everywhere.

The Burden of Deaths and Disease within Countries

As you consider causes of death and the burden of disease globally and by region, age, and sex, it is also important to consider how deaths and DALYs would vary within countries, by gender, ethnicity, and socioeconomic status. In most low- and middle-income countries, the answer to this is relatively simple:

- Rural people will be less healthy than urban people
- Disadvantaged ethnic minorities will be less healthy than majority populations
- Women will suffer a number of conditions that relate to their relatively weak social positions
- Poor people will be less healthy than better-off people
- Uneducated people will be less healthy than better educated people

In addition, people of lower socioeconomic status will have higher rates of communicable diseases, illness, and death related to maternal causes and malnutrition than will people of higher status. Lower socioeconomic status people will also suffer from a larger burden of disease related to smoking, alcohol, and diet than would be the case for better-off people. These points are fundamental to understanding global health and will also be highlighted throughout the book.

RISK FACTORS

As we discuss the determinants of health and how health status is measured, there will be many references to "risk factors" for various health conditions. A risk factor is "an aspect or personal behavior or life-style, an environmental exposure, or an inborn or inherited characteristic, that, on the basis of epidemiologic evidence, is known to be associated with health-related condition(s) considered important to prevent."[39] Risks that relate to health can also be thought of as "a probability of an adverse outcome, or a factor that raises this probability."[40] We are all familiar with the notion of risk factors from our own lives and from encounters with health services. When we answer questions about our health history, for example, we are essentially helping to identify the most important risk factors that we face ourselves. Do our parents suffer from any health conditions that might affect our own health? Are we eating in a way that is conducive to good health? Do we get enough exercise and enough sleep? Do we smoke or drink alcohol excessively? Are there any special stresses in our life? Do we wear seat belts when we drive?

If we extend the idea of risk factors to poor people in low- and middle-income countries, then we might add some other questions that relate more to the ways that they live. Does the family have safe water to drink? Do their house and community have appropriate sanitation? Does the family cook indoors in a way that makes the house smoky? Do the father and mother work in places that are safe environmentally? We might also have to ask if there is war or conflict in the country, because they are also important risk factors for illness, death, and disability.

If we are to understand how the health status of people can be enhanced, particularly poor people in low- and middle-income countries, than it is very important that we understand the risk factors to which their health problems relate. Table 2-9 shows the relative importance of different risk factors to deaths and DALYs in low- and middle-income countries, compared to high-income countries. These are shown in the table in order of their importance by category of risk.

When we consider low- and middle-income countries, the most striking factor is the extent to which malnutrition is a risk factor. Another important point is the extent to which other nutrition related risk factors are important for deaths and DALYs, such as high blood pressure and high cholesterol. Deaths and DALYs attributable to the risks of smoking and unsafe sex make up the other most significant risk factors in low- and middle-income countries.[41]

TABLE 2-9 The Leading Risk Factors for the Burden of Disease, 2001, Low- and Middle-Income and High-Income Countries, Ranked in Order of Percent

Low- and Middle-Income Countries		High-Income Countries	
Deaths	**DALYs**	**Deaths**	**DALYs**
High blood pressure (12.9)	Childhood underweight (8.7)	Smoking (12.7)	Smoking (12.7)
Childhood underweight (7.5)	Unsafe sex (5.8)	High blood pressure (17.6)	High blood pressure (9.3)
Smoking (6.9)	High blood pressure (5.6)	High cholesterol (10.7)	Overweight and obesity (7.2)
High cholesterol (6.3)	Smoking (3.9)	Overweight and obesity (7.8)	High cholesterol (6.3)
Unsafe sex (5.8)	Unsafe water, sanitation, and hygiene (3.7)	Physical inactivity (4.8)	Alcohol use (4.4)
Low fruit and vegetable intake (4.8)	Alcohol use (3.6)	Low fruit and vegetable intake (4.2)	Physical inactivity (3.2)
Alcohol use (3.9)	High cholesterol (3.1)	Urban air pollution (1.0)	Low fruit and vegetable intake (2.7)
Indoor smoke from household use of solid fuels (3.7)	Indoor smoke from household use of solid fuels (3.0)	Illicit drug use (0.5)	Unsafe sex (0.6)
Overweight and obesity (3.6)	Low fruit and vegetable intake (2.4)	Unsafe sex (0.4)	Iron-deficiency anemia (0.5)
Unsafe water, sanitation, and hygiene (3.2)	Overweight and obesity (2.3)	Alcohol use (0.3)	Child sexual abuse (0.5)

Source: Data with permission from The World Bank, Lopez AD, Mathers CD, Ezzati M, Jamison DT, Murray CJ, eds. *Global Burden of Disease and Risk Factors*, 1990–2001. New York: Oxford University Press; 2006:10.

In high-income countries, there is little undernutrition but a considerable amount of overweight and obesity. It is not surprising, therefore, that three of the most important risk factors for both deaths and DALYs in high-income countries are high blood pressure, high cholesterol, and overweight and obesity. Nor is it surprising that, despite important progress in reducing the prevalence of smoking in some countries, tobacco remains the leading risk factor for both deaths and DALYs in high-income countries.[41]

THE DEMOGRAPHIC AND EPIDEMIOLOGICAL TRANSITIONS

The previous discussion has already suggested several very important trends that occur in total fertility, which is the number of children born alive to a woman over her lifetime,[42] in mortality, and in patterns of disease. The first trend is a change over time from patterns of high fertility and high mortality to a pattern of low fertility and low mortality. This is called the "demographic transition." The second, and closely related, trend that occurs is called the "epidemiological transition," and refers to the changing pattern of disease,

from a burden of disease profile that is dominated primarily by communicable diseases to one that it dominated primarily by non-communicable diseases. Both of these important transitions are discussed further below.

Demographic Transition[43]

When we look back historically at the countries that are now high-income, we can see that they had long periods historically when fertility was high, mortality was high, and population growth was, therefore, relatively slow, or which might even have declined in the face of epidemics. Beginning around the turn of the nineteenth century, however, mortality in those countries began to decline as hygiene and nutrition improved and the burden of infectious diseases became less. In most cases, this decline in mortality went before much decline in fertility. As mortality declined, the population increased and the share of the population that was of younger ages also increased. Later, fertility began to decline and, as births and deaths became more equal, population growth slowed. As births and deaths stayed more equal, the share of the population that was of older ages increased.

The demographic transition is shown graphically in Figure 2-7.

The first population pyramid reflects a country with high fertility and high mortality. The second population pyramid is indicative of a country in which mortality has begun to decline but fertility remains high. This would be similar to the demographics one would find, for example, in a number of countries in Sub-Saharan Africa that are undergoing demographic transition. The third pyramid looks more like a cylinder than a pyramid. This reflects a population in which fertility has been reduced and in which there is a larger share of older people in the population than in the first and second pyramids. This would be similar to the demographics that one would find in a number of low fertility, aging populations in Western Europe.

The Epidemiologic Transition[44]

The epidemiologic transition is closely related to the demographic transition, as suggested throughout the previous discussion. Historically there has been a shift in the patterns of disease that follows the trends noted below:

- First, high and fluctuating mortality, related to very poor health conditions, epidemics, and famine

- Then, progressive declines in mortality, as epidemics become less frequent
- Finally, further declines in mortality, increases in life expectancy, and the predominance of non-communicable diseases

Figure 2-8 shows examples of two sets of countries. The first has a burden of disease profile that is pretransition. The second is of a developed country that has completed its epidemiological transition.

You can see in Figure 2-8 how the pattern of disease differs between the two types of countries. You can also see the changes that will occur over time, as the low-income country develops and the burden of disease moves from one that is predominantly communicable diseases to one that is predominantly non-communicable diseases.

The pace of the epidemiological transition in different societies depends on a number of factors related to the "determinants of health" that were discussed earlier. In its early stages, the transition appears to depend primarily on improvements in hygiene, nutrition, education, and socioeconomic status. Some improvements also stem from advances in public health and in medicine, such as the development of new vaccines and antibiotics.[45] Most of the countries that

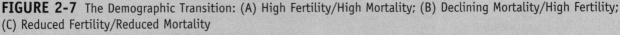

FIGURE 2-7 The Demographic Transition: (A) High Fertility/High Mortality; (B) Declining Mortality/High Fertility; (C) Reduced Fertility/Reduced Mortality

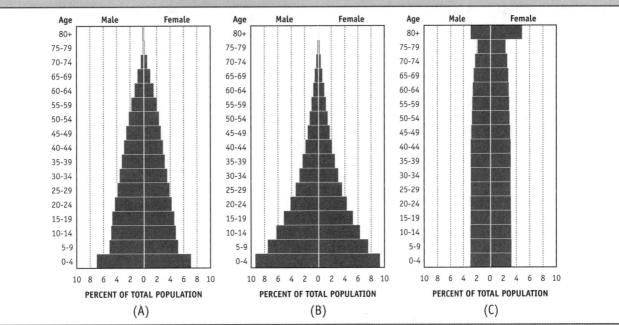

Source: Reprinted from U.S. Census Bureau. International population reports WP/02. *Global Population Profile: 2002.* Washington, DC: U.S. Government Printing Office; 2004:35.

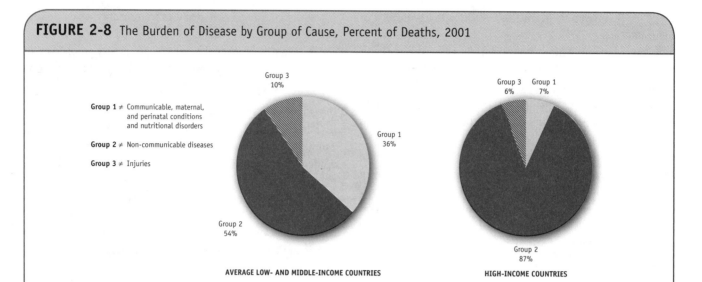

FIGURE 2-8 The Burden of Disease by Group of Cause, Percent of Deaths, 2001

Group 1 ≠ Communicable, maternal, and perinatal conditions and nutritional disorders

Group 2 ≠ Non-communicable diseases

Group 3 ≠ Injuries

AVERAGE LOW- AND MIDDLE-INCOME COUNTRIES

HIGH-INCOME COUNTRIES

Source: Data with permission from The World Bank, Lopez AD, Mathers CD, Murray CJL. The burden of disease and mortality by condition: data, methods, and results for 2001. In: Lopez AD, Mathers CD, Ezzati M, Jamison DT, Murray CJL, eds. *Global Burden of Disease and Risk Factors.* New York: Oxford University Press; 2006.

are now high-income went through epidemiologic transitions that were relatively slow, with the exception of Japan. Most developing countries have already begun their transition. However, it is still far from complete in most of them.

Implications of the Demographic and Epidemiological Transitions

There are several especially important points about these transitions that one must keep in mind.

- The large share of the population that is younger in relatively poor societies with high fertility has an enormous implication for the funds that countries must spend on education, health, and some other key investments.
- As countries age, they face pressure to fund the health of their older population, who tend to suffer from non-communicable diseases. They also face pressure on the funding of pension schemes for their older workers, because there is a large share of workers who have retired but a relatively smaller share of young people who pay taxes into the pension fund. This is now the case, for example, in much of Western Europe.
- Most low-income countries are in an ongoing epidemiologic transition and many of them, therefore, face significant burdens of communicable and non-communicable diseases, and injuries at the same

time. This strains the capacity of the health system of many of these countries. It is also expensive for countries that are resource poor to address a substantial burden of all three of these types of diseases simultaneously.

In fact, the demographic and epidemiological transitions have many important implications for public policy, some of which were noted earlier. From the point of view of this text, however, one especially important question that policy makers in low-income countries face concerning these transitions is: "How can public policy help to speed the demographic and epidemiological transitions in our country at lowest possible cost, in a manner consistent with the social values of the country?"

Figure 2-9 shows national income of a sample of countries, plotted against life expectancy at birth for females in those countries.

From this figure, one can see that, generally, the health of a country does increase as national income rises. However, one can also see that there are some countries, such as China, Costa Rica, Cuba, and Sri Lanka, that have achieved higher average life expectancies at birth than one would have predicted for countries at their level of income.

To a large extent, countries like those above achieved these important health gains as a result of:

- Focusing on investing in nutrition, health, and education, particularly of their poor people

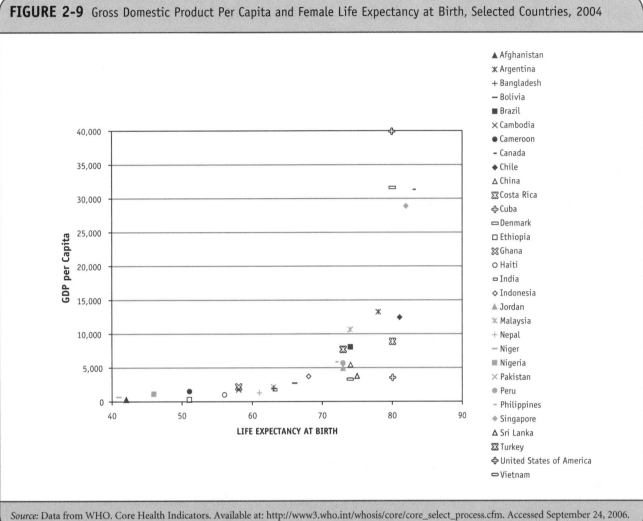

FIGURE 2-9 Gross Domestic Product Per Capita and Female Life Expectancy at Birth, Selected Countries, 2004

▲ Afghanistan
✳ Argentina
+ Bangladesh
− Bolivia
■ Brazil
✕ Cambodia
● Cameroon
- Canada
◆ Chile
△ China
▧ Costa Rica
✧ Cuba
▭ Denmark
□ Ethiopia
▨ Ghana
○ Haiti
▭ India
◇ Indonesia
▲ Jordan
✳ Malaysia
+ Nepal
− Niger
■ Nigeria
✕ Pakistan
● Peru
- Philippines
◆ Singapore
△ Sri Lanka
▧ Turkey
✧ United States of America
▭ Vietnam

Source: Data from WHO. Core Health Indicators. Available at: http://www3.who.int/whosis/core/core_select_process.cfm. Accessed September 24, 2006.

- Improving people's knowledge of good hygiene
- Making selected investments in health services that at low cost could have a high impact on health status, such as vaccination programs for children and TB control

These themes will also be discussed throughout this book.

Indeed, in the long run, economic progress *will* help to bring down fertility, reduce mortality from communicable diseases, and help to produce a healthier population. However, at the present rates of progress in improving health in most low-income countries, these changes will take a very long time to occur. One great public policy challenge for these countries and their governments, therefore, is how they can "short-circuit" this process and reach reduced levels of fertility, lower mortality, and better health for their people, even as they remain relatively poor.

CASE STUDY

The State of Kerala

Having begun to review health status and how countries can speed improvements in health, it will be valuable to end this chapter by examining a well-known case of a place that improved health status considerably, even at relatively low levels of income. One of the best known of such success stories concerns Kerala State in India.

Introduction

Kerala is a coastal state in Southwestern India with a population of more than 31 million people.[46] Despite having only slow rates of economic growth and a state per capita income lower than that of many other states in India, the health indicators for Kerala are the best in India and rival those in developed countries. What approach did Kerala take historically to produce such high levels of health, even in the face of relatively low income? What factors contributed to improvements in health status? What lessons does the Kerala experience suggest for other countries and for other states within India?

The Kerala Approach

One of the primary reasons why people in Kerala have such high levels of health has been the emphasis that the state put on education and the exceptionally widespread access to education in Kerala. The state introduced free primary and secondary education in the early part of 20th century.[47] In addition, Kerala has always put important emphasis on the education of females.

Kerala also made an early commitment to widespread health services for its people. The state created, for example, an extensive network of primary healthcare centers. This provided its citizens, throughout the state, with access to free basic health care and free family planning services. This was coupled with programs to promote exclusive breastfeeding and the improved nutrition of infants, children, and pregnant women. The central government supported the family planning program, the maternal and child health program, and the universal immunization program in all of India, but they were implemented far more effectively and efficiently in Kerala than in other states of India.[48]

The place of women in Kerala society also contributed to the uptake of education by females and improvements throughout Kerala in nutrition and health status. The role of women in many communities in Kerala differs from the roles ascribed to women in many other parts of India. In much of the rest of India, especially in parts of North India, women are regarded by families as liabilities rather than as assets. In most of India, this is partly represented in cultural terms by the fact that the family of a bride must pay a dowry to the family of the groom. In Kerala, however, women have been treated differently for over a century. They have been seen culturally much more as assets to families and they could inherit and own land, giving them a financial independence and power which was unrivalled among women elsewhere in India.[49]

It is also important to note that Kerala has historically been run by a government that has traditionally placed a premium on community mobilization on important social issues, such as education, greater empowerment of women, health, nutrition, and land reform. Many of these efforts were carried out in ways that raised social awareness about health and nutrition. In 1989, Kerala launched a total literacy campaign, for example, and by the start of the World Literacy Year in 1990, Ernakulam district in Kerala was declared India's first totally literate district.[50]

Given widespread education in Kerala and the place of women in society, it is not surprising that Kerala went through the demographic transition quite early and well before other places in India. Women with more education are more likely to work and marry later and thus have wider choice in economic and social pursuits. They also have a better knowledge of and easier access to family planning methods and lower fertility than do women with less education.[51]

The Impact

What were the impacts on health status of the emphasis that Kerala placed on education, health, nutrition, and the empowerment of women? Although it is not possible to scientifically indicate which policy contributed what share of better health, we can say that for many years the people of Kerala have enjoyed the best educational attainment of any group within India. In the last census, the literacy rates of people aged 7 years and above for India were about 65% on average, with about 76% for males and 54% for females. Kerala, however, had the highest literacy rate in the country, with about 91% overall and about 94% for males and 88% for females.[52] Kerala also boasts one of the highest newspaper readerships in the world, another feature that promotes the value of women, education, nutrition, and health. It also helps to raise political awareness and the demands of people for participation in and solutions to their concerns, such as education, health, and water.

Linked with this high level of education, especially of women and the promotion of nutrition and health, infant mortality in Kerala in 2001 was 14 per 1000, compared with 91 per 1000 for low-income countries generally and 68 per 1000 on average for India.[52] In India, about 2.1 million child deaths occur every year, which is the highest number within a single country worldwide.[53] The national under-five mortality rate is around 87 per 1000 live births with a wide variation between states. In Kerala, however, the mortality of children under five years is the best in India with an impressive rate of only 19 such deaths per 1000 births in 1998–1999.[54] In addition, maternal deaths in Kerala are much less common, at 87 per 100,000, than the Indian average of 407 per 100,000.[55] This partly reflects the extent to which deliveries take place in hospitals in Kerala. Indeed, Kerala's health care system garnered international acclaim when UNICEF and WHO designated it as the world's first "baby-friendly state." This was in recognition of the fact that more than 95% of Keralite births are hospital-delivered.[56]

Given these high health indicators, it is not surprising that nutritional status in Kerala is also much better than the Indian average, with 27% of the children younger than five years in Kerala being underweight, compared to the Indian average of 47%. Finally, one should note that life expectancy for men and women in Kerala is about the same at 73 years. This is closer to many developed countries like the United States, which had a life expectancy in 2004 of 78 years, than it is to life expectancy in most low- and middle-income countries.[57]

Lessons Learned

Kerala has long been cited, along with China, Costa Rica, Cuba, and Sri Lanka, as a model of a country or state within a country that has achieved high levels of education and health for its people, before achieving high levels of income. It appears that Kerala has achieved these impacts by politically supporting widespread access to education, nutrition, and health; mobilizing communities around the importance of these areas and of women's empowerment; and investing in low cost but high yielding areas of education, nutrition, and health. In a manner much like Sri Lanka, Kerala has also managed to achieve high levels of health status at relatively low cost.

Have the high levels of health and education in Kerala, however, been associated with high levels of growth of income in the state? The answer to that question is no. The annual per capita Gross Domestic Product (GDP) for the state in year 2001 was $469. This was close to the Indian average of $460. [58] It appears that the economic policies held by the state government over time in Kerala have not yielded high rates of economic growth or produced an environment in which domestic and foreign investors were prepared to work. Rather, the overall income of the state remains quite dependent on the money that workers from Kerala living abroad, especially in the Middle East, send back to their families in Kerala.[59]

What then are the messages to take away from Kerala in terms of the link between health and development? First, it is possible, even in the absence of high levels of income, to achieve high levels of health through political commitment, sound investments, and social mobilization. Second, however, in the absence of sound economic policies, the presence of a literate and healthy population alone will not be sufficient to promote rapid economic growth.

MAIN MESSAGES

To understand the most important global health issues, we must be able to understand the determinants of health, how health status is measured, and the meaning of the demographic and epidemiological transitions. There are a number of factors that influence health status. These include genetic makeup, sex, and age. Social and cultural issues and health behaviors are also closely linked to health status. The determinants of health also include education, nutritional status, and socio-economic status. The environment is also a powerful determinant of health, as is access to health services, and the policy approaches that countries take to their health sectors and to investments that could influence the health of their people.

It is also important to understand the most important risk factors that lead to ill health. In the low-income countries on which this book focuses considerable attention, some of the most important risk factors include nutritional status, the lack of safe water or appropriate sanitation, and tobacco smoking. Poor diets that relate to obesity, high blood pressure, high cholesterol, and cardiovascular disease are becoming increasingly important problems as well, even in low-income countries.

There are a number of uses of health data including measuring health status, carrying out disease surveillance, making decisions about investments in health, and assessing the performance of health programs. Those working in health use a common set of indicators to measure health status, including life expectancy, infant and neonatal mortality, under-five child mortality, and the maternal mortality ratio. They also use composite indices, such as DALYs, to measure the burden of disease.

Poorer countries have a relatively larger burden of disease from communicable diseases than from non-communicable diseases, compared to richer countries. As these poorer countries develop, fertility and mortality will decline, the population will age, and the burden of disease will shift toward the non-communicable diseases. These phenomena occur as countries go through what are referred to as the demographic transition and the epidemiological transition.

Life expectancy has improved in all regions of the world since 1990, except in Europe, Central Asia, and Sub-Saharan Africa. The leading cause of death worldwide has now become cardiovascular disease. However, communicable diseases remain relatively much more important in South Asia and Sub-Saharan Africa than in the rest of the world.

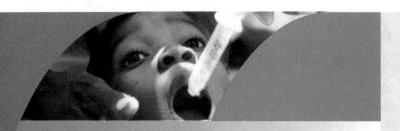

Study Questions

1. What are the main factors that determine your health?

2. What are the main factors that would determine the health of a poor person in a poor country?

3. If you could only pick one indicator to describe the health status of a poor country, which indicator would you use and why?

4. Why is it valuable to have composite indicators like DALYs to measure the burden of disease?

5. What is a HALE and how does it differ from just measuring life expectancy at birth?

6. As countries develop economically, what are the most important changes that occur in their burden of disease?

7. Why do these changes occur?

8. In your own country, what population groups have the best health indicators and why?

9. In your country, what population groups have the worst health status and why?

10. How would the population pyramid of Italy differ from that of Nigeria and why?

REFERENCES

1. A global emergency: a combined response *The world health report 2004 - changing history*. Geneva: World Health Organization; 2004:6.

2. Russia. Available at: http://www.prb.org/TemplateTop.cfm?Section=PRB_Country_Profiles&template=/customsource/countryprofile/countryprofiledisplay.cfm&Country=470. Accessed June 29, 2006.

3. Key Development Data and Statistics. Internet Resource; Computer File Available at: http://web.worldbank.org/WBSITE/EXTERNAL/DATASTATISTICS/0,,contentMDK:20535285~menuPK:1192694~pagePK:64133150~piPK:64133175~theSitePK:239419,00.html. Accessed June 17, 2006.

4. Kozik CA, Suntayakorn S, Vaughn DW, Suntayakorn C, Snitbhan R, Innis BL. Causes of death and unintentional injury among schoolchildren in Thailand. *Southeast Asian J Trop Med Public Health.* Mar 1999;30(1):129-135.

5. Public Health Agency of Canada. Population Health Approach, What Determines Health? Available at: http://www.phac-aspc.gc.ca/ph-sp/phdd/determinants/index.html. Accessed October 6, 2005.

6. World Health Organization. WHO Issues New Healthy Life Expectancy Rankings: Japan Number One in New "Healthy Life" System. Available at: http://www.who.int/inf-pr-2000/en/pr2000-life.html. Accessed January 3, 2006.

7. Hobcraft J. Women's education, child welfare and child survival : a review of the evidence. *Health Transition Review.* 1993;3(2):159-173.

8. World Bank. *Repositioning Nutrition as Central to Development—A Strategy for Large-Scale Action.* Washington, DC: The World Bank; 2006.

9. Basch P. *Textbook of International Health.* 2nd ed. New York: Oxford University Press; 2001:73-113.

10. Haupt, A, Kane, TT, Population Handbook, Washington, DC: Population Reference Bureau. 2004.

11. Haupt, A, Kane, TT, Population Handbook, Washington, DC: Population Reference Bureau. 2004.

12. WDI Data Query. Available at: http://devdata.worldbank.org/dataquery/. Accessed July 1, 2006.

13. Haupt, A, Kane, TT, Population Handbook, Washington, DC: Population Reference Bureau. 2004.

14. Zupan J. Perinatal mortality in developing countries. *N Engl J Med.* May 19 2005;352(20):2047-2048.

15. Haupt, A, Kane, TT, Population Handbook, Washington, DC: Population Reference Bureau. 2004.

16. Health Status Statistics: Mortality. Available at: www.who.int/healthinfo/statistics/indneonatalmortality/en/. Accessed June 25, 2006.

17. Haupt, A, Kane, TT, Population Handbook, Washington, DC: Population Reference Bureau. 2004.

18. Human Development Indicators 2003. Available at: http://hdr.undp.org/reports/global/2003/indicator/indic_78_1_1.html. Accessed June 25, 2006.

19. Last JM. *A dictionary of epidemiology.* 4th ed. New York: Oxford University Press; 2001:118.

20. Haupt, A, Kane, TT, Population Handbook, Washington, DC: Population Reference Bureau. 2004.

21. Last JM. *A dictionary of epidemiology.* 4th ed. New York: Oxford University Press; 2001:51.

22. Haupt, A, Kane, TT, Population Handbook, Washington, DC: Population Reference Bureau. 2004.

23. Summary Country Profile for HIV/AIDS Treatment Scale-Up: Botswana. www.who.int/3by5/support/June 2005_bwa.pdf. Accessed June 25, 2006.

24. Haupt, A, Kane, TT, Population Handbook, Washington, DC: Population Reference Bureau. 2004.

25. Country Profile: India. Available at: http://www.stoptb.org/countries/GlobalReport2006/ind.pdf. Accessed June 25, 2006.

26. Last JM. *A dictionary of epidemiology.* 4th ed. New York: Oxford University Press; 2001:35.

27. Lopez AD, Mathers CD, Murray CJL. The Burden of Disease and Mortality by Condition: Data, Methods, and Results for 2001. In: Lopez AD, Mathers CD, Ezzati M, Jamison DT, Murray CJL, eds. *Global burden of disease and risk factors.* New York: Oxford University Press; 2006:126-129.

28. Merson MH, Black RE, Mills AJ. *International public health : diseases, programs, systems, and policies.* Gaithersburg, MD: Aspen Publishers; 2000:28.

29. Health Adjusted Life Expectancy: Statistics Canada. www.statcan.ca/ennglish/fav/hale. Accessed May 25, 2006.

30. Global Burden of Disease. www.who.int/trade/glossary/story036/en/ Accessed May 25, 2006.

31. Jamison DT, Brennan J, Measham A, et al., eds. *Priorities in Health.* New York: Oxford University Press; 2006.

32. World development report 1993. New York: Oxford University Press; 1993:25-29.

33. Lopez AD, Mathers CD, Ezzati M, Jamison DT, Murray CJL. Measuring the Global Burden of Disease and Risk Factors, 1990-2001. In: *Global burden of disease and risk factors.* New York: Oxford University Press; 2006:1-15.

34. Basch P. *Textbook of International Health.* 2nd ed. New York: Oxford University Press; 2001:108-112.

35. Lopez AD, Mathers CD, Ezzati M, Jamison DT, Murray CJL. In: Lopez AD, Mathers CD, Ezzati M, Jamison DT, Murray CJL, eds. *Global burden of disease and risk factors.* New York: Oxford University Press; 2006:8.

36. Lopez AD, Mathers CD, Ezzati M, Jamison DT, Murray CJL. Measuring the Global Burden of Disease and Risk Factors, 1990-2001. In: Lopez AD, Mathers CD, Ezzati M, Jamison DT, Murray CJL, eds. *Global burden of disease and risk factors.* New York: Oxford University Press; 2006:3.

37. Lopez AD, Mathers CD, Murray CJL. The Burden of Disease and Mortality by Condition: Data, Methods, and Results for 2001. In: Lopez AD, Mathers CD, Ezzati M, Jamison DT, Murray CJL, eds. *Global burden of disease and risk factors.* New York: Oxford University Press; 2006:228-231.

38. Lopez A, Begg S, Bos E. Demographic and Epidemiological Characteristics of Major Regions, 1990-2001. In: Lopez A, Mathers C, Ezzati M, Jamison D, Murray C, eds. *Global Burden of Disease and Risk Factors.* New York: Oxford University Press; 2006:15-44.

39. Last JM. *A dictionary of epidemiology.* 4th ed. New York: Oxford University Press; 2001:160.

40. Beaglehole R, Irwin A, Prentice T. The world health report 2004 : changing history. Internet Resource] xvii, 169 p. : ill. ; 126 cm. Available at: http://www.who.int/whr/2004/en/

Materials specified: HTML VERSION http://www.who.int/whr/2004/en/Materials specified: PDF VERSION TO DOWNLOAD http://www.who.int/whr/2004/download/en/print.html

41. Lopez AD, Mathers CD, Ezzati M, Jamison DT, Murray CJL. Measuring the Global Burden of Disease and Risk Factors, 1990-2001. In: Lopez AD, Mathers CD, Ezzati M, Jamison DT, Murray CJL, eds. *Global burden of disease and risk factors.* New York: Oxford University Press; 2006:9.

42. Last JM. *A dictionary of epidemiology.* 4th ed. New York: Oxford University Press; 2001:70.

43. Lee R. The Demographic Transition: Three Centuries of Fundamental Change, Journal of Economic Perspectives. *Journal of Economic Perspectives.* 2003;17(4):167-190.

44. Omran AR. The Epidemiologic Transition: A Theory of the Epidemiology of Population Change. *The Milbank Quarterly.* 2005;83(4):731.

45. Jamison DT. Investing in Health. In: Jamison DT, Breman JG, Measham AR, et al., eds. *Disease Control Priorities in Developing Countries.* New York: Oxford University Press; 2006:3-34.

46. Registrar General & Census Commissioner. *Census of India 2001, Provisional population Totals.* New Delhi: Government of India, New Delhi; 2001.

47. Black JA. Kerala's demographic transition: determinants and consequences. *Bmj.* Jun 26 1999;318(7200):1771.

48. Zachariah K. *The Anomaly of the Fertility Decline in India's Kerala State.* Washington DC 1984.

49. Black JA. Family Planning and Kerala. *National Medical Journal of Kerala.* 1989;3:187-197.

50. Tharakan P, Navaneetham K. *Population Projection and Policy Implications for Education: A Discussion with Reference to Kerala:* Centre for Development Studies (Thiruvananthapuram) 1999.

51. Ratcliffe J. Social justice and the demographic transition: lessons from India's Kerala State. *International Journal of Health Services.* 1978;8(1):123-144.

52. United Nations Development Programme. Kerala—Human Development Fact Sheet. Available at: http://www.undp.org.in/programme/undpini/factsheet/kerala.pdf. Accessed July 21, 2006.

53. UNICEF. *State of the World's Children.* New York: Oxford University Press; 2004.

54. International Institute for Population Sciences and OrcMacro. *National Family Health Survey (NFHS-2) 1998-1999.* Mumbai: International Institute for Population Sciences and OrcMacro; 2000.

55. United Nations Economic and Social Commission for Asia and the Pacific. India: National Population Policy. Available at: http://www.unescap.org/esid/psis/population/database/poplaws/law_india/indiaappend3.htm. Accessed July 21, 2006.

56. Kutty VR. Historical analysis of the development of health care facilities in Kerala State, India. *Health Policy Plan.* Mar 2000;15(1):103-109.

57. Centers for Disease Control and Prevention. Life Expectancy. Available at: http://www.cdc.gov/nchs/fastats/lifexpec.htm. Accessed January 3, 2007.

58. Tsai KS. Debating Decentralized Development: A Reconsideration of the Wenzhou and Kerala Models. *India Journal of Economics & Business, Special Issue China & India;* 2006.

59. Joseph K. *Migration and Economic Development of Kerala.* New Delhi: Mittal Publications; 1988.

Health, Education, Poverty, and the Economy

VIGNETTES

Savitha lived in a poor village in north India. When she first became sick, she visited an unlicensed "doctor." She did not recover and then went to a practitioner of Indian Systems of Medicine. After another two weeks of illness, she went to the outpatient clinic of the main hospital. By the time Savitha had begun to recover, she had spent $20 equivalent on health services and on the transport to get to them. She had also missed two weeks of work, during which she lost another $20 of income. The total cost of this illness was about 10% of Savitha's annual earnings.

Mohammed was in first grade in a small town in northern Nigeria. Mohammed's family was poor. Mohammed was very small for his age, was very thin, and got sick more often than most children. Because of his poor health, Mohammed was unable to attend school regularly and was forced to quit school after only 1 year. Unfortunately, he could not read or write, had little knowledge of how to work with figures, and was most likely destined for a life of limited job prospects at very low pay.

Birte was born in Denmark to a middle class family. She was exclusively breastfed until she was six months old, when appropriate complementary foods were introduced. Her family took her regularly for "well baby" check-ups and she received all of her scheduled childhood immunizations. Her hearing and her eyesight were checked before she enrolled in school. Birte attended school regularly, she was attentive in class, and she performed well there. She was able to complete high school and medical school and today is a physician.

ABC company was looking for investments in forest products and examined in detail the possibility of investing in Africa. After carefully considering the potential costs and returns to such an investment, the company decided, however, not to invest in Africa but to invest instead in Asia. In the end, the company believed that they were unlikely to make an acceptable profit on any business in Africa because so many of their workers would be infected with HIV and malaria.

INTRODUCTION

Health and economic matters are intimately linked in a number of ways. First, health is an important contributor to people's ability to be productive and to accumulate the knowledge and skills they need to be productive, known as "human capital." Second, health status is also a major determinant of one's enrollment in and success in school, which itself is an important contributor to future earnings. Third, the costs of health care are also extremely important to individuals, especially to poor people, because large out-of-pocket expenditures can have a major impact on their financial status and can push them into poverty. Fourth, the costs of health care are also very important because health is a major item of national expenditure in all countries. Finally, the approach that different countries take to the financing and carrying out of health services raises important issues of equity.[1]

The objective of this chapter is to help you gain an introductory understanding of the two-way relationship between health and development. The chapter examines the connection between health and education. It then reviews the link between health and poverty and health and equity. Lastly, the chapter explores the link between health and income at the level of individuals and the connections between health and development more broadly. As it reviews these themes, the chapter will introduce you to some of the basic concepts of both global health and of health economics.

HEALTH, EDUCATION, PRODUCTIVITY, AND POVERTY

Health and Education

Essentially, there are three ways that health and education are connected. First, there are intergenerational links; the health and education of parents affects the health and education of their children. Second, malnutrition and disease affect the cognitive development and school performance of children. Lastly, education contributes to the prevention of illness.

The AIDS epidemic worldwide shows how the poor health of one generation can affect the schooling prospects and future earnings of the next generation. When mothers die of HIV, for example, children are more likely to be poorly fed, malnourished, and in ill health. As a result, they are also more likely to attend school less frequently and to perform poorly in school when they are there. During the period that a mother is sick with AIDS, it is also likely that one or more of her children will stay out of school to attend to the mother's health and the chores that the mother is no longer able to do.

Malnutrition or illness can limit schooling and school performance in a number of ways. First, families sometimes delay the enrollment of a sick or malnourished child in school. In addition, malnutrition and illness can also reduce attendance at school and, thereby, reduce an individual's performance in school. Malnutrition and illness can also decrease mental ability. All of these factors ultimately constrain what children will learn in school, decrease the number of years of schooling they complete, and, thereby, reduce future earnings.

However, there is also a powerful connection between health and education in the other direction—the impact of education on health. We already know that education and knowledge of appropriate health behaviors are important determinants of health and, indeed, that the education of a child's mother is an important predictor of the health of a child. Studies like one done in Guatemala have consistently shown, in fact, that the higher the level of education of a mother, the more likely she is to immunize her child, as noted in Figure 3-1.[2]

Another study done in the Philippines illustrated how better educated mothers are able to keep their children healthy, even in locations without a safe water supply.[3] In a study of a large number of developing countries, it was shown that every 10% increase in the level of education of mothers led to a reduction in the infant mortality rate by 4.1 deaths for every 1000 live births.[3] In addition, there is evidence from many countries that education affects the extent to which people make use of health services and better education discourages people from engaging in unhealthy behaviors. This will be referred to in a number of places in this book.

Health, Productivity, and Earnings

Health has an important impact on labor productivity and earnings, separate from its link with education. First, good health increases longevity and the longer that one lives, the longer one can earn, and the higher one's lifetime earnings. Second, a number of studies have shown that healthy workers are more productive than unhealthy workers. Among the most cited of such studies was one done on men who tapped rubber trees in Indonesia, many of whom were anemic due to hookworm infection. When the workers were treated for their infections, they became less anemic and their productivity increased by about 20%.[4] Third, many people when ill cannot go to work, and when they are absent from work, they often do not earn.

Health, the Costs of Illness, and Poverty

The costs of illness to individuals and their families can be high, can force them to lose or dispose of assets, and can cause them to fall into poverty. When people become ill in poor countries, as noted in the vignette about Savitha at the start of this chapter, they usually do seek health care and they often seek care of different types. They frequently have to pay for treatment and for drugs, the costs of which can be a very substantial share of their income. In addition, illness often leads to a decline in earnings, because people miss work. There are also other indirect costs that people bear when they are ill, such as the costs of transportation to and from a health service provider.

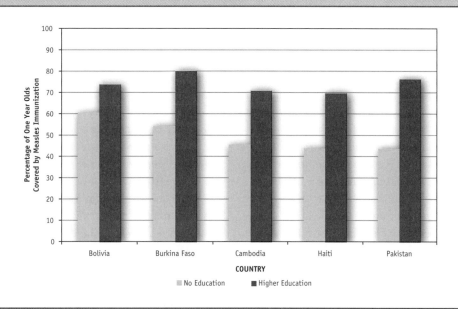

FIGURE 3-1 Percentage of One Year Old Children Receiving Measles Immunization, by Mothers with No Education and Mothers with Higher Education, for Selected Countries

Source: Data from WHO Statistical Information System (WHOSIS). Available at: http://www3.who.int/whosis/core/core_select_process.cfm. Accessed July 10, 2006.

Beyond the costs of either a short-term or a chronic illness, we must also remember the cost to individuals of living with the disability that comes from different health conditions. Measles or meningitis, for example, could lead to severe disability. Polio can lead to paralysis, and leprosy can lead to deformity. A number of mental health conditions are associated with long-term disability, as discussed further in Chapter 12. There is an increasing number of people with diabetes in rich and poor countries alike, and diabetes is often associated with a variety of disabilities. Long lasting disabilities generally require considerable expenditure on health services. They usually also lead to a significant decline in the earnings of the disabled person, compared to what they could earn if they were not disabled.

The costs of illness can be devastating for poor families. A study done in Bangladesh, for example, showed that a Bangladeshi lost the equivalent of four months of income from getting TB.[5] Surveys done in India showed that hospitalization was a major contributor to people and families falling into poverty. Of the patients who were hospitalized at some time during a 1 year period that was surveyed, almost 25% of the people hospitalized were pushed below the official Indian poverty line because of the costs of their hospitalization, related expenditures, and lost wages. Moreover, more than 40% of those hospitalized borrowed money or sold assets to pay for their health care.[6]

Indeed, in a study of the poor that was carried out as a background to the preparation of the 2000 World Development Report of the World Bank, the poor consistently noted the importance to them of maintaining good health. In addition, that report noted that ill health is an important contributor to poverty and to the economic vulnerability that also is at the foundation of poverty problems.[7] Indeed, we know that a certain segment of the population in many countries that do not have adequate health insurance are at risk that catastrophic costs of health care will drive them to poverty or bankruptcy. In Chapter 5, you will read about how different health systems try to protect the poor from the costs of health care.

HEALTH AND EQUITY

There are a number of equity issues that arise when considering global health matters, especially when examining the health, social, and economic status of poor people, disadvantaged ethnic groups, and women. The most important of these are access to health services, the manner in which health systems are responsive to the needs of people, and the extent to which the financing of health systems is fair, when taking the income of the health system users into account.[8]

One important theme that runs throughout this book is the fact that poor people, disadvantaged groups such as poor ethnic minorities, people who dwell in distant locations from health services, and women often have less access to health services than do better off groups. Sometimes, especially for the poor and for minority groups, this reflects the fact that there are fewer health services available in the areas in which they live because those places may be distant from larger towns and cities. We would expect, for example, in most countries, that rural areas will have fewer health services than urban ones. If we look at the Andean region, for example, we will see that indigenous groups often live in highland areas that are relatively lacking in health services compared to more urban areas. The same would be true in the mountainous areas of Asia, such as in Nepal, in which the western part of the country has an extraordinarily limited supply of health services and people may have to walk for days to access health services.

A related issue, however, is that the poor, women, and other groups that lack social and political power or "voice" generally seek and are accorded less access to health services than those who are better off, more powerful politically, and have more voice in the allocation of resources.[7] Figure 3-2, for example, shows the coverage of basic childhood immunization, by income group, in a set of selected countries.

As you can clearly see, the higher the income of the child's family, the greater is the likelihood that the child will be immunized. This pattern will be common in almost all low- and middle-income countries.

All better off countries, except the United States, have some type of mandatory and universal health insurance system that is meant to ensure that access to health services is not dependent on income. Many middle-income countries also have such insurance systems. However, most low-income countries do not have formalized health insurance systems, outside of the free or low cost provision of some health services by the public sector or nongovernmental sectors. Thus, many low-income countries fail to protect their poor from potentially catastrophic health costs that higher income individuals could afford. In addition, the relative cost of those health services is much greater for the poor than for better off people, which also raises important equity issues.

FIGURE 3-2 Immunization Coverage Rates by Income Quintile, for Selected Countries, by Region, 2000

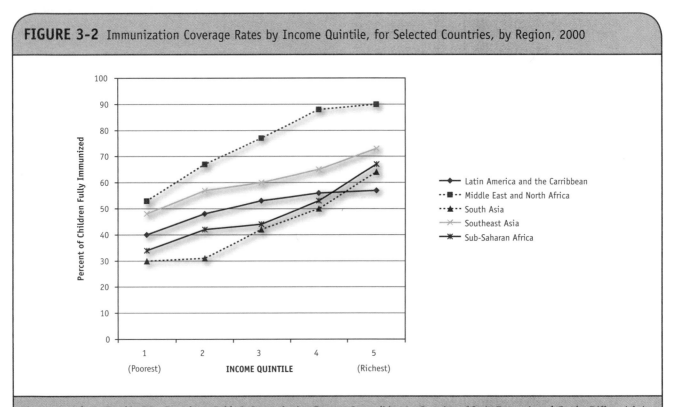

Source: Data from Gwatkin DR, Devashwar-Bahl, G. *Immunization Coverage Inequalities: An Overview of Socio-Economic and Gender Differentials in Developing Countries.* Washington, DC: World Bank; 2001.

Another set of important equity concerns that is related to the financing of health deals with the question of the extent to which different income groups benefit from public subsidies for health services. This can be a complicated issue to assess.[6] Nonetheless, it is clear that there are many countries in which public subsidies for health are disproportionately received by better off people, as shown in Figure 3-3, for India.

It is easy to imagine, for example, a country in which poor people use basic health services that are financed by the public sector which are relatively inexpensive, while better off people in the urban areas disproportionately use publicly supported hospital services that are relatively expensive. Under these circumstances, better off people, who will have higher rates of non-communicable disease, will get most of the expensive surgeries. Those surgeries will cost hundreds of times what basic health care costs, and the country would be providing a disproportionate share of public subsidies to the better off, rather than to the poor. There is no justification on clinical, economic, or equity grounds for this being the case.

HEALTH EXPENDITURE AND HEALTH OUTCOMES

One of the reasons why health is so important to countries is that they spend a lot of money on it. In addition, as noted earlier, they are also trying, in principle, to get the most for the money they spend, consistent with national values. Figure 3-4 shows the relationship between gross domestic product (GDP) per capita and health expenditure as a share of GDP.

The main themes that emerge from this figure are clear:

- The higher a country's income per person, the more money it is likely to spend per person on health.
- Most high-income countries cluster around an expenditure of 9–12% of their national income on health.
- Most countries that are low income cluster around an expenditure of 3–6% of their national income on health. This can be seen in the figure in Bangladesh, Ghana, and Nigeria.
- Despite the clustering, there are countries that are outliers and that sit significantly away from the general relationship between income per capita and percentage of national income spent on health. The United States spends more than any other country on health as a share of GDP. Cambodia and Cuba spend relatively more than one would expect for countries with their income.

Having seen what countries spend on health, it is now important to ask what they get in return for that expenditure. Do countries that spend higher shares of their national income on health have better health outcomes? Figure 3-5

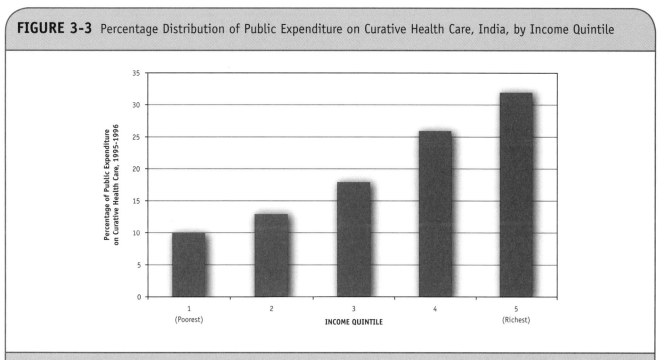

FIGURE 3-3 Percentage Distribution of Public Expenditure on Curative Health Care, India, by Income Quintile

Source: Modified with permission from Peters DH, Preker AS, Yazbek AS, et al. *Better Health Systems for India's Poor.* Washington, DC: World Bank; 2002:4.

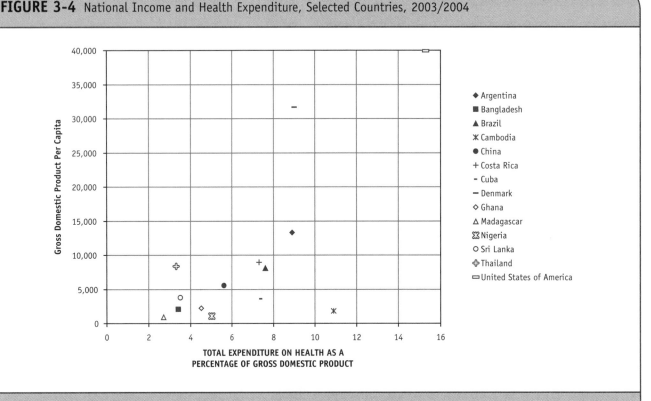

FIGURE 3-4 National Income and Health Expenditure, Selected Countries, 2003/2004

Source: Data from World Health Organization. Core Health Indicators, 2006. Available at: http://www3.who.int/whosis/core/core_select_process.cfm. Accessed July 8, 2006.

plots health expenditure as a share of GDP against life expectancy for selected countries.

We can see from this figure that:

- Many low-income countries spend a relatively low share of their GDP on health and also have low life expectancy. This is seen in Ghana, Kenya, and Mali.
- Most high-income countries spend a relatively high share of their GDP on health and have high life expectancy. This can be seen from Germany and Iceland.
- Some low-income countries spend relatively little on health but still have relatively higher life expectancy than many countries that spend a lower share of GDP on health. This can be seen in Cuba, Costa Rica, China, and Sri Lanka.
- Some high-income countries spend relatively high shares of GDP on health but still have lower life expectancy than countries that spend a lower share of GDP on health than they do. This is best shown by the United States, which is an outlier on this figure as

well as on the figure that portrays public expenditure on health as a share of GDP.

Why is it that some countries are outliers when considering their health outcomes related to health expenditure? First, we know that health status depends on a number of genetic, social, and economic factors and those factors vary across countries. Second, however, health outcomes depend not only on how much expenditure countries make per capita on health, but they also depend on the particular investments they make with that money. In colloquial terms we could say, "It is not just how much money per capita they spend on health, but it is also how they spend it that is important." This theme will also be explored throughout this book.

PUBLIC AND PRIVATE EXPENDITURE ON HEALTH

Another important concept is the distinction between public and private expenditures on health. Public expenditure refers to expenditure by the any level of government or of a government agency. Expenditure by a city government, a state government, or a national government would be public

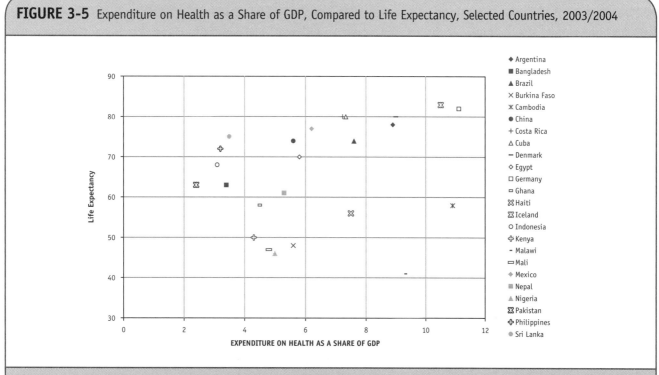

FIGURE 3-5 Expenditure on Health as a Share of GDP, Compared to Life Expectancy, Selected Countries, 2003/2004

Source: Data from World Health Organization. Core Health Indicators, 2006. Available at: http://www3.who.int/whosis/core/core_select_process.cfm. Accessed July 18, 2006.

expenditure. Expenditure on health by government agencies such as a social security system, as in many countries in Latin America, the national insurance agency, as in most countries in Western Europe, or of a specialized agency, such as a National Commission on HIV/AIDS, would also be considered public expenditure.

Private expenditure is that expenditure that comes from sources other than governments. One such source is the money that individuals spend on health. When this money is not covered or reimbursed by an insurance program, it is also called out-of-pocket expenditures on health. Other sources of private expenditure on health include expenditure by nongovernmental organizations, such as by the Bangladesh Rural Advancement Committee or the Self Employed Women's Association in India. In addition, private expenditure on health includes expenditure by the private for-profit sector. Private sector firms, for example, might contribute to the cost of health insurance or health services for their employees. They might also make contributions to the health work of other organizations.

There is some debate about what are legitimate focuses of public expenditure on health.[9] However, there is widespread agreement that public expenditure on health is war-

ranted when the investment benefits society as a whole, such as an immunization program, when health investments promote equity, and when such expenditure provides financial protection to the poor from expenditures on health that they can not afford.[9]

THE COST-EFFECTIVENESS OF HEALTH INTERVENTIONS

Most governments have a limited amount of money for health, and that money is rarely enough to finance all of the health interventions that a country would like to carry out. Thus, governments have to decide what share of their total budget will go to health and how much of the health budget will be allocated to different health interventions. All governments have to set priorities for expenditure on health, just as they have to set priorities for expenditure in other sectors.

One important tool for setting priorities for public expenditure on health is cost-effectiveness analysis. This is a method for comparing the cost of an investment with the amount of health that can be purchased with that investment. The cost of the investment can be thought of as the price of the investment. The amount of health that can be purchased could be measured in life years saved or DALYs. The cost-effectiveness of an investment in health will depend, among other things, on the incidence and prevalence of the health condition being considered, the cost of the intervention, the extent to which it can reduce morbidity, mortality, and disability, and how effectively it can be implemented.

One important example of the use of cost-effectiveness analysis is to set priorities among different ways of achieving the same health goal. Important studies were conducted, for example, on the cost-effectiveness of alternative approaches to treating tuberculosis. These studies examined the cost-effectiveness of 6 months of treatment with direct supervision of people taking their medicines, compared to treatment that was not supervised. The supervised method led to a higher rate than the unsupervised approach of people taking all of their medicine and being cured. As a result, it proved to be more cost-effective than the traditional approach that had been used. These studies strengthened the case for the World Health Organization recommending the supervised approach to therapy, which continues to be the global standard of TB treatment.[10]

It is easy to imagine how important this type of cost-effectiveness analysis can be when considering different ways of delivering the same health services. In fact, there are many important issues in delivering health services in low-income countries in which such questions remain critical. In Haiti, for example, there is a program operated by Partners in Health. Those carrying out the program had to assess whether or not the services would be delivered as effectively by volunteer workers as they would be by workers who were paid a small amount for their efforts. Although it cost more to deliver the program when the workers were paid, the outcomes were superior to those when the workers were not paid, and Partners in Health has continued to use the approach of paid workers.[11] Another issue of great importance today is the extent to which antiretroviral drugs for HIV/AIDS can be delivered effectively by nurses and community health workers, instead of physicians, because physicians are in such short supply in many countries that have high rates of prevalence of HIV/AIDS. This question is one of many concerning the delivery of services for HIV that is in need of careful cost-effectiveness analysis.

The second manner in which cost-effectiveness analysis is used is to compare the costs and the gains of different health interventions so that investment choices can be made among them. For every $100, for example, that a government has to spend on health, what allocation of government

expenditure on health will buy the most DALYs averted? What is the cost per disability adjusted life year saved from different interventions? In a relatively poor country, with a high burden of communicable diseases, such as TB and malaria, is it more cost-effective to invest in infectious disease control or in coronary bypass surgery? In a richer country, will it be cost-effective to invest in vaccination against TB?

Even if we examine the first question above in a somewhat exaggerated and simplistic manner, it will still help us to understand some of the value of cost-effectiveness analysis. Let us say, for example, that the cost of coronary bypass surgery in a low-income country is about $5000. Let us also say that the costs of such surgery are covered completely by the public sector. This surgery would benefit one individual, who will live an additional 20 years in perfectly good health because of the surgery. In the same country, we can assume an entire course of treatment for TB costs about $100. In addition, we can assume that people who get TB will all be 40 years of age and that they will live an additional 20 years in perfectly good health if they are treated for TB. What this means, in principle, is that if these were the only choices for the investment of $5000 in health that a country faced and that if this were the only type of analysis that would be done to assess investment choices, then the choice would be between saving one life or saving 50 lives. In addition, the choices would be between saving 20 additional years of healthy life of the coronary bypass patient or 2000 additional healthy years of life of the TB patient. Figure 3-6 illustrates the cost-effectiveness of a selected number of health interventions.

One can see in the figure that the cost of avoiding ill health caused by TB, malaria, and hookworms, for example, is low, while the cost of saving a life through cancer treatment is high. It is very cost-effective to get people to use seat belts in cars, but much less cost-effective to save the lives of people after they have had car accidents. As discussed further in Chapter 8, it is cost-effective to enhance the nutritional and health status of young children through supplementation with Vitamin A. However, it is much less cost-effective in health centers and hospitals to deal with the additional morbidity and mortality that occur from measles and pneumonia for children who are deficient in Vitamin A.[12]

It is important to note that cost-effectiveness analysis is rarely the sole means for determining choices among investments and generally should not be used in that way.[13] However, it is one valuable tool in making such choices. It will always be important, however, to consider such analyses in light of a number of other factors, including:

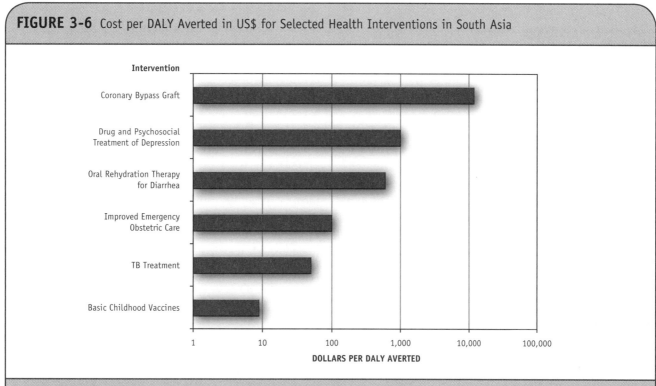

FIGURE 3-6 Cost per DALY Averted in US$ for Selected Health Interventions in South Asia

Source: Data with permission from The World Bank. Laxminarayan R, Chow J, Shahid-Salles SA. Intervention cost-effectiveness: overview of main messages. In: Jamison DT, Breman JG, Measham AR, et al., eds. *Disease Control Priorities in Developing Countries.* New York: Oxford University Press; 2006:51.

- Equity considerations
- The burden of disease
- The extent to which the investment serves society as a whole
- The extent to which the investment produces benefits that are additional to its usual ones
- The impact of the intervention on the provision of insurance

In addition, those who set priorities for health investments will also have to take account of:

- The capacity to deliver the proposed services
- The links between the proposed services and other important services
- The ability to change budget priorities in favor of the proposed investment
- Any transitional costs associated with making the proposed changes in priorities[13]

In this book, most of the assessments of cost-effectiveness will relate to DALYs averted. This is because examining the cost of life years saved from death would fail to capture the morbidity and disability that are also important aims of health interventions. In addition, it is important to note that there is no unique cut-off, below which interventions are "cost-effective" and above which they are not. Rather, it is preferable to group the cost-effectiveness of different interventions into ranges and to use cost-effectiveness analysis to explore the relative extent to which various interventions will lead to DALYs averted. In other words, it is not so important to think of TB control as cost-effective, *per se,* as it is to understand that in a county with a high prevalence of TB, control of TB using directly observed therapy will be one of the most cost-effective investments in health that can be made.[14]

HEALTH AND DEVELOPMENT

An important question at the core of thinking about global health concerns the links between health and development, at the individual, community, and society levels. Does individual health produce more individual wealth and higher levels of economic development at the community and societal levels? Or, are the effects in the opposite direction: Does more economic development at the level of society produce better health for individuals, communities, and societies? What we find when we examine these questions is that the effects of health and development go in both directions.

There is no question that good health promotes economic development at the level of societies. First, we know that when countries have to spend money to address health problems, they can not use that money for other purposes. Countries that have to spend substantial resources treating malaria, for example, have less money to spend not only on other areas of health, but also on schools, roads, and other investments outside of the health sector that could spur economic growth.

In addition, investment in economic activities, by local and foreign investors, is an essential ingredient to the economic growth prospects of low-income countries. Yet, as seen in one of the vignettes that opened this chapter, countries that have high burdens of communicable diseases do not appear to be good investment choices. In fact, in a study of the impact of malaria on economic development that is frequently cited, it was found that "a high prevalence of malaria is associated with a reduction of economic growth of 1% per year or more."[15]

There is also growing evidence of the importance of health to economic development from a number of other studies done by economists. Some have shown that higher life expectancy at birth is associated with faster economic growth rates. These studies suggest that a country with a life expectancy at birth of 77 years would be expected to grow economically 1.6% faster each year than a country with a life expectancy at birth of 49 years.[16] Another study showed that poor health was an important contributor to the slow pace of economic growth in Africa, compared to other countries with better health.[17] Another series of studies showed that improvements in nutritional status and related health status improvements were very important historically in boosting labor productivity and spurring economic growth in the United Kingdom and Europe.[12; 18–20]

It is also true that higher levels of economic development do promote better health at the level of both individuals and of society. In fact, studies that have been done on the impact of income on the health of different societies suggest that higher income is associated with better health and longer life expectancy.[21] However, more recent analyses of this question suggest that while income growth is associated with better health indicators for a country, the effect of income alone on health indicators is less than previously thought. Rather, these analyses suggest that a considerable share of the improvements in health indicators stem from technical progress such as the development of new vaccines or new drugs, or simple life saving approaches such as the use of

oral rehydration for young children with diarrhea, rather than stemming from income growth.[22]

In this light, we should ask: Is income growth necessary or sufficient for enhancing health status at the individual, community, or societal levels? Over the long run, increases in income will improve health. However, they will not improve it fast enough in most settings to achieve the health status objectives that many countries have set for themselves or that are necessary to achieve the MDGs in the time that has been set for them. What low- and middle-income countries must do, therefore, is adopt public policy choices that will allow them to speed the achievement of their health aims, even in the face of constrained income, as Kerala did. As indicated earlier, and as will be repeated throughout the book, this is the approach that has been taken by the small number of countries that have been particularly successful in meeting their health aims.

THE COPENHAGEN CONSENSUS

The importance of good health to economic development *has* increasingly been recognized. A panel of economic experts was convened in 2004 to try to identify the most cost-effective investments that would advance global welfare. Their work was referred to as "The Copenhagen Consensus," and Table 3-1 indicates the rank order of the investments that they considered. Of the four investments that were ranked as "very good," three were investments in health: treatment for HIV/AIDS, micronutrient supplementation, and control of malaria. Five investments were ranked as "good," and the first among them was to combat malnutrition by developing new agriculture technologies. Four investments were ranked "fair." The second and third of these were addressing malnutrition through improving infant and child nutrition and reducing the prevalence of low birthweight. The fourth was the scaling up of basic health services. The economists who forged the Copenhagen Consensus were clearly convinced of the important link of health to development, the relatively inexpensive ways of addressing a number of key health concerns, and the high returns that would come from doing so.[23]

CASE STUDY

Having read about the high returns to some investments in health and the need to prioritize investments in health, it will be valuable to end this chapter with a case study of another public health success story. This one concerns Guinea worm. Those interested in more detail in the case should consult *Case Studies in Global Health: Millions Saved.*

TABLE 3-1 The Copenhagen Consensus 2004

Very good projects	Fair projects
1. Diseases: Control of HIV/AIDS	**10. Migration:** Lowering barriers to migration for skilled workers
2. Malnutrition: Providing micronutrients	**11. Malnutrition:** Improving infant and child nutrition
3. Subsidies and Trade Barriers: Trade liberalization	**12. Malnutrition:** Reducing the prevalence of low birthweight
4. Diseases: Control of Malaria	**13. Diseases:** Scaled-up basic health services
Good projects	**Bad projects**
5. Malnutrition: Development of new agricultural technologies	**14. Migration:** Guest-worker programs for the unskilled
6. Water and Sanitation: Small-scale water technology for livelihoods	**15. Climate:** Optimal carbon tax
7. Water and Sanitation: Community-managed water supply and sanitation	**16. Climate:** The Kyoto Protocol
8. Water and Sanitation: Research on water productivity in food production	**17. Climate:** Value-at-risk carbon tax
9. Governance and Corruption: Lowering the cost of starting a new business	

Source: Adapted with permission from Copenhagen Consensus 2004. Available at: http://www.copenhagenconsensus.com/default.aspx?ID=158. Accessed July 8, 2006.

The Challenge of Guinea Worm in Asia and Sub-Saharan Africa

Background

Dracunculiasis, or Guinea worm disease, is an ancient scourge that once afflicted much of the world. Today, it is truly a disease of the poor, persisting in many of the world's most remote and disadvantaged regions with limited access to potable water, despite being one of the most preventable parasitic diseases. In the 1980s, an estimated 3.5 million people in 20 countries in Africa and Asia were infected with Guinea worm disease, and an estimated 120 million were at risk of becoming infected.[24]

The disease is contracted by drinking stagnant water from a well or pond that is contaminated with tiny fleas that carry Guinea worm larvae. Once inside the human, the larvae can grow up to three feet long. After a year, the grown female worm rises to the skin in search of a water source to release her larvae. A painful blister forms, usually in the person's lower limbs. To ease the burning pain, infected individuals frequently submerge the blister in water, causing the blister's rupture and the release of more larvae into the water. This contaminated water, when it is drunk, perpetuates the cycle of reinfection. Worms, usually as wide as a match, can take up to 12 weeks to emerge from the blister. They are coaxed out by being slowly wound around a stick a few centimeters each day. Debilitating pain from this process can linger for as long as 18 months.

Although rarely fatal, the disease takes a heavy toll by causing low productivity that makes it both a symptom and perpetrator of poverty—in Mali, it is called the "disease of the empty granary." Because water in contaminated ponds is widely consumed during peak periods of cyclical harvesting and planting, an entire community can be left debilitated and unable to work during the busiest agricultural seasons. The economic damage is severe: annual economic loss in three rice-growing states in Nigeria was calculated at $20 million.[25] While the disease afflicts all age groups, it particularly harms children.[25] School absenteeism rises when infected children are unable to walk to school and when children forego school to take on the agricultural and household work of sick adults. The likelihood of a child in Sudan being malnourished is more than three times higher when the adults in the child's home are infected with the disease.

The Intervention

In 1980, when the U.S. Centers for Disease Control and Prevention (CDC) first proposed an eradication campaign, the three interventions that would be required to address the disease effectively did not seem feasible: construction of expensive water sources; controlling the vector that spread the disease through the use of larvicides in water sources; and health education campaigns promoting the filtration of water with a cloth filter, self-reporting of infestations, and avoidance of recontamination of public water sources. The absence of a vaccine or cure made success seem even more improbable.

The International Drinking Water Supply and Sanitation Decade was launched the following year, however, and the CDC's Dr. Donald Henderson seized the opportunity to include the eradication of Guinea worm disease as a subgoal of the Water Decade program. Nonetheless, progress against Guinea worm disease remained slow until 1986, when three key events occurred: WHO declared eradication of Guinea worm disease a goal, public health ministers from 14 African nations met to affirm their commitment to the eradication effort, and U.S. President Jimmy Carter became a powerful advocate, personally persuading many leaders to launch national eradication efforts. He also recruited the help in the eradication program of two former popular heads of state of Mali and Nigeria, General Touré and General Gowon, respectively, thereby consolidating political commitment in Africa.

Meanwhile, technical and financial resources of the donor community were marshaled, and by 1995, eradication programs had been established in 20 countries. Water sources were provided, mainly through the construction of wells; in southeast Nigeria alone, village volunteers hand-dug more than 400 wells.[26] Larvicide was added to water sources to kill the fleas. People were taught to filter drinking water using a simple cloth filter. However, these filters were found to clog up and were used as decoration items instead.[25] A newly developed nylon cloth was then donated by the Carter Center, Precision Fabrics, and DuPont. Public education campaigns, including intensive efforts during so-called worm weeks, encouraged people to use the nylon filters, avoid recontaminating ponds, and report infestations.[27] Most of the eradication staff were volunteers trained by the ministries of health, but they pioneered a monthly reporting system for tracking and monitoring that is now hailed as a model for disease surveillance.[28]

The Impact

The campaign led to a 99% drop in Guinea worm disease prevalence. In 2005, fewer than 11,000 cases were reported, compared with an estimated 3.5 million infected people in 1986. By 1988, the campaign had already prevented between 9 million and 13 million cases of Guinea worm disease.[29] The Asian countries that were targeted, India, Pakistan, and Yemen, are now free of the disease. Most remaining cases are in Sudan where civil conflict impeded progress against the disease over many years.

Costs and Benefits

The total cost of the program between 1986 and 1998 was $87.5 million, with an estimated cost per case averted of $5 to $8.[29] The World Bank determined that the campaign has been highly cost-effective and cost-beneficial. In addition, the program had a very high economic rate of return, even when basing the calculation of economic benefits only on increases in agricultural productivity that accrued from people having avoided the disease.[29]

Lessons Learned

Success of the program has been attributed to three factors. The first is the exemplary coordination between major partners and donors. The second is the power of data, gathered through the monthly reporting system, to monitor national programs and to help keep countries focused and motivated on the program goals. The third is the high-level advocacy and political leadership from current and former heads of state, especially President Jimmy Carter and General Gowon, who visited and revisited villages in Nigeria to check on progress. The program drew on a truly global partnership between the CDC, UNICEF, WHO, the Carter Center, governments, NGOs, the private sector, and volunteers that was able to motivate changes in individual and community behaviors and successfully control a disease.

MAIN MESSAGES

The aim of this chapter was to introduce you to some of the basic concepts of economics as they relate to the global health arena. One important message of the chapter is that education and health are closely linked. Good health encourages the enrollment of students in school at the appropriate age, enhanced student attendance at school, better cognitive performance of students, and more completed years of schooling. Education and knowledge are consistently correlated with people's engagement in more appropriate health behaviors and living healthier lives than those with less schooling. In addition, education promotes greater opportunities for income earning, which itself is an important determinant of health.

We also learned that health is strongly associated with productivity and earnings. Healthier people can work harder, work more hours, and work over a longer lifetime than can those who are less healthy. Related to this in many ways, we also saw that health has an important relationship with poverty. If people work fewer hours because of ill health, then there is a risk that their income status will decline, perhaps below the poverty line. In addition, there is evidence from many countries that the direct and indirect costs to people of getting health services can itself push people into poverty.

Health is an important subject for all countries for many reasons, among the most important of which is the amount of money they spend on health. High-income countries spend more money on health than do low-income countries. However, health outcomes depend not just on how much money is spent, but also on how the money is used. One way that countries set priorities for health expenditure is by using cost-effectiveness analysis, a tool that is used in the health sector to compare how much health one can buy for a given level of expenditure. All countries, of course, face the question of how they can maximize the health of their population for the minimum cost.

There are also many strong relationships between the health of a population and the economic development of the society in which they live. Better health does promote wealth in a variety of ways, including enhancing labor productivity, reducing the amount countries have to spend on health, and enabling a more attractive investment climate. In addition, the negative impact of some diseases on economic development, such as TB, HIV/AIDS, and malaria, can be very significant. Economic development does improve health; however, many gains in health stem from technological progress, such as on vaccines, and low-income countries in particular have to develop approaches to improving health that will promote better population health faster than economic development alone will do.

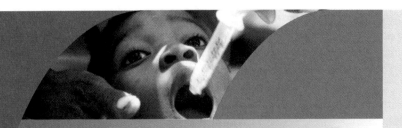

Study Questions

1. How does poor health status impact a person's income?

2. What is the relationship between health and the productivity of individuals?

3. Why might the health of some culture groups be different from the health of others?

4. What is the relationship between a country's expenditure on health as a share of national income and its health status?

5. In your country, is expenditure on health from the public sector, private sector, or both?

6. In using cost-effectiveness analysis, why should you also take into account issues such as equity?

7. How could you ensure that public subsidies on health care appropriately benefit the poor?

8. Does "health make wealth," or does "wealth make health?"

9. Why would Guinea worm disease have remained so prevalent for so long?

10. What impact would the health status of a country have on the likelihood that people will invest in economic activity in that country?

REFERENCES

1. Ruger JP, Jamison DT, Bloom DE. Health and the Economy. In: Merson MH, Black RE, Mills AJ, eds. *International Public Health, Diseases, Programs, Systems, and Policies.* Gaithersburg, MD: Aspen; 2001:617-666.

2. Pebley A, Goldman N, Rodriguez G. Prenatal and Delivery Care and Childhood Immunization in Guatemala: Do Family and Community Matter? *Demography.* 1996;33:197-210.

3. Glewwe P. *How does schooling of mothers improve child health? Evidence from Morocco.* Washington, DC: World Bank; 1997.

4. Basta SS, Soekirman, Karyadi D, Scrimshaw NS. Iron deficiency anemia and the productivity of adult males in Indonesia. *Am J Clin Nutr.* Apr 1979;32(4):916-925.

5. Croft RA, Croft RP. Expenditure and loss of income incurred by tuberculosis patients before reaching effective treatment in Bangladesh. *Int J Tuberc Lung Dis.* Mar 1998;2(3):252-254.

6. Peters DH, Preker AS, Yazbek AS, et al. *Better Health Systems for India's Poor.* Washington, DC: The World Bank; 2002.

7. Bank W. *World Development Report 2000/2001: Attacking Poverty.* New York: Oxford University Press; 2001.

8. World Health Organization. *The World Health Report—Health Systems: Improving Performance.* Geneva: World Health Organization; 2000.

9. Preker AS, Harding A. *The Economics of Public and Private Roles in Health Care.* Washington, DC: The World Bank; 2000.

10. Murray CJ, DeJonghe E, Chum HJ, Nyangulu DS, Salomao A, Styblo K. Cost effectiveness of chemotherapy for pulmonary tuberculosis in three sub-Saharan African countries. *Lancet.* Nov 23 1991;338(8778):1305-1308.

11. Walton DA, Farmer PE, Lambert W, Leandre F, Koenig SP, Mukherjee JS. Integrated HIV prevention and care strengthens primary health care: lessons from rural Haiti. *J Public Health Policy.* 2004;25(2):137-158.

12. Laxminarayan R, Chow J, Shahid-Salles SA. Intervention Cost Effectiveness: Overview of Main Messages. In: Jamison DT, Breman JG, Measham AR, et al., eds. *Disease Control Priorities in Developing Countries.* New York: Oxford University Press; 2006.

13. Yazbek AS. *An Idiot's Guide to Prioritization in the Health Sector.* Washington, DC: The World Bank; 2002.

14. Public Health Agency of Canada. Population Health Approach, What Determines Health? Available at: http://www.phac-aspc.gc.ca/ph-sp/phdd/determinants/index.html. Accessed October 6, 2005.

15. Comission on Macroeconomics and Health. *Macroeconomics and Health: Investing in Health for Economic Development.* Geneva: World Health Organization; 2001.

16. Comission on Macroeconomics and Health. *Macroeconomics and Health: Investing in Health for Economic Development.* Geneva: World Health Organization; 2001.

17. Bloom DE, Sachs J. Geography, Demography, and Economic Growth in Africa. *Brookings Papers on Economic Activity.* 1998;2:207-295.

18. Fogel R. *New Sources and New Techniques for the Study of Secular Trends in Nutritional Status, Health, Mortality and the Process of Aging* 1991.

19. Fogel R. New Findings on Secular Trends in Nutrition and Mortality: Some Implications for Population Theory. In: Rosenzweig M, Stark O, eds. *Handbook of Population and Family Economics Vol. 1a.* Amsterdam: Elsevier Science; 1997:433-481.

20. Fogel R. *The Fourth Great Awakening and the Future of Egalitarianism.* Chicago and London: The University of Chicago Press; 2000.

21. Pritchett LH, Summers LH. Wealthier is Healthier. *Journal of Human Resources.* 1996;31(4):841-868.

22. Jamison DT, Sandbu M, Wang J. *Why has Infant Mortality Decreased at Such Different Rates in Different Countries.* Bethesda, MD: Disease Control Priorities Project; 2004.

23. Copenhagen Consensus 2004: The Results. www.copenhagenconsensus.dk. Accessed July 21, 2006.

24. Carter J. The Power of Partnership: The Eradicaion of Guinea Worm Disease. *Cooperation South.* 1999(2):140-147.

25. Cairncross S, Muller R, Zagaria N. Dracunculiasis (Guinea worm disease) and the eradication initiative. *Clin Microbiol Rev.* Apr 2002;15(2):223-246.

26. Hopkins DR. Perspectives from the dracunculiasis eradication programme. *Bull World Health Organ.* 1998;76 Suppl 2:38-41.

27. Hopkins DR, Ruiz-Tiben E, Diallo N, Withers PC, Jr., Maguire JH. Dracunculiasis eradication: and now, Sudan. *Am J Trop Med Hyg.* Oct 2002;67(4):415-422.

28. Hopkins DR. The Guinea worm eradication effort: lessons for the future. *Emerg Infect Dis.* Jul-Sep 1998;4(3):414-415.

29. Kim A, Tandon A, Ruiz-Tiben E. *Cost-Benefit Analysis of the Global Dracunculiasis Eradication Campaign.* Washington, DC: World Bank; 1997.

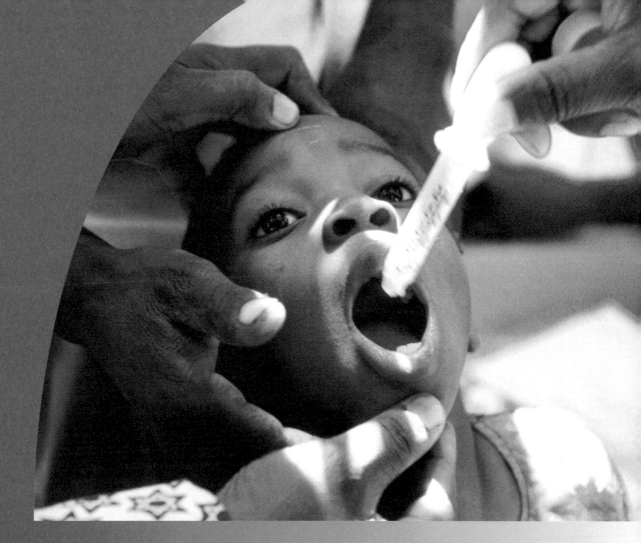

PART II

Cross-Cutting Global Health Themes

CHAPTER 4

Ethical and Human Rights Concerns in Global Health

VIGNETTES

Suraiya was a 21-year-old woman in Kabul, Afghanistan. Her sister recently died in childbirth at the age of 16 years. She had taken her sister to a health center when she was having trouble with her labor. However, the health center was 50 miles away from their house. In addition, partly because of the neglect of the last government and its discrimination against women, the health center was dilapidated. It had no equipment and the midwife there was unable to save Suraiya's sister. The baby died a few days later.

John Williams was a 21-year-old office clerk in a small country in Africa. For 3 months, he had experienced weight loss, continuous fever, and chronic fatigue. He finally got up the strength to visit the local hospital. When he got there, the staff was not welcoming. They did not treat him kindly. They did not offer to help him. They did not arrange for him to be seen by a doctor. They knew that he had HIV and did not want to treat him in their hospital.

Nandita, like many newborns, died in her first week of life in a small village in the highlands of Nepal. She had been born to a poor family in an area that was very underdeveloped and dominated by large landlords. The area around their home had almost no health workers. Her mother had no formal education, had received no prenatal care or counseling about the birth, and could not get medical help when the baby fell ill. There are international agreements about "the right to health" to which Nepal is a signator. Therefore, it is important to ask questions, such as: Was Nepal unable to provide the health services needed to save lives like Nandita's or were the political and social forces in Nepal unwilling to make such services a priority? Is this failure a matter of health policy, human rights, or both?

A potential microbicide against HIV was being tested on women in 10 cities in Africa. The women were to apply the microbicide before any sexual encounter. The developers of the microbicide were hopeful that it would be at least partially effective in stopping the transmission of HIV. However, there was still a risk that some of the women using the microbicide would become HIV positive while participating in the study. There was an important debate among those working on the microbicide about their ethical obligations to anyone who became HIV positive. Did they have to provide them with AIDS drugs for the remainder of their life, as some were suggesting?

THE IMPORTANCE OF ETHICAL AND HUMAN RIGHTS ISSUES IN GLOBAL HEALTH

Ethical and human rights issues are extremely important in global health because they cut across many areas of both human endeavor and government responsibility. In addition, there is a strong complementarity between good ethical and human rights practices on the one hand and good health outcomes on the other.[1] The previous vignettes touch only a very small sample of the many areas in global health that relate to ethical and human rights matters.

The importance of human rights issues to global health is highlighted by the fact that there are international conventions and treaties that recognize access to health services and health information, among other health areas, as human rights. Yet, there are remarkable gaps in many countries in access to health services. In addition, the poor and the disenfranchised suffer from those gaps the most.

Moreover, the failure to respect human rights is often associated with harm to human health. This has often been the case, for example, concerning diseases that are highly stigmatized, such as leprosy, TB, and HIV. If leprosy patients are not provided with the best standards of care because some health workers are afraid to work with them, the leprosy patients cannot stop the progression of their disease. If TB patients are shunned by health workers, they will die, after infecting many other people. There are many examples, such as in the vignettes about Suraiya and John, that show how the failure to respect the right to health of women or of HIV positive people can lead to poor health outcomes.

There are also a number of critical ethical issues that relate to global health. Some concern ensuring that decisions about health investments are fair, are made in fair ways, and take sufficient account of equity across groups. Another set of ethical matters is associated with appropriate ways to carry out research on human subjects.

Finally, efforts to maintain public health while dealing with new and emerging diseases, such as SARS or a potential avian influenza, raise an array of ethical and human rights issues. When we face a potential health threat, for example, what are the rights of individuals compared to the rights of society to protect itself from illness? Is it acceptable to quarantine a city? It is fair to ban travel to and from certain places? Should patients with TB who refuse to take their medicines be kept in a hospital and forced to take them? These are real issues with which health practitioners and policy makers must wrestle.

This chapter will provide an overview of some of the most critical links between human rights and global health. It will also examine how some of those links have evolved. It will briefly review the most important charters and conventions that set the foundation for the health and human rights concerns we have today. It will also touch upon a number of ethical issues that are central to global health. The chapter will conclude with comments on key challenges to enhancing ethical and human rights interests in global health activities.

The chapter is meant to be introductory. Nonetheless, it is very important as you review this chapter that you get a sense of key concerns about ethics and human rights as they relate to global health. It is also critical that you keep these concerns in mind both as you read this book and as you do further reading, writing, or working in the field of global health. More detailed information can be found in the materials that are referenced in this chapter.

THE FOUNDATIONS FOR HEALTH AND HUMAN RIGHTS

There are a number of treaties and conventions that set the foundation for human rights concerns. The most significant international declaration which focuses on human rights is the Universal Declaration of Human Rights (UDHR), which was promulgated in 1948. The UDHR is generally regarded as the cornerstone on which most of the later treaties and documents pertaining to human rights are based. The UDHR is also considered to set the standard for human rights globally, despite the fact that it does not have the force of law.

With respect to health, the UDHR states in Article 25:

> (1) Everyone has the right to a standard of living adequate for the health and well-being of himself and of his family, including food, clothing, housing and medical care and necessary social services, and the right to security in the event of unemployment, sickness, disability, widowhood, old age or other lack of livelihood in circumstances beyond his control.

> (2) Motherhood and childhood are entitled to special care and assistance. All children, whether born in or out of wedlock, shall enjoy the same social protection. [2]

Since 1948, more than 20 multilateral treaties that relate to health have been formulated which are legally binding on the countries that sign them. The European Convention on the Protection of Human Rights was signed in 1950. In 1966, two important treaties were adopted, The International Covenant on Economic, Social, and Cultural Rights (ICESR) and The International Covenant on Civil and Political Rights (ICCPR).[2-4] The ICESR has been ratified and signed by 155 countries and the ICCPR by 160 countries.[5,6] The ICESCR focuses on the well-being of individuals, including their right to work in safe conditions, receive fair wages, be free from hunger, get an education, and enjoy the highest attainable standard of physical and mental health. The ICCPR discusses rights of equality, liberty, security, and "freedom of movement, religion, expression, and association."[2–4]

In addition, under the auspices of the United Nations, a number of other important international conventions have been written, especially on specialized topics. The Convention on the Elimination of all Forms of Discrimination Against Women, for example, was adopted in 1979 by the United Nations General Assembly. It has been ratified by 83 countries. The Convention commits states to legally promote equality between men and women, ensure effective protection against discrimination against women, and to eliminate discriminatory practices aganst women. The Convention also affirms the reproductive rights of women.[7] A number of regional treaty arrangements on human rights, the most extensive of which are European and Latin American, are complementary to the UN human rights treaty system.

Many international human rights documents, including the ICCPR, have specific clauses for protecting the rights of children. Most articles in the general human rights instruments also apply equally to both adults and children. The Convention on the Rights of the Child (CRC), however, which was agreed upon in 1989, is the first human rights document which focuses specifically on the rights of children.[8] This document, which defines a child as "every human being below the age of 18 years," accords rights to be free of discrimination due to ethnicity, disability, or any other cause. It also grants the right to health and education. In addition, it includes the premise that children must have a say in decisions affecting their lives. The CRC also puts the rights of children on the same plane as the rights of adults.[8]

In its own words, the Convention on the Rights of the Child says the following, among other things, concerning health and education:

> States Parties recognize the right of the child to the enjoyment of the highest attainable standard of health and to facilities for the treatment of illness and rehabilitation of health. States Parties shall strive to ensure that no child is deprived of his or her right of access to such health care services.
>
> States Parties recognize the right of the child to education, and with a view to achieving this right progressively and on the basis of equal opportunity, they shall, in particular:
>
> (a) Make primary education compulsory and available free to all;

> (b) Encourage the development of different forms of secondary education, including general and vocational education, make them available and accessible to every child, and take appropriate measures such as the introduction of free education and offering financial assistance in case of need;
>
> (c) Make higher education accessible to all on the basis of capacity by every appropriate means;
>
> (d) Make educational and vocational information and guidance available and accessible to all children;
>
> (e) Take measures to encourage regular attendance at schools and the reduction of drop out rates.[8]

THE "RIGHTS BASED APPROACH"

"Human rights" is a term with which most people are familiar but which many people find difficult to define. It *is* generally accepted, however, that the "International Bill of Rights" is made up of the Universal Declaration of Human Rights, the International Covenant on Civil and Political Rights, and the International Covenant on Economic, Social, and Cultural Rights. It is also accepted that governments have an obligation to respect these rights, take measures to enforce them, and take steps to prevent others from violating them.[9]

In simple terms, if we were to apply the human rights concepts discussed above to global health, this would mean, among other things that we would:

- assess the impact of health policies, programs, and practices on human rights
- take account of the health impacts resulting from violations of human rights
- see health and human rights as inextricably linked and bring this notion to consideration of the determinants of health and ways in which health issues may be addressed.[1]

If we took this perspective, it would also cause us to pay particular attention in the design and implementation of global health efforts to:

- the participation in program design and planning of affected parties and communities
- equity across groups

- the empowerment of individuals over their own lives
- holding people accountable for engaging in health efforts in a manner that respects human rights.[10]

In addition, this approach to work in health would cause us to ask the following questions about different health interventions:

- Who is being served?
- How are they being served?
- Are they being served fairly?
- Are they being served with dignity and respect for their culture?
- Are they participating in decisions about these services?
- Are decisions made in open and transparent ways, in conjunction with the community?
- Who is not being served, and why are they not being served?
- Is there clear accountability for the services being rendered appropriately or not?[10]

SELECTED HUMAN RIGHTS ISSUES

There are a variety of human rights issues that relate to health that could be discussed here. In the section that follows, however, four selected topics are examined briefly because they are indicative of some of these human rights issues. These include: health as a human right, HIV/AIDS and human rights, some matters related to patents and access to medicines, and the extent to which human rights in health are absolute.

Health as a Human Right

The preamble to the constitution of the World Health Organization, which was formulated in 1946, states, "The enjoyment of the highest attainable standard of health is one of the fundemantal rights of every human being."[11] In addition, as noted above, a number of treaties signed after 1946 have further promoted the principle that health is a fundamental human right. One very important question, however, is the extent to which countries are able or willing to honor this right.

The simplest answer to this question is that, while there is increasing attention globally to the links between health and human rights, there is no mechanism for holding countries accountable for ensuring that they honor or even try to honor the right to health. The international mechanism now in place for reviewing compliance with treaties and conventions that include the right to health is voluntary reporting by countries. In addition, there are provisions in human rights treaties and conventions that recognize that resource poor countries will not be able to help all of their people to "achieve the highest standard of health possible."[9] There is also no clear definition of the meaning of the right to health or indicators agreed among countries for measuring progress against that goal.[12] Although there is considerable attention to the MDGs and the progress of meeting them, the discussion that surrounds the MDGs globally frequently does not explicitly take human rights issues into account.

Nonetheless, several countries, including Brazil, Thailand, and South Africa have recently incorporated human rights important to health into national legislation and new constitutions.[13] In addition, a 1999 court case in Venezuela has interesting relevance to the matter of health and human rights. In this case, the court held that the Venezuelan government violated the constitutional right of its people to health by failing to guarantee people living with HIV/AIDS access to antiretroviral therapy. The court ruled that this right is both part of the Venezuelan constitution and also a part of the ICESCR, to which Venezuela is party.[14]

Human Rights and HIV/AIDS

As much as any health condition in history, HIV/AIDS raises a host of human rights issues. These issues arise partly from the fact that HIV/AIDS is a health condition that is associated in most cultures with significant amounts of stigma and discrimination. Many people see HIV/AIDS, for example, as a disease that people bring on themselves by engaging in what they consider to be promiscuous behavior. This could include engaging in homosexual sex, injecting drug use, having multiple sex partners, or participating in commercial sex work. In addition, in places that are not familiar with how the disease is spread, there is often great fear of catching the disease. Although an entire book could be written about this subject, some brief comments are given on a small number of the human rights issues related to HIV/AIDS.

An important question that has arisen in many societies is how to protect the rights of people who are HIV positive to employment, schooling, and full participation in social activities. When the epidemic was first recognized in a number of developed countries, there was considerable discrimination against people who are HIV positive, some of whom lost their jobs or were not allowed to enroll in school. Such discrimination continues in many places, which raises fundamental questions of the rights of people who are living with HIV/AIDS.

Another matter that has arisen, as suggested earlier, is the access of people with HIV to health care. At least at the early stages of an HIV epidemic in a country, most health workers are poorly informed about HIV, not aware of how it is spread, and have serious fears about caring for people who are HIV positive. There are examples of many settings in which people living with HIV/AIDs have been denied care or treated with discrimination and stigma when they did receive care.

There are also a number of questions concerning HIV testing. For many years, a cardinal principle of work on HIV has been that testing for it should be voluntary and confidential. This is to ensure that people are not forced against their will to get tested and then discriminated against if people find out that they are HIV-positive. More recently, however, an increasing number of people involved in HIV activities have come to believe that in settings with high rates of prevalence of HIV, every adult should be tested for it. People promoting this approach want to encourage much greater testing for HIV because it is spread largely by people who are HIV positive, do not know their status, and have unprotected sex with multiple partners.

In line with this, Botswana has become the first country to have a policy of testing for HIV that is based on "opting out" of testing, rather than volunteering to get tested. In this case, any adult having contact with the health system is asked to take an HIV test. They have to opt out and ask not to get a test or one will be given. Despite the increasing calls for this type of approach, there remains considerable concern among a substantial number of those involved in HIV efforts that even a well-organized country like Botswana will not be able to implement such a program without *de facto* coercion of people to get tested.[15]

Other human rights issues that relate to HIV/AIDS concern the issue of patient confidentiality. For many years, there has been widespread agreement that HIV information about patients needed to be kept confidential to ensure that those who are HIV positive would not be discriminated against. Yet, the healthcare settings in many resource-poor countries that have high rates of HIV are poorly organized, do not operate very efficiently, and are not accustomed to treating patients and patient records confidentially. They also may not have the physical space to treat their patients privately and confidentially.

In addition, and also related to concerns about privacy, there are important questions about disclosure of HIV status. Should the healthcare system notify spouses or sexual partners of the HIV status of patients? Should the patients do that? What are the risks, for example, if a husband is notified about the status of his wife that he may harm her, reject her, or that his family will throw her out of the house?

Those issues are just a small sample of the many rights related questions that arise in relation to HIV/AIDS. While these questions may be more prominent when thinking about HIV/AIDS, many of them are relevant to health more generally, such as treating people with respect, treating patients and their records confidentially, not discriminating against people because of their health conditions, and being sensitive to the social and cultural milieus within which patients live.

Human Rights Are Not Always Absolute

The importance of protecting human rights related to health is widely acknowledged. Yet, it is also widely understood that there are exceptional circumstances under which these rights may be temporarily suspended, such as to protect the interest of the public during an influenza epidemic when governments might suspend for a certain time the right of people to leave their homes, to go to work, to travel, or to participate in mass gatherings, such as sporting events. Few people would deny the obligation of governments to have laws that govern public health actions. However, most of those working in public health also believe that any suspension of rights must be carried out with due process. They also believe that it is very important to monitor rights during the suspension period and make all efforts to reinstate rights as soon as possible.[16]

Intellectual Property Rights and Global Health

Any discussion of global health and human rights brings up the question of access to medicines and how this is affected by patent rights. This has become an especially important and contentious matter in the last decade, as the World Trade Organization has been formed and agreements concerning patents have been negotiated, as part of the TRIPS Agreement (Trade-Related Aspects of Intellectual Property Rights). This question has also come to the forefront because of the high costs of drugs to treat AIDS, the inability of most HIV-affected people in low-income countries to pay for those drugs, and the concern of many people that it is not ethical or just to allow so many people to die of AIDS in developing countries when medicines are available to treat them. The challenge with respect to patents for medicines needed by the poor in the developing world is how to encourage scientific discovery of diagnostics, drugs, and vaccines while ensuring the affordability of medicines by poor people in poor countries.

The basic principle behind granting intellectual property rights is to provide incentives for research, development, and use of new technologies. Patents give the inventor the right to exclude others from making, selling, or importing his invention for a fixed time period. The quasi-monopoly granted to the patent holder allows the setting of prices without regard to ordinary market forces and, therefore, allows higher prices than would be the case in the event of competition.

Many people believe that the possibility of getting a patent on a discovery, such as a drug, is essential to ensuring the continued search for new drugs. This is certainly the position of the major pharmaceutical manufacturers and is embedded in international trade agreements to a large extent. On the other hand, WHO has pointed out that in spite of the incentives of patents, only 11 out of the 1223 chemicals developed between 1975 and 1996 were to treat some of the most important diseases that affect poor people in low- and middle-income countries.[17] In fact, a recent WHO commission on intellectual property rights and innovation concluded that patents are only one of a number of factors that encourage innovation of pharmaceutical products and that financial and other incentives are also important. The commission also said that it was important that mechanisms be adopted to ensure access to pharmaceutical products when they are developed.[18]

Some countries have historically refused to grant patents or have granted only process patents on what they regard as "essential drugs," because they believe that their people have a right to these drugs at affordable prices. In principle, the human rights approach to health does not reject the concept of intellectual property rights. However, it does focus on the effect that granting such rights has on the more marginalized and disadvantaged sections of people. It is with this in mind that those advocating a human rights approach to health, as well as others concerned about the price of medicines, insist on safeguard mechanisms to ensure access to medicines by all who need them, and on special exceptions to intellectual property rights for least developed countries.[19]

THE FOUNDATIONS FOR RESEARCH ON HUMAN SUBJECTS

The foundations for research on human subjects developed out of concerns about unethical and inhumane Nazi experimentation on human subjects during World War II. These concerns grew as people learned more about the medical experiments that the Nazis conducted on prisoners during the war. The first set of guidelines for the ethical conduct of research on human subjects was issued in 1948 and others have followed since then.

The Nuremberg Code

The Nuremberg Code was formulated in 1948, following the verdict of an American military war crimes tribunal that conducted proceedings against 23 Nazi physicians and administrators for their willing participation in what were deemed to be war crimes and crimes against humanity. This group had conducted research studies and experiments on concentration camp prisoners that resulted in death or permanent deformity. The Nuremberg Code sets specific requirements which physicians are supposed to follow when conducting experiments on human subjects.[20] (See Table 4-1.)

The Declaration of Helsinki

In 1964, the World Medical Association developed a set of ethical principles for biomedical research with human subjects. The main purpose of the Declaration of Helsinki was to ensure adequate protection of the rights of individuals who participated in such research. The Declaration of Helsinki was revised in 1975, 1983, 1989, 1996, and 2000.[21]

TABLE 4-1 The Standards of the Nuremburg Code

- Those who participate in the study must freely give their consent to do so. They must be given information on the "nature, duration, and purpose of the experiment." They should know how it will be conducted. They must not be forced or coerced in any way to participate in the experiment.
- The experiment must produce valuable benefits that can not be gotten in other ways.
- The experiment should be based on animal studies and a knowledge of the natural history of the disease or condition being studied.
- The conduct of the research should avoid all unnecessary physical and mental suffering and injury.
- The degree of risk of the research should never exceed that related to the nature of the problem to be addressed.
- The research should be conducted in appropriate facilities that can protect research subjects from harm.
- The research must be conducted by a qualified team of researchers.
- The research subject should be able to end participation at any time.
- The study will be promptly stopped if adverse effects are seen.

Source: Data from Regulations and Ethical Guidelines—Directives for Human Experimentation—Nuremberg Code. Available at: http://ohsr.od.nih.gov/guidelines/nuremberg.html. Accessed August 3, 2006.

The basic principles of the Declaration of Helsinki are noted in Table 4-2.

On July 12, 1974, the U.S. National Commission for the Protection of Human Subjects of Biomedical and Behavioral Research was created via the United States National Research Act. The mandate of the Commission was to help identify basic ethical principles for the conduct of biomedical and behavioral research in human subjects and to develop guidelines that researchers would be required to follow so that all human research is in line with the ethical principles identified. The Commission prepared what has come to be known as the Belmont Report. The research principles in that report are outlined in Table 4-3.

These principles are to be put into practice by getting informed consent from any study participant, ensuring that the research is grounded in a rigorous assessment of risks and benefits, and being certain that participants are selected fairly.[22]

KEY HUMAN RESEARCH CASES

There are a number of cases of research on human subjects historically which have helped to raise ethical concerns about such research and encouraged the development of guidelines for such research, as well. Among the best known of these is the Tuskegee Study that took place in the United States. Several other U.S. cases have also been instrumental in establishing guidance on carrying out research on human subjects. These are discussed briefly below. It is important to note that these took place at times when guidelines for such research were not nearly as developed as they are today.

The Tuskegee Study

In 1932, the United States Public Health Service, in collaboration with the Tuskegee Institute, began a study in Macon County, Alabama, to record the natural history of syphilis. One of the aims of this study was to justify syphilis treatment programs for African Americans, at a time of considerable discrimination against such people and the lack of such programs. This study was called the "Tuskegee Study of Untreated Syphilis in the Negro Male."[23]

Six hundred African-American men took part in the study, 399 with syphilis and 201 who did not have the disease. The men were told by researchers that they were being treated for "bad blood," a term that was used locally to describe a number of ailments, including syphilis, anemia, and fatigue. Those participating in the study received free medical exams, meals, and burial insurance. The study was originally projected to last 6 months but went on for 40 years.[23]

TABLE 4-2 The Declaration of Helsinki—Basic Principles

- A physician's duty in research is to protect the life, health, privacy, and dignity of the human participant.
- Research involving humans must conform to generally accepted scientific principles and be based on a thorough knowledge of scientific literature and methods.
- Such research must be governed by research protocols and those protocols should be reviewed by an independent committee.
- Research should be conducted by medically/scientifically qualified individuals.
- The risks and burdens to the participants should not outweigh benefits.
- A researcher should stop a study if risks are found to outweigh potential benefits.
- Research is justified only if there is a reasonable likelihood that the population participating in the study will benefit from the results.
- Participants must be volunteers and give their informed consent to such participation.
- Every precaution must be taken to respect privacy, confidentiality, and participant's physical and mental integrity.
- Tests of medicines must be against the best available medicine that already exists.
- Study participants should get access to any diagnostics or medicines that are developed as a result of the study.
- Investigators are obliged to preserve the accuracy of results; negative and positive results should be publicly available.

Source: Data from World Medical Association, Declaration of Helsinki. Available at: http://www.wma.net/e/policy/b3.htm. Accessed August 12, 2006.

In July 1972, a front-page story appeared in the New York Times about the Tuskegee study. This article caused immense public concern and led the Assistant Secretary for Health and Scientific Affairs to appoint an advisory panel to review the study. The panel found that the men had never been properly informed of the real purpose of the study, that they had been misled, and that they lacked the information needed to give informed consent to participate in the study. In addition, the panel found that the men were never given adequate treatment for their disease even when penicillin became the drug of choice for syphilis in 1947. The panel further found that the participants were never given the choice

TABLE 4-3 The Belmont Report

Basic Ethical Principles
- Respect for Persons: The autonomy of individuals must always be respected and persons with diminished autonomy are entitled to protection.
- Beneficence: Research subjects should be protected from harm at all times. Efforts must also be made to maximize possible benefits and minimize possible harms.
- Justice: The benefits and risks of research must be distributed fairly.

Applications of the Principles
- Informed Consent—Persons must be given an opportunity to choose what shall or shall not happen to them. This must be based on the disclosure to them of sufficient information, in a manner that they can thoroughly understand. This consent must also be given completely voluntarily.
- Assessment of Risks and Benefits—There must be a careful and data based assessment of the magnitude of possible harm and anticipated benefits. This assessment must take account of many possible types of harms and benefits. Inhumane treatment of research subjects is never allowed. Risks must be reduced as far as possible. Special attention should be paid if vulnerable populations will be involved in the research.
- Selection of Subjects—There must be fair procedures and outcomes in the selection of those participating in the research.

Source: Data from Regulations and Ethical Guidelines—The Belmont Report Ethical Principles and Guidelines for the Protection of Human Subjects of Research. Available at: http://ohsr.od.nih.gov/guidelines/belmont.html. Accessed Auguust 3, 2006.

of quitting the study, even when this new, highly effective treatment became widely used.[23]

These findings led the advisory panel to conclude that the knowledge gained from the study was limited when compared to the risks to the study participants and that the study was, therefore, "ethically unjustified." The panel advised that the study immediately be stopped and in November 1972, the Assistant Secretary for Health and Scientific Affairs ended the Tuskegee study.[23]

In the summer of 1973, the study participants received more than $9 million as part of a settlement to a class-action lawsuit filed by the National Association for the Advancement of Colored People (NAACP). As part of the settlement, the U.S. government promised to give free medical and burial services to all living participants, as well as health services for wives, widows, and children who had been infected because of the study.[23]

The manner in which the Tuskegee study was carried out and the important ethical questions it raised are known to almost all researchers who conduct research on human subjects. It has had a profound impact on the carrying out of human subjects research in the future.

The Willowbrook School Study

The Willowbrook State School, situated in New York state in the United States, was an institution for mentally handicapped children. Physicians associated with the institution wanted to do a study of hepatitis, which was rampant at the school. From 1956 to 1972, as part of the study, children were intentionally infected with the hepatitis virus. The study leaders believed that this was ethical because almost all children at the school were likely to become infected within 6 to 12 months after entry to the school and the study leaders did ask the parents of the children to give informed consent for their children's participation in the study. The study design was approved by the funding agency and the Executive Faculty of the New York University School of Medicine. The study was started, however, before there was an appropriate review committee for human experimentation related to the school, but when such a committee was established, it also approved the study design.

The study was halted after public concern about the manner in which it was being conducted. There were two main criticisms of the study. The first concern was that there was no real gain to be had from intentionally infecting the children with hepatitis. Rather, they could have studied the disease in children who became naturally infected. In addition, the school was short on space and it appeared that the only space available was on a ward in which the research was being carried out, which suggested that unless parents consented to their children participating in the study, they could not be admitted to the school. This was thought by critics of the study to be unethical because it essentially coerced parents to participate in the study so that they could get their severely handicapped children into the school.[24,25]

Jewish Chronic Disease Hospital

Studies were conducted at the Jewish Chronic Disease Hospital in New York City in 1963 to better understand the processes involved when the body rejected human transplants. This was done by injecting chronically ill patients who did not have cancer with live human cancer cells. The physicians who managed the study did not inform the patients that they would be injected with live cancer cells. Their rationale in not doing this was that they could safely assume that the patients would reject the cells, and if they were informed they would not have given consent for the live cancer cells to be injected in them. Later review of the study led to the censure of the study investigators, but this was later dropped.[26]

Milgram Obedience Study

Stanley Milgram, a social psychology researcher at Yale University, designed studies to learn about conditions of obedience and disobedience. He asked a group of "teachers," paired to a group of "learners," to give electric shocks of increasing intensity to the learners when the learners made mistakes. Milgram told those serving as teachers that he was studying the effect of punishment on learning behaviors. In fact, he was studying the willingness of the teachers to follow his instructions about shocking the learners. In fact, the learners were not being shocked at all.

In carrying out this experiment, Milgram wanted to understand better what could drive people to be willing to exert pain on others, as was done in World War II during the genocide, when many participants said they harmed others because they were just following orders. Milgram did not reveal the true study design to the teachers, because he wanted to see if they would really give 450 volts of shock to the learners.

Milgram's study was criticized as unethical because it caused great stress to those who thought they were administering the shocks. This raised questions about the extent to which study participants should be subjected to stresses, especially when they were not really told the true design of the study.[27-29]

Institutional Review Boards and Human Subjects Research Today

It is important to reiterate that the studies indicated above were conducted at a time when approaches to research on human subjects were not nearly as well developed as they are today. There are now committees within various organizations that conduct research that review all proposed research on human subjects. These are called Institutional Review Boards (IRBs). As they review proposed research today, they bring to their reviews the lessons and experience that have been generated from research done earlier and some of the problems with such research, such as those indicated above. Individual countries also have organizations that oversee the work of IRBs and help to disseminate knowledge about best practices for their work.

ETHICAL ISSUES IN MAKING INVESTMENT CHOICES IN HEALTH

As noted earlier, one central issue in global health is the need to make choices among investments that can enhance the health of the population. This is necessary, especially in low- and middle-income countries, because resources will always be less than needed to meet all health needs. We have also discussed earlier how cost-effectiveness analysis is one important tool for making such choices. In addition to the issues raised by the application of cost-effectiveness analysis that were covered in Chapter 3, such analysis also raises some interesting ethical issues. A number of these are noted hereafter.

First is the question of the priority that should be given in cost-effectiveness analysis to the worst-off members of society. Many of those who work on health take a view that "benefiting people has greater moral value, the worse off those people are."[30] However, especially in developing countries, there are so many poor people that those carrying out the analysis of health investments and making policies in health will have to consider carefully how much priority they attach to the worse off. Related to this is the question of how such people are defined. Are these people, for example, those who are in ill health today, or are they people who are the most vulnerable to being in ill health in general?[30]

Another interesting question is how one makes choices between providing a small benefit to a large number of people or a large benefit to a small number of people. One case cited in the literature that occurred in the state of Oregon in the United States was an analysis that showed that society would get greater health gains by investing in capping the teeth of 100 people, compared to carrying out the removal of one appendix that was needed because of acute appendicitis. In the end, the state decided that it would have to choose the appendectomy, given that this is life threatening. Consideration of this type of issue caused the state to change its overall approach to the analysis of potential investments in health.[30]

Another ethical issue concerns the choice between "fair chances and best outcomes."[30] Let us say that one has a choice between screening two groups of women for breast cancer. In one group are poor women in a city. In the other group are better-off women in the suburbs. The best outcomes might be achieved by focusing on the better-off women, because they are much more likely to go for follow-up on any findings and have successful outcomes than the poorer women. However, would that be fair? Would it be fairer to give each group an equal chance to get screened? Would it be most fair to focus on the poorer women, given the priority one wants to accord to the disadvantaged? Even if one agreed to put a priority on fair chances, should they be organized by equal proportion, by lottery, or by another method?[30]

There are also interesting questions that arise over the extent to which societal resources should be used to address the health needs of people whose health problems may relate to their own health behaviors. Would you want tax money that you pay to help take care of the health needs of people who smoke? Would you be willing to use your tax money to help meet the health needs of people addicted to heroin? What about someone injured on a motorcycle while not wearing a helmet?[30]

The medical profession provides care only on the basis of need and not on the basis of the actions that have led to that need. Generally, those considering the ethical issues involved in these decisions believe that it would be fair to deny care or give a lower priority to the care of individuals whose behaviors appear to have caused the need for care only if "the needs must have been caused by the behavior; the behavior must have been voluntary; the persons must have known that the behavior would cause the health needs and that if they engaged in it their health needs would receive lower priority."[31] These are rarely, if ever, the case, even when dealing with cigarette smoking, both because it is addictive and because it usually begun by adolescents who are not well-informed.[31]

There are other questions that arise when considering investment choices in health and the use of cost-effectiveness analysis. These might include decisions about the cut-off value of investments one would be willing to make or the manner in which one should consider people with disabilities, because the methodology for DALYs inherently values a condition of disability less highly than a condition of good health. One could thoughtfully consider these and other related issues at great length. The important point of this section, however, is that it is critical, when considering investment choices and the tools that one will use to make decisions about them, that one should explicitly identify and assess ethical choices and how they relate to the aim of social justice that is at the core of public health work.

KEY CHALLENGES FOR THE FUTURE

Efforts to incorporate ethical and human rights concerns into global health work face a number of challenges. Some of these are briefly indicated here.

One very important point is that many students of public health and global health get insufficient exposure in their training to ethical and human rights issues. Normally, they do have to understand the core concepts of research on human subjects and how an IRB functions. However, they may have few opportunities to take courses that cover broader issues of human rights and health or give them fuller opportunities to cover ethical issues in research and in policy making. This chapter is a small attempt to correct that gap.

Second, as indicated earlier, there are enormous gaps in holding countries accountable for meeting their obligations under international conventions that refer to the right to health. On the one hand, there has been increasing pressure, largely brought on by HIV/AIDS, to hold countries accountable for providing AIDS drugs to their people. On the other hand, as indicated earlier, compliance with human rights norms is self-reported by countries. There are really no indicators for measuring such compliance, and there are really no enforcement mechanisms either. Perhaps the movement to focus attention on global health needs, which is discussed in greater detail in Chapter 15, can serve as a platform for having civil society increasingly holding countries accountable for enhancing the right of their people to health, particularly their poorest people.

Third, there is also a lack of explicit review of the fairness of many of the investment choices that are being made, both by countries and by the development assistance agencies with which they work. If one reviews the documents that relate to investments in health in low- and middle-income countries, one will generally see that particular attention is paid to ensuring that project benefits go to disadvantaged people. However, it is rare that there will be explicit reviews or articulation of how investment choices are made, the ethical choices that were a part of them, and the basis for the investment decisions. With respect to HIV/AIDS, for example, what criteria will be used to allocate drugs if there are more people clinically eligible for drugs than the amount of drugs available? Will it be access to the health center, so that there is a greater likelihood that the person will comply with treatment? Will it be pregnancy, so that one can reduce maternal to child transmission?[32] If there were a greater need to articulate these choices more openly, then these decisions might be made more fairly.

In addition, though there has been important progress in establishing IRBs and ensuring that proposed research on human subjects is reviewed before being carried out, there is little review of how the IRBs themselves have been functioning. Such a review and the strengthening of IRBs in relatively weaker or less well endowed settings is important to ensuring that research on human subjects is done properly.[33]

There are also some interesting issues on the agenda of human subjects research that are still being wrestled with internationally. One concerns the standard of care.

The Declaration of Helsinki says that vaccines, diagnostics, and therapeutics, for example, must be tested against the best available standard of care that already exists. We may wish to ensure that there is no deviation, even in developing countries, from such standards. However, does this requirement prohibit the development of new drugs, diagnostics, or vaccines that might not be as effective as the existing standard of care but which, nonetheless, might be more cost-effective than that standard in some developing countries?[34]

In addition, considerable attention is being paid to the rights of communities that are participating in research. Some people have suggested that such communities should be given compensation for their participation. Such compensation might include training or cash. It has also been proposed that communities should have access to the products that the study eventually leads to. Thus, if they participated in a study on the effectiveness of AIDS drugs, for example, they would be entitled to such drugs in the future at the expense of those managing the study. There is no clear outcome to such discussions as of yet.[34]

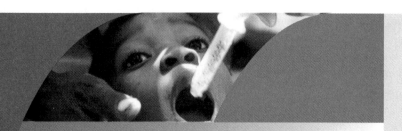

Study Questions

1. What is meant by "the right to health?"

2. What are the key features concerning health of the Universal Declaration of Human Rights?

3. What are the most important points of the Convention on the Rights of the Child?

4. How might one carry out a "human rights approach" to health in global health efforts?

5. What are some of the concerns with the impact of patents on the availability of affordable medicines in the developing world?

6. What steps might be taken internationally to encourage the development of drugs, while ensuring their affordability in developing countries?

7. What are some of the key ethical concerns in carrying out research on human subjects?

8. What are some of the most important ethical issues that deserve attention when choices are being made about investments in health?

9. How could one encourage countries and their development partners to pay greater attention to human rights issues in health?

10. What rights and compensation do you think should be given to communities that participate in research on human subjects that is trying to find new drugs?

REFERENCES

1. Mann J, Gostin L, Gruskin S, Brennan T, Lazzarini Z, Fineberg H. Health and Human Rights. *Health and Human Rights.* Fall 1994 1994;1(1):6–23.

2. United Nations General Assembly. Universal Declaration of Human Rights. Available at: http://www.un.org/Overview/rights.html. Accessed September 10, 2006.

3. International Covenant on Economic SaCRI. Unofficial Summary. Available at: http://www.cehat.org/rthc/summary.htm. Accessed September 10, 2006.

4. Office of the United Nations High Commissioner for Human Rights. International Covenant on Civil and Political Rights. Available at: http://www.ohchr.org/english/law/ccpr.htm. Accessed September 10, 2006.

5. Office of the United Nations High Commissioner for Human Rights. International Covenant on Economic, Social and Cultural Rights New York 16 December 1966. Available at: http://www.ohchr.org/english/countries/ratification/3.htm. Accessed January 18, 2007.

6. Office of the United Nations High Commisioner for Human Rights. International Covenant on Civil and Political Rights New York, 16 December 1966. Available at: http://www.ohchr.org/english/countries/ratification/4.htm. Accessed January 18, 2007.

7. United Nations. Convention on the Elimination of All Forms of Discrimination Against Women. Available at: http://www.un.org/womenwatch/daw/cedaw/text/econvention.htm. Accessed January 14, 2007.

8. Office of the United Nations High Commisioner for Human Rights. Convention on the Rights of the Child. Available at: http://www.unhchr.ch/html/menu3/b/k2crc.htm. Accessed August 14, 2006, 2006.

9. Gruskin S, Tarantola D. Health and human rights. In: Gruskin S, Grodin MA, Annas GJ, Marks SP, eds. *Perspectives on Health and Human Rights.* New York: Routledge; 2005:3–58.

10. Gruskin S, Grodin MA, Annas GJ, Marks SP. Introduction: approaches, methods and strategies in health and human rights. In: Gruskin S, Grodin MA, Annas GJ, Marks SP, eds. *Perspectives on Health and Human Rights.* New York: Routledge; 2005:xiii–xx.

11. World Health Organization. Constitution of the World Health Organization. Available at: http://policy.who.int/cgi-bin/om_isapi.dll?hitsperheading=on&infobase=basicdoc&jump=Constitution&softpage=Document42#JUMPDEST_Constitution. Accessed September 15, 2006.

12. Mokhiber CG. Toward a measure of dignity: indicators for rights-based development. In: Gruskin S, Grodin MA, Annas GJ, Marks SP, eds. *Perspectives on Health and Human Rights.* New York: Routledge; 2005:383–392.

13. Gruskin S, Tarantola D. Health and human rights. In: Gruskin S, Grodin MA, Annas GJ, Marks SP, eds. *Perspectives on Health and Human Rights.* New York: Routledge; 2005:23.

14. Torres MA. The human right to health, national courts, and access to HIV/AIDS treatment: a case study from Venezuela. In: Gruskin S, Grodin MA, Annas GJ, Marks SP, eds. *Perspectives on Health and Human Rights.* New York: Routledge; 2005:507–516.

15. Steinbrook R. The AIDS epidemic in 2004. *N Engl J Med.* 2004;351(2):115–117.

16. Easley CE, Marks SP, Morgan Jr. RE. The challenge and place of international human rights in public health. In: Gruskin S, Grodin MA, Annas GJ, Marks SP, eds. *Perspectives on Health and Human Rights.* New York: Routledge; 2005:519–526.

17. Cullet P. Patents and medicines: the relationship between TRIPS and the human right to health. In: Gruskin S, Grodin MA, Annas GJ, Marks SP, eds. *Perspectives on Health and Human Rights.* New York: Routledge; 2005:181.

18. World Health Organization. Public Health, Innovation, and Intellectual Property Rights. Available at: http://www.who.int/intellectualproperty/documents/thereport/ENPublicHealthReport.pdf. Accessed January 13, 2007.

19. Cullet P. Patents and medicines: the relationship between TRIPS and the human right to health. In: Gruskin S, Grodin MA, Annas GJ, Marks SP, eds. *Perspectives on Health and Human Rights.* New York: Routledge; 2005:179-202.

20. National Institutes of Health Office of Human Subjects Research. The Nuremberg Code. Available at: http://ohsr.od.nih.gov/guidelines/nuremberg.html. Accessed August 14, 2006.

21. World Medical Association. Declaration of Helenski. Available at: http://www.wma.net/e/approvedhelsinki.html. Accessed August 5, 2006.

22. U.S. National Institutes of Health Office of Human Subjects Research. The Belmont Report. Available at: http://ohsr.od.nih.gov/guidelines/belmont.html. Accessed August 13, 2006.

23. Centers for Disease Control and Prevention. The Tuskegee Timeline. Available at: http://www.cdc.gov/nchstp/od/tuskegee/time.htm. Accessed January 18, 2007.

24. Texas A&M Philosophy Department. Professional Ethics The Willowbrook Hepatitis Study. Available at: http://falcon.tamucc.edu/~philosophy/pmwiki/pmwiki.php?n=PhilosophyFaculty.WillB. Accessed September 9, 2006.

25. United States Department of Energy. The Development of Human Subject Research at DHEW. Available at: www.eh.doe.gov/ohre/roadmap/achre/chap3_2.html Accessed September 9, 2006.

26. Stanford University. History: The Jewish Chronic Disease Hospital Study. Available at: http://www.stanford.edu/dept/DoR/hs/History/his06.html. Accessed September 9, 2006.

27. Milgram S. The Perils of Obedience. Available at: http://home.swbell.net/revscat/perilsOfObedience.html. Accessed January 18, 2007.

28. University of Rhode Island. Stanley Milgram's Experiment. Available at: http://www.cba.uri.edu/Faculty/dellabitta/mr415s98/EthicEtcLinks/Milgram.htm. Accessed September 9, 2006.

29. Blass A. *The Man Who Shocked the World: The Life and Legacy of Stanley Milgram.* New York: Basic Books; 2004.

30. Brock D, Wikler D. Ethical issues in research allocation, research and new product development. In: Jamison DT, Breman JG, Measham AR, et al., eds. *Disease Control Priorities in Developing Countries.* 2nd ed. New York: Oxford University Press; 2006:259–270.

31. Brock D, Wikler D. Ethical issues in research allocation, research and new product development. In: Jamison DT, Breman JG, Measham AR, et al., eds. *Disease Control Priorities in Developing Countries.* 2nd ed. New York: Oxford University Press; 2006:265.

32. Rosen S, Sanne I, Collier A, Simon JL. Rationing antiretroviral therapy for HIV/AIDS in Africa: choices and consequences. *Public Library of Science.* 2005;2(303).

33. Brock D, Wikler D. Ethical issues in research allocation, research and new product development. In: Jamison DT, Breman JG, Measham AR, et al., eds. *Disease Control Priorities in Developing Countries.* 2nd ed. New York: Oxford University Press; 2006:267.

34. Brock D, Wikler D. Ethical issues in research allocation, research and new product development. In: Jamison DT, Breman JG, Measham AR, et al., eds. *Disease Control Priorities in Developing Countries.* 2nd ed. New York: Oxford University Press; 2006:267–269.

An Introduction to Health Systems

VIGNETTES

Uchenna lived in Nigeria. She had a high fever and suspected she had malaria. Her family took her to the local health clinic. When they arrived, at 11:00 in the morning, the clinic was not open. In addition, the community health worker who staffed the clinic was nowhere to be found. Her family knew that the clinic rarely operated as it was supposed to and took her instead to the district hospital. She waited 6 hours to be seen, but was finally examined by a doctor and given medicine for malaria.

Sajitha lived in a small village in northern India. She woke up with a rash that covered the upper half of her body. Her family lived quite far from the government health center and had little faith in the quality of the staff there. Thus, they took Sajitha to a local medical practitioner. He came from the village, he was always polite to people, he could be paid in cash or in kind, and he seemed to have a good record in curing people of their ills. He examined Sajitha, gave her an

injection of Vitamin B$_1$, and told her she would be fine. He used the same needle on Sajitha that he had used on several other people that day.

Melissa lived in the state of Virginia in the United States. She had been unemployed for some time, had little money, and had no health insurance. She also had cancer. She was thousands of dollars in debt to doctors and hospitals for the tests and treatment she had received so far; however, she needed more treatment, more drugs, and additional surgery. Several physicians would not take her as a patient because she had no health insurance. Eventually, after she became sicker, she found a physician who would do the surgery for very low cost. Unfortunately, she was so ill by the time she got the operation that she died a few months later from the cancer.

Cesar lived in San Jose, the capital of Costa Rica, and had been ill for some time. He visited his local health center, where he was referred to the national hospital because it appeared that he might have cancer. The national hospital confirmed the diagnosis of cancer and then treated him with drugs and surgery. He stayed several weeks in the hospital during his recovery. The cost of Cesar's care was covered by the Costa Rican Social Security System, part of the system of universal health insurance in that country.

INTRODUCTION

It is especially important for several reasons to learn about health systems early in one's study of global health. First, health services are provided to people through health systems. Second, many countries spend an important share of their national income on health systems. Third, individuals often spend a considerable share of their family income on health, as well. Fourth, many health systems do not function as planned. Fifth, health outcomes in many settings can only be improved if the effectiveness and efficiency of the health system is improved. Lastly, the performance of many health systems could be enhanced if they would focus more on effectively carrying out a selected number of low-cost but high-impact interventions.

In addition, if the MDGs are to be met, then health systems will have to be strengthened in many countries. People can not escape poverty and hunger if they are ill or have to spend an important share of their financial resources on health services. Nutritional status can not be enhanced if health systems can not help to de-worm children and provide some of them with selected micronutrient supplements. Moreover, the burden of malaria, TB, and HIV cannot be addressed effectively without considerable improvement in the health systems of most of the low-income countries and some middle-income countries.[1]

This chapter is about health systems. It will introduce you to what a health system is and the functions that health systems carry out. It will examine how health systems are organized. It will also review how different countries have chosen to address the main functions of a health system. It will discuss the key issues that health systems face in meeting their main aims, especially in low- and middle-income countries, and how they might be addressed. It will also look more broadly at how health systems can help to achieve better health outcomes for the poor. It will conclude with several cases about effective collaboration between the public and nongovernmental sectors in the provision of healthcare services. You should note that this chapter focuses largely on health services. This is only one of many important parts of a health system.

WHAT IS A HEALTH SYSTEM?

The World Health Organization defines a health system as "all actors, institutions and resources that undertake health actions—where a health action is one where the primary intent is to improve health."[2] A related definition of a health system is "the combination of resources, organization, and management that culminate in the delivery of health services to the population."[3]

Another way to put this would be to see the health system as:

- "All those who deliver health care—such as doctors, nurses, village health workers, and traditional healers
- The money flow that finances such care

- The activities of those who provide specialized inputs into the healthcare process, including medical and nursing schools and drug and device manufacturers
- The financial intermediaries, planners, and regulators, who control, fund, and influence those who provide care—including ministries of health, finance, and planning, social and private insurance institutions, and regulatory bodies
- The activities of organizations that deliver preventive services, such as immunization, family planning, infectious disease control, and 'health education' including on topics such as nutrition, smoking, and substance abuse."[4]

It is important to remember when considering health systems that they are composed of a set of interdependent parts. The organizations, money, and people that comprise health systems may be public, private for-profit, or private not-for-profit.

THE FUNCTIONS OF A HEALTH SYSTEM

The World Health Organization produces a report each year on a special topic of interest and the *World Health Report 2000* focused entirely on health systems.[5] That report has been widely read and has been the basis for considerable analysis of the goals of health systems, their functions, how they are organized, and how well they perform.

The World Health Report 2000 suggests that there are three goals for every health system:

- Good health
- Responsiveness to the expectations of the population
- Fairness of financial contribution[6]

The report further suggests that if these are the goals of health systems, then each health system has four functions to play:

- Provide health services
- Raise money that can be spent on health, referred to as "resource generation"
- Pay for health services, referred to as "financing"
- Govern and regulate the health system, referred to as "stewardship"[6]

Elaborating somewhat on those ideas, one could say that all health systems should do the following:

- Provide access to a comprehensive range of health services, including prevention, diagnosis, treatment, and rehabilitation
- Protect the sick and their families against the financial costs of ill health and disability through the estab-

lishment and operation of some type of insurance scheme

- Improve the health of populations through appropriate governance of the health system, regulation of that system, promotion of good health, and the carrying out of key public health functions, such as surveillance, the operation of public health laboratories, and food and drug administration[7]

HOW ARE HEALTH SERVICES ORGANIZED?

Health systems are generally organized into three levels of care that are usually referred to as primary, secondary, and tertiary. In most high-income countries, primary care is provided by a physician who is the first point of contact with the patient. Secondary care is usually provided at a general hospital, which is usually located in towns and cities. At these hospitals, one would get treatment for certain illnesses and conditions, including medical procedures and surgery that the primary care physician can not do. Tertiary care is provided in highly specialized hospitals that are generally located only in major cities. These specialized hospitals are staffed with a wide range of physicians and can address a diverse array of illnesses with high-level diagnostics, treatments, and surgeries.

In most low- and middle-income countries, governments have set up a health system that, in principle, has established primary, secondary, and tertiary facilities in different geographic zones by population. These countries, for example, might have a primary healthcare center for every 5000 to 10,000 people, a secondary hospital in each district, and a tertiary hospital in the nation's capital and, perhaps, other large cities. In many low-income countries, nurses, nurse-midwives, or medical assistants would staff the lowest level of the health system. The first level, where there might be trained physicians, would be at large primary healthcare centers or at district hospitals. Table 5-1 shows the types of services that one might typically expect to find at the primary, secondary, and tertiary levels in low-income countries.

As will be discussed later, it is important to note that particular attention has been paid to primary health care in low- and middle-income countries as the foundation of health system activities in prevention of illness, promotion of good health, and treatment of disease. Special attention has also been paid to the district hospital as the platform for the organization and oversight of primary health care in specified geographic areas.

THE PUBLIC, PRIVATE, AND NGO SECTORS

It is important to distinguish between the different sectors that participate in health systems and the different func-

TABLE 5-1 Typical Health System Services in a Low-Income Country, By Level

Primary Level
- Well baby care
- Sick baby diagnosis
- Maternal health care
- Family Planning
- Diagnosis and treatment of TB

Secondary Level
- As above, plus:
- Treatment of sick children
- Emergency obstetric care
- Diagnosis and treatment of adult illness
- Basic surgical services
- Some emergency care

Tertiary Level
- As above, plus:
- Treatment of complicated pediatric cases
- Treatment of complicated adult cases
- Treatment of HIV
- Specialist surgical services
- Advanced emergency care

Source: The Author

tions that they play. The public sector is the first actor in most health systems. The involvement of the public sector could be at the national, state, or municipal level, depending on the country. The public sector is responsible for the "stewardship" of the system, meaning its governance, policy setting, rulemaking, and enforcement of rules. The public sector is also responsible for raising the funds for the health system, making decisions about allocating those funds, and establishing approaches to financial protection for health. In addition, the public sector is responsible for managing and financing key public health functions, such as setting public health policies, enforcing regulations and laws related to health, disease surveillance, and food and drug administration. In some countries, as noted further hereafter, the public sector provides health services through facilities that it owns and operates. However, the public sector can also purchase health services from the private for-profit or private not-for-profit sectors.

Although some people believe that health is a right that should not be "for sale," the private for-profit sector is involved in the provision and financing of health systems in many countries. In some countries, for example, physicians operate in the private for-profit sector. In some countries, the private sector may operate health clinics, hospitals, and health services linked to an insurance scheme. Private sector health insurers are also involved in health in many countries. The private sector might also operate laboratories. The private for-profit sector can operate on its own financing, it can sell selected services to the government, or it can operate under contract to the government for a range of services. The private for-profit sector can play a very important role for those people who wish to make use of it and can either afford to make use of it or whose care is paid for by others, such as employers.

When one thinks about the private not-for-profit sector, particularly in low- and middle-income countries, one is often thinking about nongovernmental organizations, or NGOs. Broadly defined, an NGO is:

> A non-profit group or association organized outside of institutionalized political structures to realize particular social objectives, such as environmental protection, or serve particular constituencies, such as indigenous peoples. NGO activities range from research, information distribution, training, local organization, and community service to legal advocacy, lobbying for legislative change, and civil disobedience.[8]

NGOs may be large or small, may be local, national, or international, and may work in one area of activity or many. Some examples of NGOs are given in Table 5-2.

TABLE 5-2 Selected Examples of NGOs Involved in Health

International NGOs
  CARE
  Christian Children's Fund
  Doctors without Borders
  OXFAM
  Save the Children
Local NGOs
  Bangladesh Rural Advancement Committee—Bangladesh
  PHILCAT—Philippine Coalition Against Tuberculosis
  Profamilia—Dominican Republic
  Tilganga Eye Center—Nepal
  Voluntary Health Services—India

Source: The Author

NGOs are actively involved in many areas of health in a large number of countries. Typical examples would be in community-based efforts to promote better health through health education and improved water supply and sanitation. NGOs are also very involved in carrying out selected health services. Like the private for-profit sector, NGOs can operate with their own financing or they can sell services to the government.

A critical issue in designing and operating health systems is the role in the health system that ought to be assigned to the public, private for-profit, and NGO sectors and how those roles should be paid for. It is particularly important to consider carefully the extent to which the public sector should provide services, compared to the extent to which it would be more cost-efficient for the public sector to buy certain services from the private for-profit and NGO sectors. It could be the case that public sector health services at the primary level are not as effective and efficient as similar services operated by the NGO sector. As Afghanistan engaged in reconstruction after its recent civil war, for example, it contracted out a package of primary health care to the NGO sector.[9] In Bangladesh, the Bangladesh Rural Advancement Committee (BRAC), a large NGO with a presence throughout the country, is carrying out an array of nutrition programs under contract to the government of Bangladesh.[10] You will see many examples of this type of effort in this book.

SELECTED EXAMPLES OF HEALTH SYSTEMS

There are a number of ways in which health systems in high-income countries can be categorized.[11] One way to do so would be on the manner in which they raise funding; whether or not the government provides services or they are purchased from the private sector; and how the health system pays for services. Following these criteria could lead one to characterize health services as one of three types: the tax-financed system, like the National Health Services of the United Kingdom; a premium-based system, such as the German healthcare system; and, a system largely based on private finance, such as in the United States. This typology is represented in Table 5-3.

The section that follows provides an outline description of some of the main features of each of these types of health systems for a developed country. It then gives some examples of how the health system is organized in several low- and middle-income countries. It is important to note that although there are some common themes in different health systems, each country has its own system built from its own historical and political experience.

TABLE 5-3 Overview of Health Systems and Their Management

Characteristic/Properties	Tax-financed system (Beveridge)	Premium-financed system (Bismarck)	Private insurance system
Type	National health service	Social insurance	Pluralistic
General Definition	Government-regulated care with health services	Health care as guaranteed basic right	Health goods are largely consumer goods
Finance	Taxes (every taxpayer contributes)	Contributions from employee/employers	Largely private finance
Service Organization	Public	Private/public	Largely private
State Intervention	Strong/direct	Mostly indirect	Weak/indirect

Source: Adapted with permission from Southby R. Unpublished Presentation. Washington, DC: 2001.

High-Income Countries

Germany

Germany was the first country in the world to have a universal program of health insurance, which started in the 1880s.[12] The German health system is organized largely around "sickness funds." These are insurance funds that are financed by equal contributions from employers and employees, based on the salary of the worker. The government makes contributions to the sickness funds for people who are unemployed and for people who are retired. The government also regulates the health system. There are more than 200 sickness funds, which are organized by region and by occupation. The sickness funds operate on a non-profit basis. They do not provide services but rather serve as an intermediary to help organize and pay for health services.

In the German healthcare system, associations of physicians get contracts from the sickness funds to provide care to people who do not require hospitalization. The sickness funds also make arrangements for hospital services for their insured people by entering into agreements with hospitals about how many services they will be able to render at a certain price that the sickness fund will pay. Many health services are free, but there are co-payments for some services.[13,14] The sickness funds cover about 90% of the population. About 10% of the population has private insurance. Most health systems in high-income countries are based on the model of Germany, which is called a "social insurance scheme."[15]

The United Kingdom

The United Kingdom (UK) established a system of universal healthcare coverage in 1946, following World War II.[16] It aimed to provide a comprehensive set of health services to all people in the UK, without regard to their ability to pay for such services. The health services part of the healthcare system of the UK is called the National Health Service (NHS). Money for the NHS is raised from general taxes and used to make an annual NHS budget. The NHS purchases primary healthcare services for the population from groups of physicians who are trained as general practitioners who work as independent contractors to the NHS. Patient visits to these general practitioners are free. Hospitals are owned and managed by "NHS Trusts" which receive a budget each year from the NHS for agreed amounts and types of healthcare services. Private health insurance and the private provision of health care in the UK are growing, but still constitute less than 15% of the value of all care provided.[17]

The United States

The healthcare system of the United States is based on a combination of public and private financing, with overwhelmingly private provision of care. Close to 50% of health care financing relates to four publicly financed programs:

- Medicaid—for people below a certain income level
- Medicare—for people above a certain age
- The Veterans Administration—for people who served in the military

- Worker's Compensation—for illnesses and disabilities related to people's occupation

Another 50% of the financing of health care comes from individuals and their employers. Most people who are insured receive health insurance through their work, with both the employer and the employee contributing to the cost of that insurance. People who do not receive such insurance or who are self-employed or not employed can purchase insurance themselves. Most health insurance companies operate on a for-profit basis.

Health service providers work independently of the healthcare system, except for the Veterans Administration and some public health clinics. Some patients have insurance plans that allow them to visit any doctor. Others have plans that require that they use only doctors that have arranged to charge lower fees to those people in a particular insurance plan. Some people get their services from health maintenance organizations, which provide a set of agreed services to their members for an agreed annual charge. Most insurance plans and health maintenance organizations have varying co-payments for different types of services.

The United States is the only high-income country that has a healthcare system that is not founded on the principle that everyone has the right to health care, without respect to their ability to pay. Linked to this, more than 40 million people, or about 15% of the population, is not covered by insurance.[18]

Middle-Income Countries

Costa Rica

The health system of Costa Rica resembles the National Health Service of the United Kingdom in many ways. In Costa Rica, the federal government controls most of the health sector directly. The Costa Rican Social Security Administration (CCSS) owns most hospitals. Most doctors are employed by the public sector, even if they also have private practices. People who work in the formal sector of the economy are obliged to participate in the Social Security Administration, which derives its financing from taxes on wages and from funding from the government's general tax revenues. Salaried workers and their employers both contribute to the CCSS, as does the government. Informal sector workers may also join the CCSS, with fees that depend on their income. Participants in the CCSS receive most services for free but do have co-payments for some services. The government has divided the country into Health Areas, each of which has nine health teams serving 4000 people each. The health teams focuses on primary healthcare services.[19]

Brazil

The Brazilian healthcare system has three main parts. The first is services at the federal, state, and municipal level, as well as for the military, that are publicly owned and publicly financed. The second consists of private sector services that are contracted by the public sector. These two parts of the system operate under the auspices of the Unified Health System (Sistema Unico de Saude). The third part of the healthcare system is made up of private sector services that are paid for by individuals or corporate health insurance. The municipalities are responsible for primary and secondary care and the states for tertiary level care. The municipalities offer a package of basic care. They also operate programs for particular health conditions, such as the infectious diseases.[20]

Low-Income Countries

India

India has a tiered network of health services in the public sector. At the lowest level is a health sub-center, which serves 3000 to 5000 people, depending on whether or not it is in a difficult geographic area or serves tribal people. Sub-centers are staffed by one female and one male multi-purpose worker. Primary health centers serve 20,000 to 30,000 people and are staffed with a physician, a nurse, a female multipurpose worker, a health educator, a laboratory technician, and assistant level staff. Community health centers serve 80,000 to 120,000 people and are staffed with a physician, a pediatrician, a gynecologist, and a surgeon, as well as a number of paramedical staff. It operates as a small hospital with 30 beds and a laboratory and X-ray facilities. At the top of the Indian publicly provided healthcare system are fully-fledged hospitals of varying sizes and complexities. Most primary healthcare services are free in public facilities but there are charges on other services, although exemptions are supposed to be given for people of limited incomes.

In addition to having an extensive array of public facilities, India also has a very large private healthcare sector. In fact, about 80% of all healthcare expenditures are private out-of-pocket expenditures. There are two large government insurance schemes. One serves federal government employees. The other is open to public and private sector organizations and both the employer and employee make contributions to the scheme.

India has a federal political system and state governments provide most of the financing of public services. However, the federal government contributes about 10% of total expenditure by the public sector on health. Federal financing focuses on "public goods," including family planning, maternal and child health, such as immunizations, and the prevention and control of infectious diseases.[21,22]

Tanzania

Like many low-income countries in Africa, Tanzania has a health system that is largely managed and provided by the public sector. This stems partly from the fact that after gaining independence, Tanzania prohibited the provision of for-profit health services.[23] It also stems from the relatively low number of healthcare workers per person and the relative lack of income of much of the population for expenditure on private health care.

The public healthcare system has several levels. At the lowest level, there are village health posts. These are staffed by two members of the community who are given short training courses and who focus on working with the community on prevention of disease and promotion of good health. Dispensaries are the next level of primary care and serve 6000 to 10,000 people. These are staffed by a clinical officer, nurse midwife, maternal and child health aide, nurse assistant, and a laboratory assistant. Secondary care starts at the level of health centers, which are staffed by a number of physicians, clinical officers, nurse midwives, maternal and child health aides, and a public health nurse, nurse assistant, laboratory and pharmaceutical technicians, and a medical records clerk. Each health center serves approximately 50,000 people. It is intended that each district should also have a district hospital. When possible, these are public. However, when there is no public hospital, the government assists in the financing of a hospital from the NGO sector that can serve the functions of a district hospital. Regional hospitals perform many of the same functions of district hospitals but have some additional physicians in areas such as pediatrics, obstetrics and gynecology, and surgery. Tanzania has four tertiary hospitals that provide the highest level of services available in the country. A basic package of primary healthcare services is provided free in Tanzania.[23] The health systems in many countries in Sub-Saharan Africa are organized in a manner similar to the organization of the healthcare system in Tanzania.

Health Sector Expenditure

The health sector is an important part of the economy in all countries and a matter on which government and private individuals spend a substantial amount of resources. Table 5-4 shows the total expenditure on health as a share of GDP for selected countries organized by income group. The table also shows the share of total expenditure that is private.

Table 5-4 highlights a number of important points. First, we note that total expenditure on health as a percentage of GDP has a very wide range. At the low end, it appears that total expenditure on health as a share of GDP in the year 2000 was only about 1% in Afghanistan, for example, and about 1.5% in the Democratic Republic of the Congo. At the high end, however, total expenditure on health as a share of GDP on health in the year 2000 was almost 11% in Switzerland, almost 12% in Lebanon, and about 13% in the United States. In general, what we find is that the total expenditure on health as a share of GDP increases as the income of a country goes up, but it does not increase uniformly.[24]

We can also see a very wide range in the share of total expenditure on health that is private sector expenditure. Only about 20–30% of total expenditure on health is private sector expenditure in a number of high-income countries that have substantial programs of social insurance, such as France, Israel, and Ireland. On the other hand, in a number of relatively poor countries such as Sudan, Kenya, India, Bangladesh, and Vietnam, which lack a formal system of social insurance, private sector expenditure on health as a share of total expenditure on health is between 60–80%.[24]

In some respects, these data are contrary to what one might expect: poorer countries, in which people can least afford to spend for health out of their pockets, have the highest private expenditure. Better-off countries, in which people can most afford out-of-pocket expenditure, spend relatively less out-of-pocket, because their public insurance scheme is so well developed. Of high-income countries, only the United States has more than 50% of total expenditure in the private sector.[24]

KEY HEALTH SECTOR ISSUES

When we consider the extent to which various health systems meet the criteria WHO has set for measuring health system performance, it is clear that some health systems produce better outcomes than others. Table 5-5 indicates for a selected group of countries how they fared in the 2000 WHO ranking of health system performance.

The WHO ranking suggests that, in general, the health systems in high-income countries perform better than do the health systems in middle- and low-income countries. However, the ranking also confirms a point noted earlier: the health systems of a small group of middle-income countries, such as Sri Lanka, Cuba, and Costa Rica rate higher in the WHO ranking than a number of countries with higher incomes. [25]

As we explore health systems in greater detail, however, it becomes clear that all systems wrestle with a variety of challenges and constraints, no matter how high they rank on the WHO scale. Some of the most important of such chal-

TABLE 5-4 Total Health Expenditure as a Percentage of GDP and Private Expenditure on Health as a Percentage of Total Expenditure of Health, Selected Countries, 2003

Country	Health Expenditure as % of GDP	Private Health Expenditure as % of Total Health Expenditure
Afghanistan	6.5	60.5
Australia	9.5	32.5
Bangladesh	3.4	68.7
Brazil	7.6	54.7
Cambodia	10.9	80.7
Cameroon	4.2	71.1
Costa Rica	7.3	21.2
Cuba	7.3	13.2
Denmark	9.0	17.0
Dominican Republic	7.0	66.8
Egypt	5.8	57.4
Ghana	4.5	68.2
Haiti	7.5	61.9
India	4.8	75.2
Indonesia	3.1	64.1
Jordan	9.4	54.8
Nepal	5.3	72.2
Nigeria	5.0	74.5
Pakistan	2.4	72.3
Peru	4.4	51.7
Philippines	3.2	56.3
South Africa	8.4	61.4
Sri Lanka	3.5	55.0
Thailand	3.3	38.4
United States of America	15.2	55.4
Vietnam	5.4	72.2

Source: Data from WHO. WHO Statistical Information System. Core Health Indicators. Available at: http://www3.who.int/whosis/core/core_select_process.cfm. Accessed September 20, 2006.

lenges have to do with how to address changing epidemiological and demographic patterns, governance of the health sector, having an appropriate number and disposition of healthcare personnel, the financing of health care, and the role of the private sector in the overall health system. In addition, the quality of care poses many issues, as does providing financial cover for the poor from the cost of health services, and the extent to which people have access to and get covered by the most appropriate health services for their needs. As was discussed earlier and will be discussed further throughout the book, the health systems in many countries face critical issues of equity. Finally, health systems face a number of problems concerning their design and the overall

achievement of health outcomes, some of which have been the subject of "health sector reform" efforts. These themes are explored briefly here.

Demographic and Epidemiological Change

Demographic and epidemiological changes raise critical challenges for the health systems of most countries. In high-income countries, and in many low- and middle-income countries, people are living longer. As they do so, societies face higher burdens of non-communicable diseases. Many of these conditions are chronic and the cost of treating these conditions is high compared to conditions that occur at younger ages or the cost of acute bouts of communicable dis-

TABLE 5-5 Overall Health System Performance Ranking, Selected Countries

Country	Overall Performance Ranking	Country	Overall Performance Ranking
Afghanistan	173	Haiti	138
Argentina	75	India	112
Bangladesh	88	Jordan	83
Bolivia	126	Mexico	61
Cambodia	174	Morocco	29
Cameroon	164	Nepal	150
Canada	30	Niger	170
China	144	Pakistan	122
Costa Rica	36	Peru	129
Cuba	39	Philippines	60
Denmark	34	South Africa	175
Dominican Republic	51	Sri Lanka	76
Egypt	63	Turkey	70
France	1	United States of America	37
Germany	25	Vietnam	160
Ghana	135	Zambia	182

Source: Data from WHO. The World Health Report 2000. Geneva: WHO; 2000:Annex Table 1.

eases. As a result, relatively poor countries, with few resources to spend on health and weak institutions to address health issues, face a "triple burden" of disease simultaneously—the burdens of non-communicable disease, communicable disease, and injuries.[26]

Stewardship

The quality of governance is an important determinant of outcomes in the health sector, as in many other sectors, as well. In high-income countries, the health sector will tend to be governed in relatively open and transparent ways. These countries will tend to have clear rules and regulations for the management and operation of the health sector, and high-income countries can enforce those regulations. There is usually relatively little corruption in the health sectors of high-income countries.

Unfortunately, however, there are major problems of governance in many low- and middle-income countries. These problems often affect the performance of the health-care system and penalize poor people more than other people, because the poor have fewer choices about where they can go for their health care and less power in dealing with healthcare personnel. Governance in these settings will tend to be weak across all sectors and governments in low- and middle-income countries are often unable to enforce health

sector rules and regulations. This may be especially true with respect to the inability of the health sector to oversee the work of the private healthcare sector.[27]

The management of human resource matters is often especially weak, with staff sometimes being recruited by virtue of their connections, rather than their merit or fit with existing hiring rules. In addition, some staff that are recruited have to "pay off" the people who are recruiting them by giving them an up-front payment for their post or a percentage of their salary each month. Healthcare personnel are often absent from their jobs without sanction. When health services procure goods or construct facilities, they frequently do not get the best prices available, because they are engaging in corrupt practices with the providers of those goods or construction or because they do not have the capacity to engage in sound procurement practices. In many countries, healthcare personnel arrange to get payments from patients for services that are intended to be free.[27]

Other Human Resource Issues

The most severe human resource issues in better-off countries will tend to be imbalances in the number of certain types of healthcare personnel. Some countries do not produce enough physicians. Others do not produce enough nurses, and they tend to make up these shortages through the recruitment of healthcare personnel from other countries, particularly low- and middle-income countries. This greatly contributes to the problem of "brain drain" in the healthcare sector of lower income countries, as discussed later in the chapter. [28]

The human resource issues in low-income countries are considerable and consistent. The very poorest countries, especially in Sub-Saharan Africa, will not have enough healthcare personnel to operate a health system effectively. They will face shortages of physicians, nurse midwives, nurses, and laboratory and other technicians. Despite their needs for better stewardship, they will also face important gaps in qualified health service managers, both clinical and non-clinical. In addition, the quality of training, knowledge, and skills of many of their healthcare staff will be deficient. Those staff who are well-trained will usually be clustered in major cities, and there are often important shortages of appropriately trained healthcare personnel everywhere else in the country, especially in rural and poor areas. Public sector salaries of staff will be very low compared to salaries in the private sector. As a result, many staff members lack the incentive to perform their jobs properly, often practice in the private sector, as well as in the public sector, even if this is not allowed, and are frequently absent from work. In the face of poor salaries and working conditions in which they often lack the facilities, equipment, and materials needed to perform their work well, many healthcare personnel move to other countries, particularly higher income countries, in which salaries and working conditions are much better.[27,29]

The Financing of Health Systems

The health systems in many countries battle continuously for sufficient financing to meet their highest priorities in effective and efficient ways. Better-off countries face issues of rising costs because of aging populations and the ever-increasing demands for the use of new technologies and new drugs. All health systems ration services in some ways. In many high-income countries, a critical issue is how to find the funding that is needed, even with increased efficiency, to reduce the waiting times for certain medical procedures that are financed through the national insurance program. This has been a highlight of the healthcare debates, for example, in the United Kingdom and Canada. A few of the high-income countries, such as Switzerland and the United States, also face important economic questions about the share of their total GDP that they are devoting to health and the implications of this for the rest of the economy.

As you would expect, the financing issue in most low- and middle-income countries revolves around the absolute lack of public sector financial resources for health. It is true

that many low-income countries do not spend effectively or efficiently the financial resources that they do have for health. However, it is also true that most low-income countries do not provide the health sector with the public funds needed to ensure that an appropriate basic package of health services is available to all people without respect to their ability to pay. The costs of such a basic package has been estimated to range in the low-income countries between the equivalent of US$12 and US$50.[30] We have already seen, however, that the very poorest countries allocate from public funds only between 1–3% of their GDP for health, which would give them only about $3 to $10 per year to finance such a basic package.[31]

Quality of Care

The United States Institute of Medicine (IOM) defines quality as "the degree to which health services for individuals and populations increase the likelihood of desired health outcomes and are consistent with current professional knowledge."[32] Six elements comprise quality of care, according to the IOM approach, as noted in Table 5-6.

There is good evidence from high-, middle-, and low-income countries that many health systems suffer from important problems of quality and that quality varies considerably within health systems. Studies in the United States, for example, showed that "physicians complied with evidence based guidelines for at least 80% of patients in only 8 of 306 hospital regions."[33] In a study in Papua New Guinea, a low-income country with rampant malaria, only 24% of health workers could indicate correct treatment for malaria.[34] In a similar study in another low-income country, Pakistan, only 35% of the health workers could indicate the proper treatment for a certain type of diarrhea.[35] In another study of clinical practices in 7 developing countries, 75% of the cases were "not adequately diagnosed, treated, or monitored and . . . inappropriate treatment with antibiotics, fluids, feeding, or oxygen occurred in 61% of the patients."[36]

There are many causes of poor quality health services in low-income countries, including poor management, a lack of financial resources, poorly trained and inappropriately deployed staff, a failure of staff to do their work as intended, and unempowered patients, as discussed throughout this chapter. Many health systems also provide very little supervision of healthcare personnel and have only weak systems for monitoring the performance of their health system.[33]

Financial Protection

As also discussed earlier, one measure of the performance of a health system is "fairness of financial contribution," as

WHO calls it. This refers to financing health care in a way that does not cause people to be denied access to health care or to become impoverished because of their need to spend money on health.[37]

The ability of people to pay for health services *is* a barrier to their access to health care and catastrophic health costs impoverish people in many settings. In most high-income countries, this is not a significant problem because they have social insurance schemes and essentially offer health insurance to all of their people. However, this is a common problem in poorer countries. Studies in India have shown that expenditure on health is a leading cause of families falling below the poverty line and a major cause of families selling assets to pay their bills for health care.[22] Household surveys done in a large number of countries showed that more than 1% of the families surveyed had to spend on health half or more of their income that was left after paying for food. Other studies have shown a decline in the use of TB medicines and hospital deliveries of babies when charges were levied on these services.

Access and Equity

You read in Chapters 2 and 3 about the extent to which health disparities are an important feature of many health systems. You have also seen how important it is to always assess health status, the provision of health services, and health outcomes by sex, age, income, education, and location. In low- and middle-income countries, disparities in access to services and in equity are often reflected in the following ways, among others:

- a lack of coverage of basic health services in areas where poor, rural, and minority people live
- service coverage with a lower level of inputs in the areas previously noted, compared to other areas, such as fewer trained personnel and less equipment and drugs
- service coverage that varies, such as already illustrated for immunization programs, with income and education levels, as well as by location, with urban dwellers getting preference
- better-off people getting access to relatively expensive services that are generally less available to the lower-income groups

It is very important as we assess the performance of health systems that we examine the coverage of health programs for different types of people. It is also important that we examine how services which are accessible to lower-income and other disadvantaged groups compare to the services available to higher-income groups.

TABLE 5-6 Institute of Medicine Elements of Quality

Safe: avoiding injuries to patients
Effective: providing services based on scientific knowledge
Patient-centered: providing care that is responsive to individual patient preferences, needs, and values
Timely: reducing waits and sometimes harmful delays for those who give and receive care
Efficient: avoiding waste, including waste of equipment, supplies, ideas, and energy
Equitable: providing care that does not vary in quality because of personal characteristics such as gender, ethnicity, geographic location, or socio-economic status

Source: Adapted with permission from the IOM Quality Initiative: A Progress Report at Year Six. Available at: http://www.iom.edu/Object.File/Master/7/612/News_issue1_final.pdf. Accessed November 3, 2006.

Making Health Systems Work

In light of the previously mentioned and generally weak management of health systems in developing countries, it is not surprising that many health systems in low- and middle-income countries operate at low levels of effectiveness and efficiency. Considerations of how such health systems might be improved generally have to address a common set of questions, often related to what people call "health sector reform." Some of the most important of these questions include:

- On what aspects of the health system should the government focus?
- What services should the government provide compared to the services it might finance but purchase from others?
- How can health providers be paid in a way that maximizes their incentive for performance?
- What kind of insurance mechanisms can be established to protect the poor, even in a low-income country?
- On what services should expenditure be focused to get the maximum gains in health, with a particular focus on the poor?

ADDRESSING KEY HEALTH SECTOR CONCERNS

There are few easy answers to addressing effectively the most critical health sector issues, particularly in low-income countries. Nevertheless, there is an increasing body of evidence about measures that can be taken to deal with some of the specific problems noted above and to design and manage heath systems more effectively and efficiently. These are discussed briefly here.

Demographic and Epidemiological Change

There are only a limited number of steps that the very poorest countries can take to deal with the multiple burdens of communicable and non-communicable diseases and injuries. Yet, most of these countries will face an increasing burden from non-communicable disease, particularly cardiovascular disease, as discussed in Chapter 12, and road traffic accidents, as discussed in Chapter 13.

Perhaps the single most important step that developing countries can take today to reduce the burden of cardiovascular disease later will be to reduce the disease burden that is related to tobacco use. There is very good evidence that even in low-income settings, measures to make it harder and more expensive to buy cigarettes can reduce tobacco smoking.[38] Even with their limited financial resources and management capacity, low-income countries need to start now to take these steps. They can also take other measures including better engineering of roads, safer cars, and more traffic enforcement to reduce road traffic accidents.[39]

Governance

It will also be difficult to improve the governance of the health system in countries in which overall governance is weak and corruption is high. Nonetheless, a number of measures are proving to be useful in addressing key governance issues in health. Corruption has been reduced, for example, in countries like Poland that have launched national anticorruption programs with strong political backing. In addition, reforming procurement systems and making them more open and transparent has been associated with reducing corruption in contracting in countries like Chile and Argentina. Increasing audits of the health system and enforcing penalties to deal with adverse findings has assisted Madagascar in reducing corruption. There are an increasing number of efforts at reducing corruption and enhancing management through oversight by communities. In a number of cases, such as in Uganda, the Philippines, and Bolivia, community boards were provided more information about the money and services that the community should have received and the authority to provide oversight of these resources in a way that could lead to the firing of corrupt officials. Contracting out some services, carrying out customer satisfaction surveys among the users of the health system, and letting communities provide services with "citizen report cards" are also proving to be helpful to enhancing governance in some settings.[27]

Human Resources

Despite the fact that many human resources issues in health relate to the overall lack of financial resources, there has still been progress in addressing them in some countries. Given the problems of migration of health workers and the number of workers dying in Sub-Saharan Africa from HIV/AIDS, many countries will have to train more healthcare workers and health service managers than they are now training. In addition, countries might be able to reduce the share of their health workers who are migrating by training them so they gain needed skills but do not get credentials for those skills that would be recognized by other countries.[40] Moreover, lower-level health personnel can be trained to carry out a number of functions often reserved for higher-level staff. In Malawi, which has an acute shortage of doctors, nurses were trained to perform cesarean sections.[41] As antiretroviral therapy is being scaled up for AIDS, community-based workers are being taught how to dispense drugs for patients who have been doing well on treatment and to recognize when the patients are having problems and need to be referred for other care. These are tasks reserved for doctors in some AIDS treatment programs.

Financial incentives are also very important to encourage better performance of healthcare personnel. These might include better salaries, additional payments for serving in hard to reach areas, providing housing for people who work in those areas, or special allowances for training. There is also good evidence that the productivity of health workers is higher when their pay is tied to services provided per patient that they actually perform, rather than just paying them a salary. The design of incentives and provider payment mechanisms, of course, has to take important account of what one is trying to achieve and of the local culture. Incentives might be different, for example, if one were trying to reduce migration, trying to get staff to serve in rural areas, or just trying to get staff to come to work in a timely way.[42]

Financing Health Services

The scope for very low-income countries to raise additional resources for health is limited, given the overall scarcity of resources. Nevertheless, there is some scope for shifting resources from other areas of the economy in some countries, given the potentially high returns to investments in health. In many cases, however, countries will need some time to work with their development partners to get assistance in financing key health activities. It is unlikely that those countries that spend the least per person on health can finance an effective package of health services without increasing per person expenditure and getting help from other countries and organizations to do so.

As can be seen in the case study on Tanzania at the end of this chapter, however, there is also some scope for enhancing health outcomes by shifting expenditure within the health sector. By focusing expenditure on a selected group of low cost investments that are known to be effective if managed properly, even very poor countries may be able to improve health outcomes of their poorest people.[31,43] To assist in raising and managing resources for health more effectively, many countries will need to enhance the data they have on health expenditure and also monitor health investments and expenditures more carefully.

Financial Protection

Very poor people in low-income countries and many middle-income countries, as well, will find it difficult for some time to pay for healthcare services and will face financial risks when they have to do so. Unfortunately, there are no "magic bullets" that can address this problem. However, greater financial protection would be offered to the poor if governments allocated a larger amount of funding to a basic package of free primary health care and targeted that to those places and people most at need. Governments could couple this with subsidized services for selected hospital services for the poor, as well, although these schemes are often difficult to manage. Second, governments could also contract a package of primary healthcare services from NGOs and the private sector and subsidize that package for the poor. This has been done with some success in Afghanistan and Cambodia. Third, governments could encourage NGOs to provide services from their own resources, as selected local and international NGOs have the resources to do. The Bangladesh Rural Advancement Committee (BRAC), which will be discussed later, is one such NGO, with a long record of involvement in primary health care for the poor. Fourth, there is some evidence that schemes in which communities raise funds for an insurance pool and purchase health services with those funds might enhance the availability of health services to communities, although there are still questions about how much the very poor can participate in them.[11,31,44]

Access and Equity

Improving access and equity of services is largely a question of political will and health systems planning. Many countries have not focused sufficient attention on the health of their disadvantaged people and have not been sufficiently aware of the kinds of gaps in health coverage and health status that these people face. There is increasing evidence, however, like that cited earlier, that the coverage of health services is inequitable and often leaves out those living in difficult regions and those with less income, less education, and less empowerment. Countries need to use the data they get from national surveys, such as the Demographic and Health Surveys[45] to identify gaps in health status and health coverage. They then need to specifically target health resources to the places and people most in need. Very substantial gains could be had in health status within many countries, for example, if the coverage of effective programs for at least childhood vaccination, TB, and malaria were increased among the poor. The enhancements in health would be even greater if carried out in conjunction with improvements in water supply, sanitation, nutrition, and overall hygiene and health caring behaviors. Some of this can be accomplished through improvements in knowledge that also need to be at the core of efforts to improve the health of the poor.

Quality

Low quality health services waste money and are dangerous to people's health. Although most of us probably believe that low quality is primarily a reflection of inadequate financial resources, there is good evidence that quality can be enhanced in a number of ways even in the absence of additional resources.

It is very important, first, that health systems carry out assessments that will help them to understand the quality gaps in their programs. Second, there is evidence that better professional oversight, supervision, and continuing training can enhance the quality of care provided by health service providers. Third, the use of clear guidelines, protocols, and algorithms for services can also improve quality, particularly where health workers are not well educated or trained. Fourth, when contracting services to the private and NGO sectors, governments can link their payments with performance against specific goals and can independently verify that they have been achieved. Finally, focusing some health staff, as noted earlier, on becoming very proficient at some services is consistently associated with better quality of care.[46]

There is also evidence that "total quality management" approaches can enhance the quality of care, even in low-income countries. In this approach, which is a continuous one, groups of health providers define goals, measure how the system is doing in achieving them, get together to decide how they might best address the gaps in their program, and then test to see how their proposed improvements are working. Even in the poorest areas of North India, this kind of effort, coupled with standard guidelines for managing certain services, produced improvements in the quality of care. The safety of anesthesia has been enhanced in Malaysia in similar ways.[47]

Delivering Primary Health Care

In the end, of course, trying to enhance health outcomes for the poor through better health services in low- and middle-income countries is not just a question of addressing the specific issues discussed previously. Rather, it is also a question of the overall orientation of the health system and how it will carry out those services that can potentially have the biggest impact on improving health outcomes for disadvantaged groups.

There is a broad consensus that a number of measures are needed to achieve this aim. First, services should be focused on the main burdens of disease. Second, health outcomes

can only be achieved if the health system is strengthened to deliver those services effectively and efficiently. Third, the core of activities to meet these goals should be at the levels of primary health care and the district hospital.[48]

There have been a number of very important declarations, studies, and reports that have suggested what the "basic healthcare package" should contain. The most important are noted in Table 5-7.

Although there are some important differences in the exact content of the packages that have been suggested, they are generally in agreement on most of the elements of such a package. To a large extent, it has been recommended that countries try to deliver the services noted in Table 5-8 as close to where people live as possible, through close work

---

TABLE 5-7 Model Primary Care Package of Essential Health Services Interventions

Key Intervention	Childhood disease-related interventions (treatment)	HIV/AIDS prevention
Maternity-related interventions	Acute respiratory infections	Youth-focused interventions
Prenatal care	Diarrhea	Interventions with sex workers and clients
Treatment of complications during pregnancy	Causes of fever	Condom social marketing and distribution
Skilled birth attendants	Malnutrition	Workplace interventions
Emergency obstetric care	Anemia	Strengthening of blood transfusion systems
Postpartum care	Feeding and breastfeeding counseling	Voluntary counseling and testing
Family planning		Prevention of mother-to-child transmission
Tetanus toxoid	**Malaria prevention**	Mass media campaigns
	Insecticide-treated nets	Treatment for sexually transmitted infections
Childhood disease-related interventions (prevention)	Residual indoor spraying	
Bacillus Calmette-Guerin		**HIV/AIDS care**
Polio vaccination	**Malaria treatment**	Palliative care
Diptheria-pertussis-tetanus vaccination		Clinical management of opportunistic illnesses
Measles vaccination	**Tuberculosis treatment**	Prevention of opportunistic illnesses
Hepatitus B vaccination	Directly observed treatment short course (DOTS) for smear-positive patients	Home-based care
Haemophilus influenza type B vaccination	DOTS for smear-negative patients	HIV/AIDS HAART provision
Vitamin A supplementation		
Iodine supplementation		
TB vaccination		**Tobacco control program (taxes, legal action, information, nicotine replacement)**
Anthelminthic treatment		
School health program (incorporating micronutrient supplementation, school meals, anthelminthic treatment, health education)		**Alcohol control program**

Source: Adapted with permission from The World Bank. Tollman S, Doherty J, Mulligan J. General primary care. In: Jamison DT, Breman JG, Measham AR, et al., eds. *Disease Control Priorities in Developing Countries.* New York: Oxford University Press; 2006:1193–1209.

between the primary healthcare level and the district hospital. The hospital would help to supervise the work in primary health care as well as serve as the referral service for activities that can not be handled adequately at the primary level, such as complications of pregnancy. Each of the components of the package is explored in greater detail in the chapters that follow, but they are outlined in Table 5-8.[48]

Ideally, these services would be delivered in an integrated manner. You should be aware, however, that because of weaknesses in the health systems of many countries, some governments and their development partners have established some "vertical" programs. These have historically been used to address problems such as smallpox, malaria, and TB for which governments set up separate management, financing, procurement, staffing, and reporting, in parallel with the regular health programs of the government.

TABLE 5-8 Selected Essential Healthcare Interventions by Level of Service in a "Close to the Client" System

Level of Care	TB	Malaria	HIV/AIDS	Childhood Diseases	Maternal/ perinatal	Smoking
Outreach services		Epidemic planning and response Indoor residual spraying	Peer education for vulnerable groups; needle exchange	Specific immunization campaign Outreach IMCI: home management of fever Outreach for micronutrients and deworming		
Health centre/ health post	DOTS	Treatment of uncomplicated malaria Intermittent treatment of pregnant women for malaria	Anti-retrovirals plus breast-milk substitutes for mother-to-child transmission Prevention of OI, and treatment of uncomplicated OI VCT Treatment of STIs	IMCI Immunization Treatment of severe anemia	Skilled birth attendance Antenatal and postnatal care Family planning post partum	Cessation advice; pharmacological therapies for smoking
Hospital	DOTS for complicated TB cases	Treatment of complicated malaria	Blood transfusion for HIV/AIDS HAART treatment of severe OI for AIDS Palliative care	IMCI: severe cases	Emergency obstetric care	

Source: Adapted with permission from Jha P, Mills A. Improving health outcomes for the poor. *Report of Working Group 5 of the Commission on Macroeconomics and Health.* Geneva; WHO; 2002:52.

Although this vertical approach may not be the most efficient and effective manner in principle in which to operate health services, in practice it is sometimes seen as the only way to accomplish urgent goals in weak health systems. There is an increasing consensus that if such approaches are going to be taken, then they should be linked with efforts to improve related aspects of the health system. The polio eradication program, for example, can be used to strengthen laboratories, surveillance, and the management of the cold chain for some medicines and vaccines.

CASE STUDIES

Many countries have undertaken efforts to address the key health sector challenges discussed earlier. One consistent theme that arises when looking at those efforts that have succeeded is the importance of community-based approaches to health services at the lowest level. Three cases are discussed below. The first is a very well-known case about the work of the Bangladesh Rural Advancement Committee (BRAC) in helping Bangladesh to reduce mortality from diarrhea. This case is complemented in Chapter 10 by a case about Egypt's efforts at spreading the use of oral rehydration therapy. The intervention started by BRAC has been shown to be replicable in other countries and has provided the world with a number of very important lessons about improving health services for the poor in developing countries. The second and third cases in this section discuss some interesting efforts in Africa to enhance the effectiveness and efficiency of health systems. They are small in size to date and have not been fully and independently evaluated. However, they do suggest opportunities for expansion of their approaches that could become important.

The case on Vitamin A and onchocerciasis reviews the attempts by a number of African countries to provide services in more effective and efficient ways by combining the delivery of several programs. This case is complemented by the case in Chapter 15 about the successes in reducing the burden of onchocerciasis in a large number of countries. The third case discusses a pilot project in Tanzania that sought to improve health outcomes by explicitly targeting a larger share of health expenditure on the diseases that most affect the poor.

Combating Diahrreal Disease in Bangladesh

Introduction

In Bangladesh, almost three out of every five infants who die during the first month of life die from diarrhea, pneumonia, and malnutrition, with diarrhea being the major cause.

Children under the age of 5, and especially those under 2, have the highest rate of diarrhea and are prone to severe illness and mortality. Diarrhea results in the loss of water and electrolytes, which causes dehydration and subsequent morbidity and mortality. Therefore, it is essential that fluids and electrolytes be replaced.

The Intervention

BRAC is an important nongovernmental organization that is active in health and community development in Bangladesh. In 1980, BRAC began to implement a large-scale intervention to make oral rehydration therapy widely available and easy to administer by nonprofessionals without special equipment. As part of this effort, BRAC taught mothers to prepare oral saline and to treat their children with it. However, because about 80% of the population were illiterate, there was concern as this activity got underway that mothers would not be able to prepare the solution accurately and that this could result in their children having high blood sodium rather than overcoming their diarrhea.

Through its Oral Rehydration Teaching Program, BRAC communicated a 10-point health message, including how to prepare the oral rehydration solution (ORS) using local ingredients and accurate measurements. ORS was prepared with a three-finger pinch of common table salt and one fistful of unrefined brown sugar in half a local container (467 cc) of water, and was stirred well. The salt–sugar solution was simple to make, cheap, safe, effective, and the ingredients were readily available.[49]

Female health workers or Oral Rehydration Workers (ORWs) as they were called, were trained in the preparation of the solution. The ORWs worked in teams to visit every household in each village. One woman/mother in every household was taught 10 critical points using a flip chart with pictorial representations of ORS preparation and diarrhea management. Questions asked on each of the points ensured that the messages were understood before the workers left. Most importantly, the mother had to prepare the solution under the direct supervision of the ORW. The ORWs ensured that the women accurately measured the right amount of water. The process of accurate measurement was reviewed and the women were asked to repeat the preparation process. The team moved from one location to another approximately every two weeks.

The Impact

Oral Rehydration Workers visited all the villages in Bangladesh, except for a few tribal districts. Twelve million households received supervised teaching, and often more than one woman in a household was taught to prepare the ORS. When tested later, over 90% of the women knew of and could prepare the solution and about 90% of the solutions they prepared were safe and effective. In addition, prior to BRAC's initiation of this program, there was very little knowledge of oral rehydration in Bangladesh, and ORS packets were not available in rural Bangladesh. However, from the mid-1980s, the sale of these packets increased. If all types of diarrhea, mild or moderate, watery or non-watery, are included, then about half the diarrhea episodes in the following decade were treated with oral rehydration therapy.[50] Furthermore, another study done in the mid-1990s showed that treatment of diarrhea by oral rehydration therapy was known to over 70% of children who were 11 to 12 years of age in Bangladesh, 10 to 15 years after their mothers were taught about this method.

The Costs and Benefits

In addition to using its own funds, BRAC also received financial support for this effort from Oxfam, the government of the United Kingdom, the Swedish Free Church Aid, the aid agency of the Swiss government, and the United Nations Children's Fund (UNICEF). The total value of this assistance was about $9.3 million. The cost of teaching one household about oral rehydration therapy was a one-time investment of $0.75.

Lessons Learned

BRAC's intervention in Bangladesh shows that mothers, regardless of their literacy level, can learn to improve health behaviors when provided with the right kind of training. When BRAC started the pilot, the general opinion was that illiterate women would not be able to learn how to measure and mix the ingredients. The strategy chosen by BRAC was not new or unknown to the women—BRAC simply built on their knowledge of cooking and feeding their children. The training was also done in familiar surroundings with ingredients that they use on a daily basis. The women were also taught in groups and found it easier to learn from each other than learning on one's own.

Evaluation of the program indicated some of the characteristics that made scaling up oral rehydration therapy possible. The intervention was relatively simple, requiring no assistance once the method was taught; it was inexpensive, requiring no household expenses, except for the purchase of the salt and sugar. The training and messages were built on existing knowledge and skills, such as childcare and cooking, and were also culturally acceptable. The performance of the ORWs was measured through the knowledge acquired by

mothers. Though the program was large, an administrative structure of checks and balances could be put into place along with rigorous supervision. Lastly, there was a clear goal with a specific outcome and an institutional commitment to the process.[50]

NGOs often focus on small populations, which are not representative, and on pilot projects that do not get scaled up. BRAC's effort showed that NGOs are capable of taking to scale pilot or demonstration projects. To do so, however, required strong supervision, supervisor accountability, and local level flexibility and autonomy. In addition, however, experience with the incentive salary system used by BRAC shows that this approach can only be used when employees who are not effective can be dismissed and not reassigned to any other position or job, as is usually the case for government workers. It is also important that there be tangible and quantifiable outcomes that are relatively easy to measure, and an independent monitoring unit is necessary. Finally, the strategic use of male and female workers allowed female workers to access households and gain the confidence of women, while male workers talked to the men in places where men congregate.

Integrating Services at the Grassroots Level

Introduction

All health systems face the question of how they can most effectively and efficiently provide health services, particularly in difficult to reach areas. Often these programs are carried out in vertical ways. In this case, the program is operated parallel to other programs and may have its own management, staff, financing, and procurement arrangements. It might even have its own facilities. In some settings, this way of operating is undertaken because of extreme weaknesses of the overall health system. However, it would be much more efficient if programs could be carried out in an integrated fashion like they are performed in the health systems of most developed countries. This case study discusses efforts to integrate the delivery of vitamin A and drugs for onchocerciasis (river blindness) in a number of countries in Africa, in hopes of improving the effectiveness and efficiency of the vitamin A program, the onchocerciasis program, and the overall health system.

As will be discussed in much greater detail in Chapters 8 and 10, vitamin A deficiency is a leading cause of under-five childhood mortality,[51] childhood blindness, and infectious disease in 95 developing countries worldwide. According to the World Health Organization in 2001, 140 million preschool children and more than 7 million pregnant women suffer from vitamin A deficiency. Vitamin A supplementation has proven effective in combating vitamin A deficiency and has therefore become a key intervention to improve child survival. More than 40% of children in Sub-Saharan Africa are at risk for vitamin A deficiency. Estimates indicate that correcting vitamin A deficiency will avert more than 645,000 child deaths per year in Sub-Saharan Africa.[52]

Onchocerciasis is the second leading infectious cause of blindness in the world and is endemic throughout much of Sub-Saharan Africa. It is caused by a parasite, the filaria *Onchocerca volvulus*. The transmission of this parasite to humans takes place through the bite of the blackfly (*Simulium* genus). According to 2005 estimates,[53] about 37 million people are infected with the disease in Africa. Two hundred and seventy thousand people are blind due to onchocerciasis, but it is more than a blinding disease; it can also cause disfiguring skin changes, musculoskeletal problems, weight loss, immune system changes, and, in some cases, epilepsy and growth arrest. Onchocerciasis is commonly found in remote regions where government health services are unavailable.

Ivermectin is the front-line drug used to treat onchocerciasis and is usually delivered through "community-directed treatment." This strategy trains community volunteers to sensitize other community members about the disease and its treatment, and to organize campaigns to distribute Ivermectin to eligible members of a community once a year for 15 to 20 years.

The Intervention

Because polio is no longer a threat in most of Africa, African governments are currently phasing out National Immunization Days (NID). This policy change leaves a gap in delivery of vitamin A supplementation to children younger than five years, which was previously included in NID campaigns. Nigeria and Cameroon sought, with the assistance of an NGO called Helen Keller International, to bridge this gap by combining vitamin A supplementation with community-directed treatment with Ivermectin for river blindness. Both countries had high vitamin A deficiency among young children at the time this program was developed. In Nigeria, 25% of the children were vitamin A deficient, and in Cameroon about 40% of the children were vitamin A deficient.[54]

Integrating the two treatments seemed logical for a number of reasons. First, both are relatively easy to deliver by trained community volunteers. Second, they target complementary beneficiary groups, thereby providing something for both young children and women who have recently delivered babies. In addition, both rely on similar supply systems and support from Ministries of Health. It has been estimated that combining the treatments has the potential to supplement over 11 million children at least once per year with high doses of vitamin A.[51]

To test the integration, pilot studies were conducted in Nigeria, beginning in 2001, and in Cameroon, beginning in 2003, where community-directed treatment with Ivermectin was well-established. Careful planning was undertaken with community representatives and Ministry of Health personnel, and training modules and materials were adapted to include vitamin A information and messages. Community volunteers were trained to discuss the practical aspects of how to integrate the two interventions in their village. Volunteers then explained to village residents the importance of vitamin A for child survival and that vitamin A doses would be given only to children from 6 to 59 months of age and to women who had given birth within the last 2 months, during the campaign period. They also discussed the need for a second vitamin A dose for children in 6 months, and the importance of exclusive breastfeeding to protect young children from malnutrition.

The Impact

A program evaluation of the Cameroon pilot showed good results, with high vitamin A supplementation and high Ivermectin coverage maintained in all pilot communities. As the project was scaled up in a 2-month campaign, from 1 health district covering under 50,000 people to 15 health districts covering over 642,000 people, vitamin A supplementation coverage was 77% among children from 6 to 59 months of age and 90% among women who had given birth in the last 2 months. In addition, Ivermectin coverage increased from 70.3% in 2003 to 74% in 2004. In 2007, national-level scale up in Cameroon is planned for delivery of at least one of the vitamin A doses during a community-directed campaign for treatment with Ivermectin.

In Nigeria, the integrated program was piloted in two states, reaching more than 300,000 children from 6 to 59 months of age and about 72,000 postpartum women. By 2003 and 2004, the strategy was replicated in an additional four states supported by the State Onchocerciasis Control Programs with assistance from UNICEF, Sight Savers International, and the Mission to Save the Helpless. During the scaling up phase, the pilot program provided supplements to about 950,000 children from 6 to 59 months of age with 80% coverage and to about 117,000 women within 6 weeks of giving birth, with 60% coverage. Ivermectin coverage did not decline in these areas, but rather was maintained at over 80% of the total population, indicating again that community volunteers are able to provide both interventions together. Because National Immunization Days for polio are continuing in Nigeria, national scale-up of the program has been delayed until 2007, when the NIDs will terminate if the polio program meets its goals.

Costs and Benefits

The cost to integrate vitamin A supplementation into community-directed treatment with Ivermectin is minimal compared to implementing two separate interventions. The cost to undertake key community-directed treatment activities, including training, supervision, distribution, and reporting, is cost-shared between Ministry of Health, non-governmental organizations, communities, and donors including the African Program for Onchocerciasis Control. Ivermectin is donated by Merck and Co. Inc, through the Mectizan® Donation Program to governments.

A recent World Health Organization cost study[55] found that the average cost of one Ivermectin treatment is $0.58, without volunteer time included, and $0.78 if volunteer time is included. In Nigeria, the study found that integrating vitamin A supplementation and Ivermectin treatment costs an extra $0.18 per vitamin A treatment but decreases to $0.15 per treatment when scaled up to six states. At the national level, the cost of integrating the two treatments would be $0.10 per vitamin A treatment.

Lessons Learned

Integration means expanding partnerships to include all stakeholders at each level. Advocacy is essential to ensure that governments are willing to bring in relevant partners and commit funding to an integrated approach. To scale-up, a strategy must be fully tested and well planned. Ongoing supervision, monitoring, and evaluation are critical during scale-ups to improve program results across a more diverse cultural and geographic area. The vitamin A–Ivermectin integrated treatment approach has been or is being adopted by other countries as well, including the Democratic Republic of Congo, Sierra Leone, and Sudan. The results in these countries will shed further light on how services can be integrated to enhance effectiveness and efficiency of services in low-income countries.

Enhancing Community Health Services in Tanzania[56]

Introduction

Tanzania is a low-income country in Sub-Saharan Africa. Most people in Tanzania live in rural areas. The burden of disease in Tanzania is typical of that for a low-income African country, with high rates of infant and child mortality, maternal mortality, and high prevalence of malaria, TB, and HIV/AIDS. Until recently, the government of Tanzania was spending about $8 per person each year on health.

The Intervention

The International Development Research Center (IDRC) of Canada and the government of Tanzania established a joint program to determine if health outcomes of poor people in rural areas could be improved by aligning health expenditure more closely with the burden of disease and increasing expenditure on selected health conditions. This effort was called the Tanzania Essential Health Interventions Project and took place in two rural districts with a total population of about 700,000 people.

The program started by trying to map the burden of disease. Given the poor database with which they had to work, this was done by a door to door survey of the involved communities to see what people said were the causes of ill health, disability, and death. The program team then calculated the burden of disease and reviewed government expenditure to see if it was being allocated in accordance with that burden.

What they found was substantial gaps between the two. Only 5% of the budget went for malaria, although it caused 30% of the DALYs lost. Only 13% went to the leading causes of DALYs lost in children, despite the fact that they caused 28% of the disease burden. In addition, some diseases received more funding than seemed reasonable, given their contributions to the burden of disease and the cost of addressing them.

An additional $2 was allocated to the two pilot communities per person to spend on areas of high disease burden. In addition, the communities began to use simple algorithms for diagnosing and treating common diseases in a standard way, such as diarrhea, pneumonia, and malaria. The health districts also began to order drugs more in line with their needs, rather than just using a common package of drugs sent by the government that did not always meet their needs. Finally, health education was undertaken to get members of the community to use insecticide-impregnated bed nets when they slept to reduce the likelihood of contracting malaria.

The Outcome

Studies showed that the infant mortality rate decreased from 100 to 78 from the year 1999 to the year 2000 in one of the districts, which was a decrease of 28%. The under-five child mortality rate decreased from 140 to 120 over the same period, which was a drop of 14%. It appears that the second district had similar results to the first. Comparable communities that did not participate in this pilot did not see drops in infant and child mortality like those that occurred in the pilot communities. People in the involved communities also decided to build their own health centers so that they do not have to travel so far for health services.

Costs

The communities could not use all of the $2 that was allocated for the program. Rather, to achieve the outcomes noted above, they used only about $0.80, which was equal to about a 10% increase in public expenditure per person on health in these two areas.

Lessons Learned

The success of this pilot program appears to have depended on a number of factors. First, the project was carefully planned. Second, the communities were involved in the planning, designing, and execution of the program. Third, the approach of the project was based on good data and evidence about the burden of disease. Fourth, the program focused on implementing low-cost interventions that are known to be highly effective and that targeted health conditions of importance. Finally, the program reflects a point noted in Chapters 2 and 3: The manner in which countries spend money on health is as important as how much they spend. These lessons are consistent with the lessons learned from a variety of other important health programs over the last several decades.

MAIN MESSAGES

A health system is "the combination of resources, organization, and management that culminate in the delivery of health services to the population."[52] The main functions of a health system are to raise money for health services, provide health services, pay for health services, and engage in governance and regulation of health activities. In line with this, health systems provide prevention, diagnosis, treatment, and rehabilitative services; protect the sick and their families against the cost of ill health; and carry out key public health functions, such as surveillance, the operation of public health laboratories, and food and drug administration. Health systems are important parts of all economies and in some cases make up as much as 15% of GDP.

Health systems have three levels of health care: primary, secondary, and tertiary. Depending on the country, the public, private, and nongovernmental sectors participate in different parts of the health system. A critical issue in the design of health systems is the roles that each of these sectors should play. There is agreement that governments must regulate and provide oversight of the health system. However, there is also a growing view that the government does not need to provide all services but, instead, should consider how they might most effectively be provided, which could mean government contracting the private or NGO sectors for some services.

High-income countries generally have a health system that can be categorized as social insurance, such as Germany; have a tax-financed national health insurance scheme, such as in the United Kingdom; or, have a system that is largely based on private finance, such as in the United States. In most low- and middle-income countries, governments have established a health system that provides each level of care on a geographic basis.

Countries spend a wide range of their GDP on health, from 1% in Afghanistan to about 13% in the United States. Countries spend a larger share of their GDP on health as they become more developed. Most of the high-income countries have health systems that are largely publicly financed, except the United States. In low-income countries that lack social insurance, most expenditure on health is private and out-of-pocket. In general, the health systems of high-income countries are more effective at meeting health system aims than are the systems in low- and middle-income countries.

The health systems of all countries, but especially those in low- and middle-income countries, face a number of important challenges, including:

- How to cope with an aging population and increasing amounts of non-communicable disease
- The quality of governance
- The number, quality, and distribution of healthcare personnel
- The mobilization of sufficient financial resources for the health sector
- How to provide health care at an appropriate level of quality
- How to ensure access to and equitable provision of services
- The creation of mechanisms to provide the poor with protection from the costs of health services

Governance is a difficult issue to address because governance issues are generally problems across all sectors, and not just the health sector. Nonetheless, by giving communities more control over health sector resources, having them openly monitor their use, enhancing the capacity of the health sector to engage in procurement functions, and contracting out services that can most effectively and efficiently be delivered by the private or NGO sectors, governance can be improved.

Ensuring that countries have the right number of trained health personnel in the right places will continue to be difficult. However, there is evidence that different kinds of incentives, such as housing, additional pay, and greater access to training can encourage health personnel to serve in underserved areas. The productivity of health providers can also be encouraged through appropriate incentives.

It will continue to be difficult for low-income countries to raise the resources they need to finance a cost-efficient package of health services. However, given the potential returns to investments in health, even very poor countries must consider allocating a larger share of their overall resources to health. In addition, existing expenditure on health is very inefficient in many countries and some financial savings can be had from improving the efficiency of existing expenditure and by allocating a higher share of resources to areas that will yield the highest returns.

The quality of services can be improved, even in low-income settings. Accreditation of services is potentially promising, but not yet a proven way of improving health outcomes. Oversight by senior health staff in structured ways has improved outcomes in some settings. Providing health personnel with clear guidelines, protocols, and algorithms for treatment of patients can also improve the quality of care. There is also increasing evidence that total quality management activities can improve health outcomes, even in very low-income settings.

Greater attention needs to be paid in most countries to enhancing the coverage by the health system of poor and marginalized populations. One way to do this is to engage these communities in the planning and design of health system interventions. Improving services to the poor and ensuring that these services do not hurt families financially will also require that greater attention be paid to various insurance schemes, including both social insurance for the poor and community-based insurance programs.

In addition, low- and middle-income countries can help to enhance the health of their poor by moving in the previously noted directions and then focusing expenditure on a package of services that at relatively low-cost will have the highest impact on preventing illness among the poor and on treating those illnesses that most effect them. As discussed further in other chapters, this would include:

- Promoting access to safe water and enhanced sanitation and encouraging improved hygiene
- Enhancing people's food habits and providing selective nutrition supplementation
- Providing a basic package of reproductive health services
- Providing a basic package of neonatal health services
- Vaccinating and de-worming young children, oral rehydration for diarrhea, and treatment of pneumonia and malaria
- Preventing and treating, as appropriate, HIV, TB, and malaria
- Preventing tobacco use

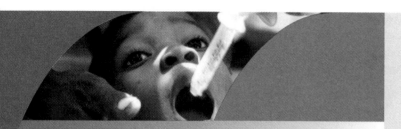

Study Questions

1. What is a health system?

2. What are the primary functions of a health system?

3. What are primary, secondary, and tertiary health care and what services are generally rendered at each level?

4. How might one compare and contrast the organizational forms of healthcare systems of the United Kingdom, Germany, and the United States?

5. What is the range of public expenditure on health as a share of their GDP that countries spend on health? Why is there such a wide range?

6. Which types of countries tend to have a larger share of private expenditure on health than public expenditure on health? Why is this so, compared to countries that have health systems that are most publicly funded?

7. What are some of the significant issues that arise in trying to govern health systems in low- and middle-income countries?

8. What are some of the key human resource challenges that low- and middle-income countries face in staffing and operating their health systems?

9. What are the most important epidemiological and demographic issues that face health systems and what are the implications of those issues for healthcare costs?

10. What are some of the most important steps that can be taken to improve the effectiveness and efficiency of weaker health systems in low- and middle-income countries?

REFERENCES

1. UN Millenium Development Goals. Available at: http://www.un.org/millenniumgoals/. Accessed March 15, 2006.

2. World Health Organization (WHO). HSP. Available at: http://www.who.int/health-systems-performance/about.htm Accessed May 6, 2006.

3. Roemer M. *National Health Systems of the World* Vol 1: The Countries. Oxford, England: Oxford University Press; 1991.

4. Roberts MJ, Et al. *Getting Health Reform Right: A Guide to Improving Performance and Equity.* New York: Oxford University Press; 2004.

5. World Health Organization (WHO). *The World Health Report 2000.* Geneva: World Health Organization; 2000.

6. World Health Organization (WHO). Overview. *The World Health Report 2000.* Geneva: World Health Organization; 2000:1.

7. Southby R. Presentation: George Washington University; 2004.

8. World Resources Institute. Biodiversity Glossary of Terms. Available at: www.edu.gov.nf.ca/curriculum/teched/resources/glos-biodiversity.html. Accessed September 22, 2006.

9. The World Bank. *Afghanistan Health Sector and Emergency Reconstruction and Development Project.* Washington, DC 2003.

10. The World Bank. *Bangladesh Integrated Nutrition Project.* Washington, DC 1995.

11. Mills A, Rasheed F, Tollman S. Strengthening Health Systems. In: Jamison DT, Breman JG, Measham AR, et al., eds. *Disease Control Priorities in Developing Countries.* 2nd ed. New York: Oxford University Press; 2006:87–102.

12. Basch P. *Textbook of International Health.* 2nd ed. New York: Oxford University Press; 2001:376.

13. Brenner G, Rublee D. Germany. In: Fried BJ, Gaydos LM, eds. *World Health Systems: Challenges and Perspectives.* Chicago: Health Administration Press; 2002:121–135.

14. Basch P. *Textbook of International Health.* 2nd ed. New York: Oxford University Press; 2001:121–136.

15. Basch P. *Textbook of International Health.* 2nd ed. New York: Oxford University Press; 2001:376–578.

16. Basch P. *Textbook of International Health.* 2nd ed. New York: Oxford University Press; 2001:380.

17. Gaydos LM, Fried BJ. The United Kingdom. In: Fried BJ, Gaydos LM, eds. *World Health Systems: Challenges and Perspectives.* Chicago: Health Administration Press; 2002:267–277.

18. Upshaw VM, Deal KM. The United States of America. In: Fried BJ, Gaydos LM, eds. *World Health Systems: Challenges and Perspectives.* Chicago: Health Administration Press; 2002:67-82.

19. Dow WH, Sáenz LB. Costa Rica. In: Fried BJ, Gaydos LM, eds. *World Health Systems: Challenges and Perspectives.* Chicago: Health Administration Press; 2002:463–473.

20. Portugal R, Abrantes AV. Brazil. In: Fried BJ, Gaydos LM, eds. *World Health Systems: Challenges and Perspectives.* Chicago: Health Administration Press; 2002:404–419.

21. Shah ON. India. In: Fried BJ, Gaydos LM, eds. *World Health Systems: Challenges and Perspectives.* Chicago: Health Administration Press; 2002:495–506.

22. Peters DH, Preker AS, Yazbek AS, et al. *Better Health Systems for India's Poor.* Washington, DC: The World Bank; 2002.

23. Health. Available at: http://www.tanzania.go.tz/health.html. Accessed September 12, 2006, 2006.

24. World Health Organization (WHO). Core Health Indicators. Available at: www.who.int/whosis/core/core_select_process.cfm. Accessed September 10, 2006.

25. World Health Organization (WHO). Statistical Annex. *The World Health Report 2000.* Geneva: World Health Organization; 2000.

26. Mathers CD, Lopez AD, Murray CJL. The Burden of Disease and Mortality by Condition: Data, Methods, and Results for 2001. In: Lopez AD, Mathers CD, Ezzati M, Jamison DT, Murray CJL, eds. *Global Burden of Disease and Risk Factors.* New York: Oxford University Press; 2006:45–93.

27. Lewis M. *Tackling Healtcare Corruption and Governance Woes in Developing Countries.* Washington, DC: Center for Global Development; 2006. Working Paper 78.

28. Physicians for Human Rights. An Action Plan to Prevent Brain Drain: Building Equitable Health Systems in Africa. Available at: http://www.physiciansforhumanrights.org/library/report-2004-july.html. Accessed January 22, 2007.

29. Hongoro C, Normand C. Health Workers: Building and Motivating the Workforce. In: Jamison DT, Breman JG, Measham AR, et al., eds. *Disease Control Priorities in Developing Countries.* 2nd ed. New York: Oxford University Press; 2006:1309–1322

30. Jamison DT, Breman JG, Measham AR, et al., eds. *Priorities in Health.* Washington, DC: The World Bank; 2006.

31. Schieber G, Baeza C, Kress D, Maier M. Financing Health Systems in the 21st Century. In: Jamison DT, Breman JG, Measham AR, et al., eds. *Disease Control Priorities in Developing Countries.* 2nd ed. New York: Oxford University Press; 2006:225–242.

32. Institute of Medicine. *Measuring the Quality of Health Care.* Washington, DC 1999.

33. Peabody JW, Taguiwalo MM, Robalino DA, Frenk J. Improving the Quality of Care in Developing Countries. In: Jamison DT, Breman JG, Measham AR, et al., eds. *Disease Control Priorities in Developing Countries.* 2nd ed. New York: Oxford University Press; 2006:1293–1307.

34. Beracochea E, Dickenson R, Freemand P, Thomason J. Case Management Quality Assessment in Rural Areas of Papua New Guinea. *Tropical Doctor.* 1995;25(2):69–74.

35. Thaver IH, Harpham T, McPake B, Garner P. Private practitioners in the slums of Karachi: what quality of care do they offer? *Soc Sci Med.* Jun 1998;46(11):1441–1449.

36. Nolan T, Angos P, Cunha AJ, et al. Quality of hospital care for seriously ill children in less-developed countries. *Lancet.* Jan 13 2001;357(9250):106-110.

37. World Health Organization (WHO). *The World Health Report 2000.* Geneva: World Health Organization; 2000:93–115.

38. Jha P, Chaloupka FJ, Moore J, et al. Tobacco Addiction. In: Jamison DT, Breman JG, Measham AR, et al., eds. *Disease Control Priorities in Developing Countries.* 2nd ed. New York: Oxford University Press; 2006:869–885.

39. Norton R, Hyder AA, Bishai D, Peden M. Unintentional Injuries. In: Jamison DT, Breman JG, Measham AR, et al., eds. *Disease control priorities in developing countries.* 2nd ed. New York: Oxford University Press; 2006:737–753.

40. Hongoro C, Normand C. Health Workers: Building and Motivating the Workforce. In: Jamison DT, Breman JG, Measham AR, et al., eds. *Disease Control Priorities in Developing Countries.* 2nd ed. New York: Oxford University Press; 2006:1312.

41. Hongoro C, Normand C. Health Workers: Building and Motivating the Workforce. In: Jamison DT, Breman JG, Measham AR, et al., eds. *Disease Control Priorities in Developing Countries.* 2nd ed. New York: Oxford University Press; 2006:1313.

42. Hongoro C, Normand C. Health Workers: Building and Motivating the Workforce. In: Jamison DT, Breman JG, Measham AR, et al., eds. *Disease Control Priorities in Developing Countries.* 2nd ed. New York: Oxford University Press; 2006:1316–1317.

43. World Health Organization (WHO). *The World Health Report 2000.* Geneva: World Health Organization; 2000:73–92.

44. World Health Organization (WHO). *The World Health Report 2000.* Geneva: World Health Organization; 2000:73–91.

45. USAID. Demographic and Health Surveys. Available at: http://www.measuredhs.com/. Accessed September 24, 2006.

46. Peabody JW, Taguiwalo MM, Robalino DA, Frenk J. Improving the Quality of Care in Developing Countries. In: Jamison DT, Breman JG, Measham AR, et al., eds. *Disease Control Priorities in Developing Countries.* 2nd ed. New York: Oxford University Press; 2006:1299.

47. Peabody JW, Taguiwalo MM, Robalino DA, Frenk J. Improving the Quality of Care in Developing Countries. In: Jamison DT, Breman JG, Measham AR, et al., eds. *Disease Control Priorities in Developing Countries.* 2nd ed. New York: Oxford University Press; 2006:1298.

48. Tollman S, Doherty J, Mulligan J-A. General Primary Care. In: Jamison DT, Breman JG, Measham AR, et al., eds. *Disease Control Priorities in Developing Countries.* 2nd ed. New York: Oxford University Press; 2006:1193–1210.

49. Chowdhury S. Educating mothers for health—output based incentives for teaching oral rehydration in Bangladesh. Available at: http://rru.worldbank.org/Documents/Other/11ch6.pdf. Accessed January 22, 2007.

50. Chowdhury A, Cash R. *A Simple Solution: Teaching Millions to Treat Diarrhea at Home.* Dhaka: University Press Ltd.; 1996.

51. Beaton, Et al. *Effectiveness of VAS in the control of young children morbidity and mortality in developing countries.* Geneva: World Health Organization; 1993. ACC / SSN nutrition policy discussion paper 13.

52. Aguayo V, Baker S. Vitamin A deficiency and child survival in sub-Saharan Africa: A reappraisal of challenges and opportunities. *Food and Nutrition Bulletin.* 2005;26(4).

53. World Health Organization. *Report of the Joint Action Forum of the African Program for Onchocerciasis Control.* Geneva: World Health Organization; December 2005.

54. Anemia. NSoVADa. *Nigeria Food Consumption and Nutrition Survey 2001-2003.* Cameroon: MOH/HKI/UNICEF/WHO; September 2001.

55. McFarland D, Et al. *Study of cost per treatment with ivermectin using CDTI strategy.* WHO/APOC; August 2005.

56. Economist T. Health care in poor countries—Better health for not much money. *The Ecomomist.* 2002(August 15).

Culture and Health

LEARNING OBJECTIVES

By the end of this chapter the reader will be able to:

- Define *culture*
- Describe the most important relationships between culture and health
- Outline some of the theories of how behavior change occurs in health
- Describe some key measures to promote behavior change for better health
- Discuss the importance of social assessments

VIGNETTES

Joshua was just older than 1 year of age and lived in eastern Zimbabwe. His mother could tell that he had a fever. She wondered what had caused it. Was it the food that he ate? Was it the mixing of the "hot" foods and the "cold" foods? Or was it possible that they had done something to offend local custom? If the fever did not get better tomorrow, then she would take Joshua to the local healer.

Siu-Hong was 80 years old and lived in Hong Kong. He had a severe toothache for more than a week. His children repeatedly encouraged him to go to the dentist, but he would not go. He did not like dentists or "western medicine." In addition, he would have to wait in line to be seen at the dentist's office and would miss work at the clothes market. His children finally convinced him to go to the dentist by giving him a "present" of $25 and offering to take him to "dim sum," the traditional South Chinese "brunch."

Dorji lived in Bhutan, just outside the capital city of Thimpu. He felt tired, weak, and dizzy for some time but had no fever. After another week of feeling this way, Dorji went to visit his local health clinic. Each clinic in Bhutan had two medical practitioners, one who practiced the indigenous system of medicine and the other who practiced "Western biomedical medicine."[1] In light of Dorji's symptoms, he visited the indigenous practitioner inside the clinic. The "doctor" gave him some herbs that he thought would help his condition. However, he also thought Dorji had an underlying infection and took him across the hall to the "other doctor" who prescribed antibiotics for him.

Arathi was a young mother in southeast India. She and the other women in her village were participating in the Tamil Nadu Nutrition Project. They were all young mothers, many of whose babies were underweight for age. Arathi nursed her baby as she had learned from her mother to do. She also gave the baby some other foods as she had learned from her mother and grandmother. Despite this, her baby was quite small for her age. As part of the project, the community nutrition workers taught all the women and children in the village songs about proper feeding and about the vitamins the children needed. They also sponsored weekly weighing parties, in which all of the babies of the village were weighed and the mothers together decided if the baby was growing properly and what could be done to make the baby healthier. They also helped the mothers to make a food supplement for the babies who were "too small."

THE IMPORTANCE OF CULTURE TO HEALTH

Culture is an important determinant of health in a number of ways, as discussed in Chapter 2. First, culture is related to health behaviors. People's attitudes toward foods and what they eat, for example, are closely related to culture. The food that pregnant women eat, birthing practices, and how long women breastfeed are also linked to their cultural backgrounds. Hygiene practices are closely tied to culture, as well. Second, culture is an important determinant of people's perceptions of illness. Different culture groups may have different beliefs about what constitutes good health and what constitutes illness. Third, the extent to which people use health services is also very closely linked with culture. Some groups may use health services as soon as they feel ill. Others, however, may visit health practitioners only when they are very sick. Fourth, different cultures have different practices concerning health and medical treatment. Chinese and Indian cultures have well defined systems of medicine. There is a long history in many other societies, as well, of local systems of medicine that include notions of illness, various types of practitioners of medicine, and different kinds of medicines.

The purpose of this chapter is to introduce you to the most important links between health and culture, particularly as they relate to global health and people in low- and middle-income countries. The chapter begins by introducing you to the concept of "culture." It then examines how views of health, illness, the use of health services, and the role of different health providers vary by culture. The chapter also reviews some of the theories of behavior change that relate to enhancing people's health. The chapter concludes with comments about how one can ensure that investments take appropriate account of health and related cultural issues.

As you review this chapter, it is important to note that some cultural values enhance health. A culture, for example, that puts a strong emphasis on monogamy in marriage should have lower rates of HIV/AIDS than cultures in which having multiple sexual partners is more tolerated. However, some cultural values may not enhance health. A cultural emphasis on heaviness in people, for example, as a sign of prosperity or wealth, may be harmful to health, because it would encourage cardiovascular disease and diabetes. Some cultures have food taboos that prevent pregnant women from getting all of the nutrients they need in pregnancy. This chapter aims to help you to understand the relationship between culture and health, identify practices helpful and hurtful to good health, and learn about approaches to promoting healthier behaviors.

THE CONCEPT OF CULTURE

The concept of culture was developed at the end of the 19th century by anthropologists. There have been many defini-

tions of culture. An early definition suggested that culture was:

> that complex whole which includes knowledge, beliefs, art, law, morals, custom and any other capabilities and habits acquired by man as a member of society."

A relatively modern definition states that culture is "a set of rules or standards shared by members of a society, which when acted upon by the members, produce behavior that falls within a range of variation the members consider proper and acceptable."[3] In the simplest terms, one may call culture "behavior and beliefs that are learned and shared."[4]

Cultures operate in a variety of domains, including:

- The family
- Social groups beyond the actor's family
- Individual growth and development
- Communication
- Religion
- Art
- Music
- Politics and law
- The economy[4]

As one thinks about the links between culture and health, it is also important to understand the term "society," which refers to "a group of people who occupy a specific locality and share the same cultural traditions."[3] Societies have social structures that are the "relationships of groups within society that hold it together."[5] In addition, we must note that there is heterogeneity within all cultures. Sometimes this is reflected in what people call subcultures. There are many shared aspects, for example, of Chinese culture. However, China is a very large country and even among the Han Chinese, there are important variations as one moves across China in language, food, wedding customs, and music, among other things. The same would be true of North India. People across North India have much in common. Yet, there are many variations of North Indian culture in different places, such as in the state of West Bengal, on the one hand, and Rajasthan, on the other. This can be seen, again, in language, music, art, and food.

When thinking about the links between culture and health, one also needs to consider that some cultural practices may be well adapted to some settings but poorly adapted to others. Alternatively, they may be well adapted to the way people have been living, but less well adapted to the way people live after important changes or developments in their communities.[6] The culture of nomadic people, for example, may be well suited to their nomadic lifestyle. However, their culture may be very ill equipped to deal with a life style after societal change that would cause them to be more sedentary.

As we consider the relationship between culture and health, we should be aware of the ways in which a culture is viewed by people from outside that culture group. First, we should distinguish between the views of outsiders to a culture and insiders to a culture. This helps us to understand when we are looking at something from our perspective, compared to looking at it from the perspective of those who live within that culture.

Especially in the early days of anthropology, those who studied cultures other than their own often viewed them solely through the prism of their own society and judged much of what they saw to be lacking. This view is called ethnocentrism. Contrary to this view is "cultural relativism," or the idea that "because cultures are unique, they can be evaluated only according to their own standards and values."[7]

The approach that will guide the rest of this chapter and, indeed, the book as a whole, is the question: "How well does a given culture satisfy the physical and psychological needs of those whose behavior it guides?"[7] For example, is female circumcision, also called female genital mutilation, a health-enhancing procedure or a harmful procedure? Is it good or bad for the health of a newborn to be given sugar water? How should one see cultural practices that discriminate against women and cause them to eat less well than men or that might lead to the disproportionate abortion of female fetuses, as in India and China? On the other hand, what about cultures that do encourage exclusive breastfeeding for six months? What about male circumcision, which is associated with reduced transmission of HIV?

You will realize as you make your way through the book that those responsible for guiding health policies and programs in different countries must have a good understanding of the cultures with which they are working if they are to be helpful in enhancing health for the members of those societies. This is also true of outsiders, including development assistance agencies. They must be very sensitive to local cultures, while simultaneously considering with their government partners and in conjunction with insiders to the culture, what behavior changes may be needed to enhance individual and population health in a particular setting.[8]

HEALTH BELIEFS AND PRACTICES

Different cultures vary in their perceptions of their bodies and their views of what is illness, what causes illness, and what should be done about it. They have different views on how to prevent health problems, what health care they should seek, and the types of remedies that health providers might offer.[4] The next section will highlight selected aspects of belief systems about health that one would see most in low- and middle-income countries and in immigrant populations in developed countries.

Perceptions of Illness

Perceptions of illness vary considerably across culture groups. What one culture may view as entirely normal, for example, another culture may see as an affliction. Worms are so common among children in some cultures that people do not see infection with worms as an illness. Malaria is so common in much of Sub-Saharan Africa that many families see it as normal. In much of South Asia, back pain among women is very common and is also seen by women as just a normal part of being a woman.[9] Schistosomiasis is very common in Egypt. It causes blood in the urine, which is referred to in Egypt as "male menstruation" and seen as normal because it is so common.[10]

Perceptions of Disease

Medical anthropologists, among others, define disease as the "malfunctioning or maladaptation of biologic and psychophysiologic processes in the individual."[11] Pneumonia is a disease. HIV/AIDS is a disease. Polio is a disease. Illness, however, is different from disease. "Illness represents personal, interpersonal, and cultural reactions to disease or discomfort."[11] People may feel like they have an illness. They can describe it and its symptoms. They may have a name in their culture for this problem. However, they may not have a "disease," which is a physiological condition. This is a very important point, because different cultures may have very different perceptions of the causes of illness.

Most people in the developed countries follow the "Western medical paradigm" in explaining the causes of disease. This will be familiar to you. You get influenza and colds from viruses. You get diabetes as an adult from an inability to control your blood sugar, although there may be a genetic component to this. You get heart disease from smoking, from being obese, or from having cholesterol that is too high.

On the other hand, many people, especially those in or from the developing world and more "traditional societies" often see illness as being caused by factors other than disease, as defined in the biomedical model. There are many cultures, for example, that believe that illness is brought on by the body being "out of balance." Among the most common of these concepts is the notion of "hot" and "cold." In this case, the body may get out of balance if one engages in certain unhealthy practices. In Chinese culture, for example, one should not drink cold liquids while eating hot food. In some cultures, some foods are regarded as "hot" and some foods are regarded as "cold" and people have to eat them in certain appropriate proportions or only at certain times to avoid illness.

Many people also believe that illness has supernatural causes. A study done among Americans of Caribbean and African descent living in the southern United States showed that many people believed that the symptoms of illness stem from supernatural causes.[12] There are many cultures in which people believe that illness comes from being affected by "the evil eye," being bewitched or possessed, losing their soul, or offending gods.[13] Some indigenous Canadians have a belief that "illness is not necessarily a bad thing, but instead a sign sent by the Creator to help people re-evaluate their lives."[14] A study of the cultural perceptions of illness among Yoruba people in Nigeria found that illness could be "traced to enemies, including witchcraft, sorcery, gods, ancestors, natural illnesses, or hereditary illness."[15]

Emotional stresses are also seen in different cultures as causes of illness. This could come about as a result of being stressed or extremely frightened. Being too envious is also viewed as a cause of illness.[13] Sexual matters are seen as causes of illness in some cultures, as well. In several cultures, for example, frequent sexual relations is believed to weaken men, by taking away their blood.[13] These beliefs are quite common in parts of India.

Folk Illness

Many cultures also have what are called "folk illnesses." These are local cultural interpretations of physical states that people perceive to be illness, but that do not have a physiologic cause. "Empacho" is an illness that is commonly described in a number of Latin American cultures. This is often discussed as a condition caused by food that "gets stuck to the walls of the stomach or intestines, causing an obstruction."[16] It is said to be caused by any of a variety of inappropriate food practices, and in children it is said to produce a number of gastrointestinal symptoms, including bloating, diarrhea, and a stomachache.

To cure empacho, families may limit some foods, give abdominal massages with warm oil, or pop the skin on the small of the back. They will also often consult a local healer, such as the *santiguadora* in the Puerto Rican community and *sobadora* in the Mexican community. Some Mexican communities in both the United States and Mexico also treat this "illness" with some powders.

To understand health problems in low- and middle-income countries, it is very important to understand the existence of folk illnesses such as empacho. It may be that the condition described by communities as empacho has no known or real biomedical basis. However, even if this condition has no biomedical basis, people believe this is an important illness and any efforts to improve the health of the community will have to consider such beliefs.[16] Table 6-1 lists some of the culturally defined causes of illness.

The Prevention of Illness

Given the wide range of views of what causes illness, it is not surprising that there are many different cultural practices that concern avoiding illness. Many cultures, for example, have taboos, or things that they forbid people to do if they are to stay healthy. A large number of taboos concern what not to eat during pregnancy, as was suggested in a study of traditional beliefs in Western Malaysia, which indicated that pregnant women should avoid certain important sources of protein.[17] A study in southern Nigeria about traditional beliefs concerning eating in pregnancy found widespread belief that pregnant women must avoid:

- sweet foods, so the baby would not be weak
- eggs, so the baby would not grow up to be a thief
- snails, so the baby would not be dull, salivate excessively, or not develop speech properly.[18]

A study in Brazil suggested that women should not eat game meat and fish during pregnancy, although both could be good sources of protein.[19] A study of poor women in South India showed that "taboos affected the intake of fruits and legumes" and legumes are among the most important sources of protein for many Indian women.[20]

There is also a wide array of ritual practices that people undergo to avoid illness. Related to this, there are traditions in some cultures to get rid of bad spirits or evil forces to ensure that one does not fall ill. There are beliefs among the Yoruba people in Nigeria, for example, that charms, amulets, scarification, or some oral potions can prevent illness that is caused by one's enemies.[15] Some tribal groups in Rajasthan, India, put charms at certain crossings to inflict harm on others, to avoid harm to themselves, to appease an evil spirit, or to leave their affliction there with the spirit.[21] In rural Senegal, a special ritual is performed for women who have lost two children, or had two miscarriages, or appear to be infertile. The ritual is intended to prevent the causes of child death and infertility.[22]

The Diagnosis and Treatment of Illness and the Use of Health Services

In many cultures, when people are ill, it is common that they first try to care for the illness themselves with home remedies. This is often followed by a visit to some type of local healer and the use of indigenous medicines from that healer. Only if the illness does not resolve after that will families seek the help of a "western doctor." Even then, it is quite common for people to use modern medicines and indigenous medicines at the same time.

Studies that were done of the treatment of diarrheal disease in Central America showed very clearly, for example, that people tried a variety of mechanisms for diagnosing and treating their illnesses.

The manner in which people and families care for illnesses is called "patterns of resort." People seek help from different healthcare providers at different times for a number of reasons.[23] One important concern is the cost of services, both direct, such as fees, and indirect, such as the cost of transportation, time en route, or waiting. Another concern is the means of payment. People with little cash may prefer to visit a healer or doctor who takes payment in kind, rather than in cash. This could be in small gifts or payment in farm products such as fruits, vegetables, or poultry. People are also driven by the reputation of the provider. They will go to a provider that is reputed in their community to have good results over a provider who does not enjoy this type of reputation.

The manner in which the provider treats them socially is also an important determinant of the use of services. People generally prefer to go to a provider who is from their community, speaks their language, is known to them, and treats them with respect, rather than an outsider who may be disrespectful. It is interesting to note that people tend to treat folk illnesses at home and then go to a local healer. As a last resort, they may go to a physician, even if they understand that the physician "does not treat empacho."[16]

It is also very important to understand the extent to which a large share of the treatment of illness in most cultures takes place first at home. People in developed countries may take some aspirin, drink plenty of water, eat a certain soup, and try to rest when they first develop symptoms. They may also take a variety of different types of herbal products or vitamins. Only if people do not feel better by a certain time will they try to see a health provider. People in more traditional societies have analogous patterns of behavior when they believe themselves to be ill. Understanding these patterns, of course, is central to any efforts to enhance their health through efforts such as maternal care, vaccination programs, or treatment of infectious diseases, such as AIDS, TB, or malaria.

Health Providers

There are a many different types of health service providers. Some of these are shown in Table 6-2. As you can see in the table, some of the providers are practitioners of indigenous systems of medicine, such as ayurvedic practitioners in India and practitioners of Chinese systems of medicine, such as herbalists and acupuncturists. Other practitioners will be part of a wide array of local health providers. These include, for example, traditional birth attendants, priests, herbalists, and bonesetters. The types of practitioners of western medicine will depend on the size and location of the place in which they work and could include, for example, community health workers, nurses, midwives, nurse-midwives, physicians, and dentists. You should also be aware that in many low- and middle-income countries, pharmacists, or stores that sell drugs, also frequently dispense both drugs and medical advice. Although prescriptions for drugs may be legally required, many low- and middle-income countries

---

TABLE 6-1 Selected Examples of Cultural Explanations of Disease

Body Balances	Emotional	Supernatural	Sexual
Temperature	Fright	Bewitching	Sex with forbidden
Energy	Sorrow	Demons	person
Blood	Envy	Spirit possession	Overindulgence in sex
Dislocation	Stress	Evil eye	
Problems with organs		Offending god or gods	
Incompatibility of horoscopes		Soul loss	

Source: Adapted with permission from Scrimshaw SC. Culture, behavior, and health. In: Merson MH, Black RE, Mills A, eds. *International Public Health: Diseases, Programs, Systems, and Policies.* Sudbury, MA: Jones and Bartlett; 2006:53–78.

TABLE 6-2 Selected Examples of Health Service Providers

Indigenous	Western Biomedical	Other Medical Systems
Midwives	Pharmacists	Chinese medical system
Shamans	Nurse-midwives	• practitioners
Curers	Nurses	• chemists/herbalists
Spirtualists	Nurse-practitioners	• acupuncturists
Witches	Physicians	Ayuervedic practitioners
Sorcerers	Dentists	
Priests		
Diviners		
Herbalists		
Bonesetters		

Source: Adapted with permission from Scrimshaw SC. Culture, behavior, and health. In: Merson MH, Black RE, Mills A, eds. *International Public Health: Diseases, Programs, Systems, and Policies.* Sudbury, MA: Jones and Bartlett; 2006:53–78.

are unable or unwilling to enforce this requirement. It is also important to note that many health providers will combine indigenous health practices with western medicine.[24]

HEALTH BEHAVIORS AND BEHAVIOR CHANGE

As you saw in Chapter 2, the leading causes of death in low- and middle-income countries are ischemic heart disease, cerebrovascular disease, HIV, and pneumonia. Malaria, TB, and diarrhea are also among the top 10 causes of death in these countries.[25] The risk factors for these diseases and conditions include nutrition (both undernutrition and over-nutrition), tobacco use, unsafe sex, and unsafe water and sanitation.[26] There are many behaviors that *are* conducive to good health. However, what is the extent to which behavior is a contributing factor to the leading risk factors for illness and premature death in the developing world? A number of examples are discussed next.

An infant's being underweight for age is the most important risk factor for premature death in the developing world. Although income and education are closely linked with nutritional status of both mother and child, cultural variables are also important determinants of their nutrition. As noted earlier, there are many cultures that have food taboos for pregnant women that are not helpful to birth outcomes, and other cultures encourage pregnant women to eat less rather than more. In addition, the extent to which women breastfeed their babies is closely linked with culture, as is the timing for the introduction of complementary foods. Undernutrition also stems from other eating practices that are also closely tied to culture. Can behaviors be changed so

that pregnant women will eat the most nutritious foods they can, given their level of income, and exclusively breastfeed their babies for six months?

Unsafe sex is the major risk factor for HIV/AIDS in low- and middle-income countries. Some people, such as commercial sex workers, may not have the bargaining power with their clients to negotiate sex with a condom. The same will often be true of women who are forced into unsafe sex by their husbands and boyfriends or because of their own economic position, as you will read about in Chapters 9 and 11. However, many people who engage in unsafe sex do have control over whether or not to use a condom. What would it take to ensure that they do so?

Hygiene is another area that closely relates to health behaviors and the lack of safe water and sanitation is a risk factor of importance for diarrheal disease. In many low- and middle-income countries hygiene may be low, and families need to learn to use water safely, dispose of human waste in sanitary ways, and wash their hands with soap after defecating. Behaviors regarding hygiene, of course, are intimately linked with culture. How can they be changed?

As you will read about later, indoor air pollution is a major risk factor for respiratory infections. This relates largely to the fact that families in many cultures cook indoors without appropriate ventilation. Some families may not be able to afford an improved stove. However, other families cook as they do because of tradition and the lack of knowledge of the health impacts of indoor air pollution. How could one change such fundamental matters as the way that people cook?

Cigarettes are the leading risk factor for cardiovascular disease and cancer, as you will read more about in Chapter 12. Most people who smoke cigarettes start smoking as adolescents. Are there measures that can be taken to change these behaviors? How would the efforts to change behavior have to differ if one tried to stop adolescents from taking up smoking, compared to helping adult smokers to quit?

Of course, behaviors are closely linked with culture and health not only in developing countries, but in developed countries, as well. Moreover, in developed, as well as in developing countries, there is a wide array of behaviors that do not promote good health. In the developed countries, for example, an increasing number of people are obese and have diabetes, associated, as you will read in Chapter 12, with poor diet and a sedentary lifestyle. Many people also continue to smoke, even though smoking is the single largest risk factor for both cardiovascular disease and cancers. Despite the widespread availability of seat belts in cars, some people still do not use them. What needs to be done to get people to change these behaviors to ones that are healthier?

Improving Health Behaviors

There are a number of models or theories that explain why people engage in certain health behaviors and what can be done to encourage changes in those behaviors. Those interested in greater detail in how to change health behaviors can review *The Essentials of Health Behavior*, another book in this series.[27] Some of the most important concepts about health behavior and models about behavior change, however, are examined very briefly here.

The Ecological Perspective

As one considers the factors that influence behaviors that relate to health, it is important to take what is called an ecological perspective. This is a concept that suggests that the factors influencing health behaviors occur at several levels. These are noted in Table 6-3.

The basic precepts concerning the ecological approach are:

- "health related behaviors are affected by, and affect, multiple levels of influence: intrapersonal or individual factors, interpersonal factors, institutional factors and public policy factors."
- "behavior both influences and is influenced by the social environments in which it occurs."[28]

You can try to imagine, for example, whether or not an adolescent male will take up smoking. This will depend on how he feels about smoking, what he thinks others think of his smoking, the setting in which he operates, how expensive

TABLE 6-3 The Ecological Perspective

Factors	Definition
Individual	Individual characteristics that influence behavior such as knowledge, attitudes, beliefs, and personality traits
Interpersonal	Interpersonal processes, and primary groups including family, friends, and peers
Institutional	Rules, regulations, policies, and informal structures
Community	Social networks and norms or standards that exist formally or informally among individuals, groups, and organizations
Public policy	Local, state, and federal policies and laws that regulate or support healthy actions and practices for disease prevention, early detection, control, and management

Source: Adapted with permission from Murphy E. *Promoting Healthy Behavior, Health Bulletin 2.* Washington, DC: Population Reference Bureau; 2005.

it is to buy cigarettes, and how easy it is to buy them. Of course, if he does start smoking, some of his own peer group may follow.

The Health Belief Model

The Health Belief model was the first effort to articulate a coherent understanding of the factors that enter into health behaviors. It was developed by the U.S. Public Health Services as they tried to understand why people did or did not avail of the opportunity to get chest X-rays for tuberculosis.[29] The premises of this model are that people's health behaviors depend on their perceptions of:

- Their likelihood of getting the illness
- The severity of the illness if they get it
- The benefits of engaging in behavior that will prevent the illness
- The barriers to engaging in preventive behavior

In this model, people's health behavior also depends on whether or not people feel that they could actually carry out the appropriate behavior if they tried, which is called "self-efficacy."[30]

One could think about how this model pertains to engaging in safe sex. The extent to which a young man uses a condom will be influenced by his fear of getting HIV/AIDS, how serious a disease he believes it to be, the extent to which a condom can prevent HIV/AIDS, and how easy it is to buy a condom and get a partner to agree to use it. The young man must also feel that he will buy the condom and use it.

Stages of Change Model

The Stages of Change model was developed in the 1990s in the United States in conjunction with work on alcohol and drug abuse.[31] The premise behind this model is that change in behavior is a process and that different people are at different stages of readiness for change. The stages of change are outlined in Table 6-4.

It is easy to see how this model might apply to alcohol and drug abuse. You can imagine an excessive drinker, as discussed in Chapter 12, who is not aware of his problem or who will not face it and needs help in doing so. Other people,

who are aware of their problem and willing to do something about it, may need help to stop. Still others, who have already broken their addictions, need positive reinforcement to maintain their health.[30]

The Diffusion of Innovations Model

The Diffusions of Innovations model had its origins in work that was done on promoting agricultural change in the United States. In this model, "an innovation is an idea, practice, service, or other object that is perceived as new by the individual or group."[32] This model is based on the notion that communication is needed to promote social change and that "diffusion" is the process by which innovations are communicated over time among members of different groups and societies.[33] This model focuses on how people adopt and can be encouraged to adopt "innovations" but does not get involved with how they might maintain what they have adopted.

Table 6-5 outlines the stages that have to be undertaken to try to diffuse a health innovation.

This model also suggests that as the innovation begins to be diffused, people will fall into six groups:

- Innovators
- Early adopters
- Early majority
- Late majority
- Late adopters
- Laggards[32,33]

In addition, the model also indicates that the pace of adoption will be influenced by:

- The gains people think they will get by adopting the innovation
- How much the innovation fits in with their existing culture and values
- How easy it is to try out the innovation
- Whether or not there are role models who are already trying out the innovation
- The extent to which potential adopters see the innovation as cost-efficient and not taking too much of their time, energy, or money[32,33]

One can imagine how the Diffusion of Innovations Model may apply to efforts to change diets in developed countries away from certain fats and toward more fruits and vegetables, fewer processed foods, and more whole grains. Some people change their diets relatively quickly. Others in the community make these shifts only as they can overcome some of their long held dietary patterns. Some people shift as they learn more from their friends, some of whom become

---

TABLE 6-4 The Stages of Change Model

Stages
- Precontemplation
- Contemplation
- Decision/Determination
- Action
- Maintenance

Source: Data with permission from Murphy E. *Promoting Healthy Behavior, Health Bulletin 2.* Washington, DC: Population Reference Bureau; 2005.

TABLE 6-5 Diffusions of Health Innovations Model

Stages of Diffusion
- Recognition of a problem or need
- Conduct of basic and applied research to address the specific problem
- The development of strategies and materials that will put the innovative concept into a form that will meet the needs of the target population
- Commercialization of the innovation, which will involve prodution, marketing, and distribution efforts
- Diffusion and adoption of the innovation
- Consequences associated with adoption of the innovation

Source: Adapted with permission from Scrimshaw SC. Culture, behavior, and health. In: Merson MH, Black RE, Mills A, eds. *International Public Health: Diseases, Programs, Systems, and Policies.* Sudbury, MA: Jones and Bartlett; 2006:53–78.

role models for change. The relatively high costs of some of the organic and other healthy foods may be a constraint to adoption of change by some people. Others may simply not be willing or able to change the way they and their families have always eaten.

UNDERSTANDING AND ENGENDERING BEHAVIOR CHANGE

As you can clearly see, in many instances, improving health requires that the behaviors of individuals, families, and communities be changed. You also see, however, that behaviors are intimately connected to culture, which is inherently not easy to change. Under these circumstances, what can be done, first to understand what behaviors need to be changed and, second, to change them? These questions are answered briefly here.

Understanding Behaviors

A first step in trying to promote behavior change must be to gain a good understanding of the behaviors that are taking place. This requires a careful assessment of:

- The behaviors that are taking place
- The extent to which they are helpful or harmful to health
- The underlying motivation for these behaviors
- The likely responses to different approaches to changing the unhealthy behaviors

By taking a look at breastfeeding, for example, we can get a sense of how one would carry out such an assessment. One can consider how infant deaths might be reduced. As part of this effort, it is important to get a better sense of the extent to which any nutritional issues are harmful to infant health and how they might be improved. One important part of this effort would be to examine breastfeeding practices. In doing so, we would try to answer the following questions, among others:

- When do women start breastfeeding?
- Do they feed on schedule or on demand?
- Do they feed male and female children the same way?
- For how long do they breastfeed exclusively?
- At what age do they introduce complementary foods?
- Until what age do they continue to breastfeed, even while the children are getting complementary foods?
- Why do they engage in these practices?
- Why do some women not breastfeed?
- Who breastfeeds and who does not?
- Who has influence over their breastfeeding practices?

The answers to these questions, of course, will vary by culture group; however, once we get answers to them, we can begin to formulate a plan for behavior change that is built on the cultural values and approaches of the people. Without understanding current practices, the rationale for them, and who has influence over them, it will be impossible to promote behavior change in the appropriate directions. When we do have a sense of the existing practices and why they take place, what can be done to change behaviors?

Changing Health Behaviors

There are many different approaches to changing health behaviors. Some operate at the level of the individual, some at the level of the community, and some at the level of society as a whole. Generally, they include some combination of communication through the mass media and more personal communication. Several approaches to behavior change are discussed briefly here.

Community Mobilization

One very important way to encourage change in health behaviors is to engage in community mobilization. In this case, the effort focuses on getting an entire community to engage in the effort at promoting more healthy behaviors. This requires considerable efforts aimed at helping people across the community to identify the problems that they face, identify potential solutions to them, and then work together to put those solutions in place. Generally, it also requires that the leaders within the community are themselves mobilized, willing to be "champions" for the needed change, and then promote that change.[34] You will read more later, for example, about the Tamil Nadu Nutrition Project which was noted in one of the vignettes at the opening of this chapter and the manner in which the affected communities were involved in promoting a variety of innovations, including weighing babies together, identifying together the babies who were not thriving, and working together to make supplementary food for their children. In addition, all of the community was involved in learning about appropriate foods and about needed micronutrients. You will also read later about a variety of community-based activities, including efforts to address diarrheal disease through oral rehydration in Egypt and polio campaigns in Latin America.

Mass Media

The mass media are often used to promote change in health behaviors. Most people in developing countries have access to radio, which is often used for this purpose. Increasingly, however, those engaged in promoting better health are using a tool referred to as "entertainment-education." Many of these efforts have focused on soap opera series in which the characters bring out the main messages about healthy behaviors. The British Broadcasting Company has a group, for example, that works with developing countries to produce soap operas on health topics of importance such as HIV/AIDS. Such a series was done on HIV in India, and one is under production on HIV for Nigeria. The government of Myanmar had a soap opera about leprosy that featured Myanmar's best known actress. The aims of the soap opera were to help people know how to diagnose leprosy, to inform them that it could be treated completely if treated early, and to get people to come forward for treatment at an early stage.

Social Marketing

Social marketing is the application of the tools of commercial marketing to try to promote behavior change and the uptake of important health actions or products. This has been used widely in family planning work. It is also being used in other fields, such as in selling bed nets for malaria control. In social marketing, a local brand of a product is often created, such as a condom, a contraceptive pill, or an insecticide-treated bed net. Mass media and other forms of communication are then used to promote the brand and the behaviors related to the product. Of course, successful marketing depends on very careful market research and a good understanding of the local culture, values, and behaviors. It also depends on what is called "the four Ps" in social marketing:

- Attractive product
- Affordable price
- Convenient places to buy the product
- Persuasive promotion[35,36]

Often the products being marketed through social marketing are sold through commercial channels but their price is subsidized by the government.

Health Education

Health education is something with which every reader of this book will be familiar. It comes in many forms, such as in the classroom, in the news media, on the radio and television, and on the Internet. Successful health education programs that were aimed at sex education have several features in common that hold lessons for other efforts at making health education effective.

- They focused on risky behaviors and were clear about abstinence and consistent condom use
- They provided accurate information
- They addressed how to deal with social pressures
- They selected teachers and peer educators who believed in the program
- They geared the content of the program to the age, sexual experience, and culture of the students[37]

Achieving Success in Health Promotion

The previous section refers to specific types of health promotion that can be used to encourage a change in health behaviors or the adoption of healthy behaviors. There are a number of lessons that have emerged both about these approaches and when looking broadly at what constitutes an effective health promotion effort. These are noted in Table 6-6.

SOCIAL ASSESSMENT

There is one additional area that it is important to cover concerning the links between health and culture. This is "social assessment" or "social impact assessment." A social impact

---

TABLE 6-6 Selected Factors for Success in Health Promotion

Identify specific health problems, related behaviors, and key stakeholders

Know and use sound behavioral theories

Research motivations and constraints to change, considering biologic, environmental, cultural, and other contextual factors

Use participatory assessment tools and include relevant stakeholders in the design, implementation, and evaluation of the intervention

Plan and budget carefully

Identify people who exhibit healthy behaviors that differ from the social norm

Create an environment that enables behavior change through policy dialogue, advocacy, and capacity building

Organize an intervention that addresses both specific behaviors and contextual factors

Work to ensure sustainability

Evaluate from the beginning

Form partnerships to scale up and/or adapt the most successful interventions for implementation in other settings.

Source: Adapted with permission from Murphy E. *Promoting Healthy Behavior, Health Bulletin 2.* Washington, DC: Population Reference Bureau; 2005.

assessment is "a process for assessing the social impacts of planned interventions or events and for developing strategies for the ongoing monitoring and management of those impacts."[38] In more expansive terms, "Social impact assessment includes the processes of analyzing, monitoring, and managing the intended and unintended social consequences, both positive and negative, of planned interventions (policies, programs, plans, projects) and any social change processes invoked by those interventions. Its primary purpose is to bring about a more sustainable and equitable biophysical and human environment."[38]

The social impact assessment looks at a variety of domains that go beyond health. These include impact, among other things, on historical artifacts and buildings, communities, demography, gender, minority groups, culture, and health. The assessment should be carried out in a way that builds on local processes, engages the community fully, and proactively tries to maximize the potential good that can come from the proposed investment. It "promotes community development and empowerment, builds capacity, and develops social capital."[38] The detailed approach of a social impact assessment is outlined in Table 6-7.

Many readers will be familiar with environmental assessment of proposed investment schemes and many countries require such assessments be done before any major physical investment. In some respects, a social assessment is the social analogue to the environmental assessment. In this case, let us suppose that a development agency and a government are going to collaborate to develop a series of health centers in a particular region of a country. If the country carried out the recommended social assessment before it designed the project, then it would aim as it carried out the design to involve the community in this work. The country would also ensure that the design took account of the needs of various groups in the community and was based on their culture and values, and it would keep in mind how programs need to be tailored to address them. The assessment would seek to identify any negative consequences that might emerge from the investment and how those consequences might be mitigated. The plan emerging from the assessment would also have an approach to monitoring and evaluation of the proposed investment to ensure that the social impacts that were foreseen were correct and that the program design really is consistent with local values and the underlying needs of the community.

Some years ago, very little attention was paid in some development assistance agencies and in some governments to social assessment. Little effort was spent on examining the social and cultural issues involved in designing appropriate interventions in health. In addition, little attention was paid

---

TABLE 6-7 Selected Focuses of Social Impact Assessment

Identifies interested and affected peoples

Facilitates and coordinates the participation of stakeholders

Analyzes the local setting of the planned intervention to assess likely impacts to it

Collects baseline data to allow for evaluation of the impact of the intervention

Gives a picture of the local cultural context, and develops an understanding of local community values, particularly how they relate to the planned intervention

Identifies and describes the activities that are likely to cause impacts

Predicts likely impacts and how different stakeholders are likely to respond

Assists in evaluating and selecting alternatives

Recommends measures to mitigate any likely negative impacts

Assists in the valuation process and provides suggestions about compensation for affected peoples

Describes potential conflicts between stakeholders and advises on resolution processes

Develops coping strategies for dealing with residual and non-mitigatable impacts

Contributes to skill development and capacity building in the community

Assists in devising and implementing monitoring and management programs

Source: Adapted with permission from Vanclay F. Social Impact Assessment: International Principles. Available at http://www.iaia.org/Members/Publications/Guidelines_Principles/SP2.pdf. Accessed on July 5, 2007.

---

to the potential impact on health or on other social areas of investments in sectors outside of health. Although the quality of social assessment may vary both within and across some agencies and governments, it is now a normal practice that social assessments are done for all major development projects.

MAIN MESSAGES

Culture is a set of beliefs and behaviors that are learned and shared. Culture operates, among other areas, in the domains of the family, social groups beyond the family, religion, art, music, and law. Culture is an important determinant of health, in many ways. It relates to people's health behaviors, their perceptions of illness, the extent to which they use health services, and forms of medicine that they have practiced traditionally. This chapter examines the links between culture and health from the perspective of the extent to which a culture satisfies the physical and psychological needs of those who follow it.

Perceptions of illness vary considerably across cultures. What is seen as normal in some societies may be seen as illness in others. Different societies also have differing perceptions of the causes of illness and of disease. In addition to perceptions related to the "western medical paradigm," diseases may be viewed, for example, as due to the body "being out of balance," supernatural causes, offending the gods, emotional stress, or witchcraft. Different cultures also take an array of steps, beyond the western medical paradigm, to prevent illness. Some of these include rituals, the wearing of charms, and the observance of certain food taboos.

When people believe themselves to be ill, they usually resort to trying "home remedies" first. Following that, people in traditional societies often visit some type of traditional healer. It may be some time before they consult a physician practicing "modern medicine," and often only when they are certain they are quite ill and other forms of treatment have not brought relief.

Many forms of traditional behavior are conducive to good health. This might include, for example, traditional practices that provide for the mother to spend some time with her baby before she returns to her normal work and household chores. Male circumcision, as practiced in many cultures, reduces the transmission of HIV/AIDS. Other traditional practices, however, are not health promoting. Feeding sugar water to infants, for example, is not good for the health of the infants, who should be exclusively breastfed for six months. How can healthy behaviors be promoted?

There are a number of "models" of how behaviors can be changed, including: "The Health Belief Model," "The Diffusions of Innovation Model," and the "Stages of Change Model." To encourage behavior change, of course, requires a good understanding of the behaviors that are taking place, how they relate to health, the underlying motivation for them, and the likely response to various approaches to changing them.

When thinking about trying to change behavior on a large scale, such as promoting an immunization program, the use of seat belts, the willingness to seek treatment for leprosy, several approaches are important. One way to engender change is to engage in community mobilization. Promoting messages about desirable and undesirable health behaviors can also be done effectively using the mass media. Social marketing and health education efforts are also important. An effective tool for any efforts at investing in health or trying to change behaviors is to carry out a social assessment, which will identify the social basis of the health issues one is trying to influence, as well as the likely social impacts of the proposed activities.

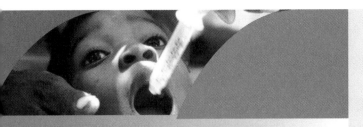

Study Questions

1. What is culture? Give some examples of aspects of culture that vary across different societies.

2. Why is it important to assess the relationship between culture and health in specific societies by the extent to which cultural practices promote or discourage good physical and mental health?

3. Name three cultural practices that are health promoting. Name three cultural practices that are harmful to health.

4. How does culture relate to people's perceptions of illness? Why would some cultures regard some illnesses as "normal?"

5. What would low-income people in traditional societies likely see as possible causes of illness?

6. What is the difference between "illness" and "disease?"

7. When an infant is ill in a traditional society in a low-income country, from whom and in what order are the parents likely to seek help?

8. Why would members of the community seek treatment for illness from traditional healers?

9. If you wanted to encourage the large scale adoption of a healthy behavior, such as giving up cigarette smoking, what information would you want to know as you plan your effort?

10. Why are social assessments important? If they are done well, what gains would they produce that might not come if there were no such assessment?

REFERENCES

1. Scrimshaw SC. Culture, Behavior, and Health. In: Merson MH, Black RE, Mills A, eds. *International Public Health: Diseases, Programs, Systems, and Policies.* Gaithersburg, MD: Aspen Publishers; 2001:53–78.

2. Tylor E. *Primitive Culture.* London: J. Murray; 1871.

3. Haviland WA. The Nature of Culture. *Cultural Anthropology.* 6th ed. Fort Worth, TX: Holt, Rinchart & Winston, Inc.; 1990:30.

4. Miller B. Culture and Health: George Washington University; 2004.

5. Haviland WA. The Nature of Culture. *Cultural Anthropology.* 6th ed. Fort Worth, TX: Holt, Rinchart & Winston, Inc.; 1990:31.

6. Haviland WA. The Nature of Culture. *Cultural Anthropology.* 6th ed. Fort Worth, TX: Holt, Rinchart & Winston, Inc.; 1990:46.

7. Haviland WA. The Nature of Culture. *Cultural Anthropology.* 6th ed. Fort Worth, TX: Holt, Rinchart & Winston, Inc.; 1990:51.

8. Scrimshaw SC. Culture, Behavior, and Health. In: Merson MH, Black RE, Mills A, eds. *International Public Health: Diseases, Programs, Systems, and Policies.* Gaithersburg, MD: Aspen Publishers; 2001:56.

9. Murphy EM. Being born female is dangerous for your health. *The American Psychologist.* Mar 2003;58(3):205–210.

10. Scrimshaw SC. Culture, Behavior, and Health. In: Merson MH, Black RE, Mills A, eds. *International Public Health: Diseases, Programs, Systems, and Policies.* Gaithersburg, MD: Aspen Publishers; 2001:57.

11. Kleinman A, Eisenberg L, Good B. Culture, illness, and care: clinical lessons from anthropologic and cross-cultural research. *Ann Intern Med.* Feb 1978;88(2):251–258.

12. Hopper S. The Influence of ethnicity on the healthcare of older women. *Clin Geriatric Med.* 1993;9:231–259.

13. Scrimshaw SC. Culture, Behavior, and Health. In: Merson MH, Black RE, Mills A, eds. *International Public Health: Diseases, Programs, Systems, and Policies.* Gaithersburg, MD: Aspen Publishers; 2001:58.

14. Letendre AD. Aboriginal Traditional Medicine: Where Does It Fit? *Crossing Boundaries - an interdisciplinary journal.* 2002;1(2).

15. Jegede AS. The Yoruba Cultural Construction of Health and Illness. *Nordic Journal of African Studies.* 2002;11(3):322–335.

16. Pachter LM. Culture and clinical care. Folk illness beliefs and behaviors and their implications for health care delivery. *Jama.* Mar 2 1994;271(9):693.

17. Bolton JM. Food taboos among the Orang Asli in West Malaysia: a potential nutritional hazard. *The American Journal of Clinical Nutrition.* August 1972 1972;25:788–799.

18. Chiwuzie J, Okolocha C. Traditional Belief Systems and Maternal Mortality in a Semi-Urban Community in Southern Nigeria. *African Journal of Reproductive Health.* August 2001 2001;5(1):75–82.

19. Trigo M, Roncada MJ, Stewien GT, Pereira IM. [Food taboos in the northern region of Brazil]. *Rev Saude Publica.* Dec 1989;23(6):455–464.

20. Sundararaj R, Pereira SM. Dietary intakes and food taboos of lactating women in a South Indian community. *Trop Geogr Med.* Jun 1975;27(2):189–193.

21. Bhasin V. Sickness and Therapy Among Tribals of Rajasthan. *Stud Tribes Tribals.* 2003;1(1):77–83.

22. Fassin D, Badji I. Ritual buffoonery: as coail preventive measure against childhood mortality in Senegal. *Lancet.* January 1986;18(1):142–143.

23. Scrimshaw SC. Culture, Behavior, and Health. In: Merson MH, Black RE, Mills A, eds. *International Public Health: Diseases, Programs, Systems, and Policies.* Gaithersburg, MD: Aspen Publishers; 2001:62.

24. Scrimshaw SC. Culture, Behavior, and Health. In: Merson MH, Black RE, Mills A, eds. *International Public Health: Diseases, Programs, Systems, and Policies.* Gaithersburg, MD: Aspen Publishers; 2001:63.

25. Lopez AD, Mathers CD, Murray CJL. The Burden of Disease and Mortality by Condition: Data, Methods, and Results for 2001. In: Lopez AD, Mathers CD, Ezzati M, Jamison DT, Murray CJL, eds. *Global burden of disease and risk factors.* New York: Oxford University Press; 2006:70.

26. Lopez AD, Mathers CD, Ezzati M, Jamison DT, Murray CJL. Measuring the Global Burden of Disease and Risk Factors 1990-2001. In: Lopez AD, Mathers CD, Ezzati M, Jamison DT, Murray CJL, eds. *Global burden of disease and risk factors.* New York: Oxford University Press; 2006:10.

27. Edberg M. *Essentials of Health Behavior: An Introduction to Social and Behavioral Therory Applied to Public Health.* Sudbury, MA: Jones & Bartlett Publishers, Inc.; 2007.

28. Murphy E. *Promoting Healthy Behavior, Health Bulletin 2.* Washington, DC: Population Reference Bureau; 2005.

29. Rosenstock IM, Strecher VJ, Becker MH. Social learning theory and the Health Belief Model. *Health Educ Q.* Summer 1988;15(2):175–183.

30. Murphy E. *Promoting Healthy Behavior, Health Bulletin 2.* Washington, DC: Population Reference Bureau; 2005.

31. Murphy E. *Promoting Healthy Behavior, Health Bulletin 2.* Washington, DC: Population Reference Bureau; 2005.

32. Scrimshaw SC. Culture, Behavior, and Health. In: Merson MH, Black RE, Mills A, eds. *International Public Health: Diseases, Programs, Systems, and Policies.* Gaithersburg, MD: Aspen Publishers; 2001:66.

33. Rogers E. *Diffusion of Innovations.* 3rd ed. New York: Free Press; 1983.

34. Murphy E. *Promoting Healthy Behavior, Health Bulletin 2.* Washington, DC: Population Reference Bureau; 2005.

35. Murphy E. *Promoting Healthy Behavior, Health Bulletin 2.* Washington, DC: Population Reference Bureau; 2005.

36. Murphy E. *Promoting Healthy Behavior, Health Bulletin 2.* Washington, DC: Population Reference Bureau; 2005.

37. Murphy E. *Promoting Healthy Behavior, Health Bulletin 2.* Washington, DC: Population Reference Bureau; 2005.

38. Vanclay F. Social Impact Assessment: International Principles. Available at: http://www.iaia.org/Members/Publications/Guidelines_Principles/SP2.pdf. Accessed October 27, 2006.

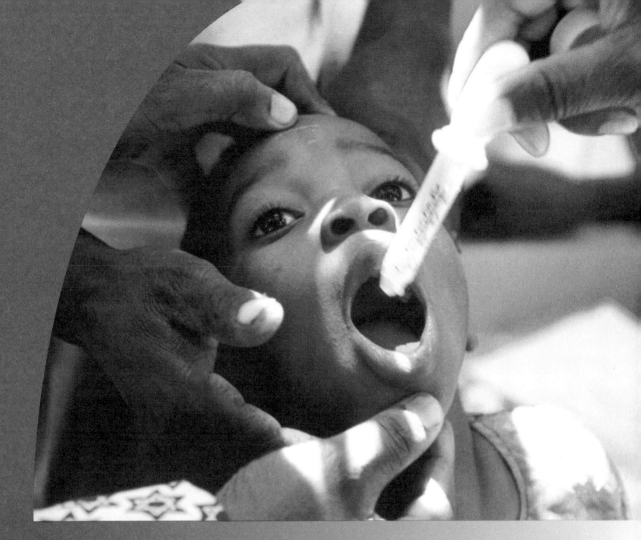

PART III

The Burden of Disease

CHAPTER 7

The Environment and Health

By the end of this chapter the reader will be able to:

- Discuss the most important environmental threats to health in low- and middle-income countries
- Review the burden of disease from indoor and outdoor air pollution and unsafe water and sanitation
- Examine the contribution of personal hygiene to reducing the burden of environmentally-related health problems
- Comment on the costs and consequences of these environmental burdens
- Describe some of the most cost-effective ways of reducing the global burden of environmental health problems

VIGNETTES

Rashmi lived in the eastern part of Nepal in a modest home. Rashmi often had difficulty breathing. This was linked to the way Rashmi cooked, with a stove inside the house that was not vented outside. She used cow dung or wood as fuel. She cooked two meals a day on the stove and she often held her new baby on her back as she did so. She heard about different stoves and about using kerosene for fuel. However, she lacked the money to buy a new stove or to fuel it with kerosene.

Sunisa was a young mother in a rural area in northern Laos. She had two children, a 1 year old and a 3 year old. Sunisa was not wealthy. Her house was simple and had no water supply. She collected water daily from the stream about half a mile from her house in containers she carried on her head. She stored the containers at the edge of her house, covered by cloth. Sunisa was not an educated woman and did nothing to purify the water. Her two daughters regularly had bouts of diarrhea, partly the result of drinking unsafe water.

Juan had lived in Mexico City his whole life and was now 70 years old. He remembered a time when the city was not so crowded, had few cars, and when the views from the city were magnificent. He lamented the fact that today the city was too crowded to enjoy, the traffic was overwhelming, and the air was often unbreathable. It was so polluted that on many days there was no view at all. Juan had a very hard time breathing, as he suffered from chronic obstructive pulmonary disease (COPD). Juan suspected that air pollution contributed to his illness.

Raj and his family lived in a slum at the edge of Patna, India. The slum was the size of a small city. Most of the houses were made of scrap wood with scrap metal roofing. The houses had no water connection and people had to walk to the edge of the slum to get their water from a standpipe or to buy it from a tanker if the standpipe did not work. There were no private toilets either. There were a few communal toilets that were shared but they were always dirty. For this reason, many people in the slum, especially the women, waited until dark and then went to defecate in fields near the slum.

THE IMPORTANCE OF ENVIRONMENTAL HEALTH

Environmental health issues are major risk factors in the global burden of disease. Using a somewhat narrow definition of what is an "environmental" cause of disease, a recent study of the global burden of disease[1] suggests that about 8.4% of the total burden of disease in low- and middle-income countries is the result of three environmental conditions: unsafe water, hygiene, and excreta disposal; urban air pollution; and indoor smoke from household use of solid fuels. Another study, which took a broader view of "environmental" risk factors, concluded that between 25–33% of the global burden of disease can be attributed to environmental risk factors.[2]

The importance of environmental risk factors to the global burden of disease should not be a surprise. The third

TABLE 7-1 Environmental Health and the MDGs

Goal 1—Eradicate Poverty and Hunger
Link—Reducing environmental risk factors is central to eradicating poverty by reducing the burden, which falls largely on the poor, of environmentally-related morbidity and mortality.

Goal 2—Achieve Universal Primary Education
Link—Children that do not have access to clean water and sanitation are more likely to suffer from undernutrition due to a vicious cycle of diarrheal disease and malnutrition. There is a correlation between nutritional status and learning. Children with poor nutritional status are not as likely to stay in school or learn as much as healthy children.

Goal 3—Promote Gender Equality and Empower Women
Link—Improving access to water can improve the lives of poor women in the developing world by reducing the amount of time required to get water. Reducing indoor air pollution can also substantially improve the lives of women since they suffer a disproportionate burden when they are cooking.

Goal 4—Reduce Child Mortality
Link—Addressing environmental risk factors can reduce the two leading causes of death in children—diarrheal diseases and pneumonia. Diarrheal disease is reduced through improved access to clean water and sanitation. Pneumonia can be reduced through improvements in indoor air quality.

Goal 5—Improve Maternal Health
Link—Diarrheal disease associated with poor sanitation and unsafe water can harm the nutritional status of the mother.

Goal 6—Combat HIV/AIDS, malaria, and other diseases
Link—Environmental improvements can reduce the breeding grounds for malarial mosquitoes and vectors of some other disease, such as shistosomiasis and dengue fever.

Goal 7—Ensure environmental sustainability
Link—Measures to improve water supply, sanitation, and personal hygiene promote sustainability, especially when they are carried out in community-based ways.

Source: Author commentary on the UN Millennium Goals. Available at: http://www.un.org/millenniumgoals/ goals. Accessed July 11, 2006.

leading cause of death in low- and middle-income countries is lower respiratory infections, the sixth is chronic obstructive pulmonary disease, and the seventh is diarrheal disease. As you know, each of these is closely linked with environmental factors. In addition, environmental risk factors are even more important when considering the causes of death of children 0 to 14 years of age in low- and middle-income countries. Lower respiratory conditions are the second leading cause of death for them and diarrheal diseases third. Together, they account for about 30% of all deaths in this age group.

Environmental health matters are also of special importance because addressing them effectively is central to the achievement of the MDGs, as shown in Table 7-1.

As you can see in the table, reducing environmental risk factors is critical to meeting the poverty and hunger goal, given the large share of ill health and resulting economic losses from these risk factors. Improving access to water can be a major improvement to the lives of poor women in the developing world, given the amount of time they have to spend getting water. Enhancing sanitation produces important social gains for women, as well, because in the absence of improved sanitation, they face major discomforts, inconveniences, and sometimes illness. Addressing environmental risk factors can clearly make a major contribution to reducing child mortality by reducing two of the leading causes of death in children. As you will read about later, reducing indoor air pollution can also lead to major improvements in the health of women and children. Finally, environmental improvements can reduce the breeding grounds for malarial mosquitoes, and many measures that reduce the health risks of the environment will increase environmental sustainability.

This chapter aims to introduce you to some of the most important links between health and the environment. Environmental health is a very broad topic. Given the introductory nature of this book, this chapter will focus largely on only three of the most important risk factors in terms of the burden of environmentally-related diseases in low- and middle-income countries. Following the recent burden of disease study, these will include unsafe water, sanitation, and hygiene; outdoor air pollution; and indoor air pollution that comes from the use of solid fuels.[3] These factors are also the focus of attention of this chapter because the risk factors that will be examined take a disproportionate toll on the health of low-income people in the developing world and the enhancement of their health status will require important gains in environmental health.

The chapter begins by covering some of the most important terms and concepts that relate to environmental health. It then explores the burden of disease related to the three risk factors noted previously. After that, it briefly reviews the costs and consequences of the selected environmental risk factors. The chapter concludes by discussing some of the most cost-effective ways to address these risk factors in low- and middle-income settings. Much has been written about environmental health. Those readers who wish to explore environmental health in greater detail are encouraged to pursue some of those writings. They might wish to begin with an introductory text on environmental health.[4,5]

KEY CONCEPTS

It is important to understand how the word "environment" will be used in this chapter. In some cases, the word environment in a health context is defined very broadly, meaning everything that is not genetic. In other cases, when considering health, the word environment includes only physical, chemical, or biological agents that directly affect health. For the purposes of this chapter, the environment will largely be defined as "external physical, chemical, and microbiological exposures and processes that impinge upon individuals and groups and are beyond the immediate control of individuals."[6] The chapter, however, also looks at some behavioral matters related to water and sanitation and indoor air pollution.

It is also valuable to understand the meaning of "environmental health." This generally refers to a set of public health efforts that "is concerned with preventing disease, death, and disability by reducing exposure to adverse environmental conditions and promoting behavior change. It focuses on the direct and indirect cases of disease and injuries and taps resources inside and outside the healthcare system to help improve health outcomes."[7]

The World Health Organization takes a broad view of the environment and says,

> Environmental health comprises those aspects of human health, including quality of life, that are determined by physical, chemical, biological, social, and psychosocial factors in the environment. It also refers to the theory and practice of assessing, correcting, controlling, and preventing those factors in the environment that can potentially affect adversely the health of present and future generations.[8]

Table 7-2 highlights some examples of environmental health issues, their determinants, and their consequences. It organizes these examples by their level of impact: the household, the community, the region, or global.

TABLE 7-2 Typical Environmental Health Issues: Determinants and Health Consequences

Underlying Determinants	Selected Adverse Health Consequences
Household	
Unsafe water, inadequate sanitation and solid waste disposal, improper hygiene	Diarrhea, and vector-related diseases, such as malaria, schistosomisasis, and dengue
Crowded housing and poor ventilation of smoke	Respiratory diseases and lung cancer
Exposure to naturally occurring toxic substances	Poisoning from arsenic, manganese, and fluorides
Community	
Improper water resource management, including poor drainage	Vector-related diseases, such as malaria and schistosomisasis
Exposure to vehicle emissions and industrial air pollution	Respiratory diseases, some cancers, and reduced IQ in children
Global	
Climate change	Injury/death from extreme heat/cold, storms, floods, and fires. Indirect effects: spread of vector-borne diseases
Ozone depletion	Aggravation of respiratory diseases, population dislocation, water pollution from sea level rise, etc. Skin cancer, cataracts. Indirect effects: compromised food production, etc.

Source: Adapted with permission from The World Bank. Environmental Health. Available at: http://web.worldbank.org/WBSITE/EXTERNAL/TOPICS/EXTHEALTHNUTRITIONANDPOPULATION/EXTPHAAG/0,,contentMDK:20656146~menuPK:2175463~pagePK:64229817~piPK:64229743~theSitePK:672263,00.html. Accessed October 27, 2006.

KEY ENVIRONMENTAL HEALTH BURDENS

The next section very briefly examines the most important health conditions that relate to the environmental issues that are discussed in this chapter. The section after that will examine the burden of disease from those conditions.

Indoor Air Pollution

WHO estimates that about half of all of the people in the world depend on solid fuel for their cooking and heating. The indoor air pollution that is discussed here is related to these uses. Such fuels include the fossil fuel coal, and the biomass fuels of cow dung, wood, logging wastes, and crop waste.[9,10] In the cases that most concern us, cooking and heating are done on open stoves that are not vented to the outside. These are generally used by poorer segments of society, as people usually move to kerosene or gas for cooking and switch to improved stoves as their family income grows.

Biomass fuels and coal do not completely combust when they are burned. Instead, they leave behind breathable particles of a variety of gases and chemical products. The amount of these substances in a poorly ventilated home can exceed WHO norms by more than 20 times.[10] Smoke from burning biomass inside the home can produce conjunctivitis, upper respiratory irritation, and acute respiratory infection. The carbon monoxide produced can lead to acute poisoning. Other gases and smoke are associated over the long term with cardiovascular disease, chronic obstructive pulmonary disease, adverse reproductive outcomes, and cancer.[11] As discussed further later, women and children are especially vulnerable to the effects of indoor air pollution.

Outdoor Air Pollution

Many pollutants can be found in the urban air. The most common effects of outdoor air pollution are respiratory symptoms, including cough, irritation of the nose and throat, and shortness of breath.[12] Table 7-3 indicates some of the most common pollutants in the outdoor air, examples of their sources, and the most important health effects. Some preexisting health factors make some people susceptible to being harmed by air pollution. Older and younger people are generally most susceptible to the health effects of outdoor air pollution.

There have been a number of instances in which severe air pollution has been associated with considerable excess mortality in a very short time. Among the most famous cases was in London, England, in 1952. Because of what is called a temperature inversion, a dense fog, full of pollutants, hung over the city center for several days. The value of certain particulates in the air was 3 to 10 times the normal value. On December 13, 1952, the city administration reported a death rate per 100,000 people that was more than four times the normal daily death rate for that period.[13]

TABLE 7-3 Selected Urban Air Pollutants

Name of Pollutant	Example of Source	Health Effects
Carbon monoxide (**criteria pollutant**)	Combustion of gasoline and fossil fuels; cars	Reduction in oxygen-carrying capacity of the blood
Lead (**criteria pollutant**)	Leaded gasoline, paint, batteries	Brain/CNS damage; digestive problems
Nitrogen dioxide, nitrogen oxides (**criteria pollutant**)	Combustion of gasoline and fossil fuels; cars	Damage to lungs and respiratory system
Ozone (**criteria pollutant**)	Variety of oxygen formed by chemical reaction of pollutants	Breathing impairment; eye irritation
Particulate matter (**criteria pollutant**)	Burning of wood and diesel fuels	Respiratory irritation; lung damage
Smog	Mixture of pollutants, esp. ozone; originates from petroleum-based fuels	Irritation of respiratory system, eyes
Sulfur dioxide (**criteria pollutant**)	Burning of coal and oil	Breathing problems; lung damage
Volatile organic compounds (VOCs)	Burning fuels; released from certain chemicals (e.g., solvents)	Acute effects similar to those of smog; possible carcinogen

Source: Adapted from US Environmental Protection Agency. The Plain English Guide to the Clean Air Act: The Common Air Pollutants. Available at: http://www.epa.gov/oar/oaqps/peg_caa/pegcaa11.html. Accessed March 28, 2005; and US Environmental Protection Agency. The Plain English Guide to the Clean Air Act: Glossary. Available at: http://www.epa.gov/oar/oaqps/peg_caa/pegcaa10.html. Accessed January 28, 2007.

Sanitation, Water, and Hygiene

Only about 65% of the people in the world have access to safe excreta disposal. This ranges from about 80% in the Latin America region to only slightly above 50% in the Africa region.[14] Many of the large cities in Africa have no modern sanitation system, and in Asia large shares of the populations in some areas also have no access to sanitary disposal of human waste.

There is good evidence that improved disposal of human waste is associated with reductions in diarrheal disease, intestinal parasites, and trachoma. Failure to dispose properly of human waste contaminates water and food sources and leads to an increase in transmission of pathogens through the oral-fecal route. Failure to improve sanitation is also associated with the spread of parasitic worms, such as ascaris and hookworm.[15] Improved sanitation reduces the burden of trachoma, because the flies that are significantly involved in the spread of that disease breed, among other places, in human waste.[16]

More than one billion people, mostly in low- and middle-income countries, lack access to safe water sources within a reasonable distance of their home.[17] Access to improved water sources ranges from below 50% in Sub-Saharan Africa to about 70% in Asia to almost universal access in developed countries.[18] It is estimated that about 400 million children lack access to safe water.[19] In addition, even the water that people do have access to and that is deemed safe in official statistics is often of low bacteriological quality and contains important pathogens. Many diseases relate to water in one of a variety of ways.

Waterborne diseases are among the most important in terms of the burden of disease and they are numerous in low- and middle-income countries. Some of the most important waterborne pathogens are shown in Table 7-4.

These pathogens are associated with diarrhea and a host of other gastrointestinal problems. As you will read about further in the chapters on child health and infectious dis-eases, they can be deadly when they lead to severe diarrhea and dehydration. Such diseases are especially risky for the very young, the very old, and people who have compromised immune systems, such as people living with HIV/AIDS.

THE BURDEN OF ENVIRONMENTALLY-RELATED DISEASES

As noted earlier, it is estimated that about 8.4% of the total burden of disease in low- and middle-income countries is due to water, sanitation, and hygiene; urban air pollution; and indoor air pollution. The relative share of each of these factors is:

- Indoor smoke from household use of solid fuels—3.7%
- Unsafe water, sanitation, and hygiene—3.2%
- Urban air pollution—1.5%[3]

These are explored more fully later.

Many people believe that the most important environmental risk factor in low- and middle-income countries is outdoor air pollution; however, this is not true. Rather, indoor air pollution is the third most important risk factor in high mortality developing countries, exceeded only by malnutrition and unsafe sex, and similar in importance to water, sanitation, and hygiene.[9] It is estimated that indoor air pollution from the use of solid fuels is responsible for 1.6 million deaths annually from pneumonia, chronic respiratory disease, and lung cancer. It is thought, in fact, that indoor air pollution is responsible for about 700,000 of the 2.7 million annual deaths from chronic obstructive pulmonary disease (COPD) and about 15% of all deaths from lung cancer.[9]

These figures include only those diseases for which there is solid evidence of a link with indoor air pollution from the use of solid fuels. However, this may be an underestimate of the real burden of disease from indoor air pollution because there is some evidence that indoor air pollution of this type is also associated with asthma, cataracts, and TB. There is also

---

TABLE 7-4 Classification of Water-Related Infections

Transmission	Water-Related infections
Waterborne	The pathogen is in water that is ingested
Water-washed (or water-scarce)	Person-to-person transmission because of a lack of water for hygiene
Water-based	Transmission via an aquatic intermediate host
Water-related insect vector	Transmission by insects that breed in water or bite near water

Source: Data with permission from The World Bank. Cairncross S, Valdmanis V. Water supply, sanitation, and hygiene promotion. In: Jamison DT, Breman JG, Measham AR, et al., eds. *Disease Control Priorities in Developing Countries.* 2nd ed. New York: Oxford University Press; 2006:775.

tentative evidence of links with adverse pregnancy outcomes, especially low birthweight, ischemic heart disease, and two types of cancer other than lung cancer.[9]

Almost all the burden of disease from indoor air pollution from the use of solid fuels is in the developing world. Women do most of the cooking in low- and middle-income countries and they are most subject to the health risks from indoor air pollution. Indeed, it is estimated that 59% of all of the deaths attributable to indoor air pollution are among females.[9] Young children in developing countries are often carried by their mothers on their backs as they attend to household and work chores, such as cooking. They also tend to spend long hours at home with their mothers. Therefore, they are also exposed more than others to indoor air pollution and it is estimated that 56% of all deaths attributable to indoor air pollution are among children younger than five years.[9]

Urban Outdoor Air Pollution

One study of the global burden of disease attributed 1.5% of annual deaths and 0.5% of the total burden of disease to outdoor air pollution.[20] The study further indicated that 81% of the deaths and 49% of the DALYs attributable to outdoor air pollution occur among people 60 years of age or more. Three percent of the deaths and 12% of the DALYs occur in children younger than five years.[20] It has also been estimated that outdoor air pollution by urban particulate matter causes about 5% of the global cases of lung cancer, 2% of the deaths from cardiovascular and respiratory conditions, and 1% of respiratory infections.[21]

India and China have major burdens of disease that relate to outdoor air pollution from particulate matter. In fact, about two thirds of the global burden of disease from outdoor air pollution is in the developing countries of Asia.[22] A number of countries in Eastern Europe also face a high burden of disease from outdoor air pollution. In some countries of that region, between 0.6–1.4% of the burden of disease is attributable to outdoor air pollution from particulate matter.[22]

Sanitation, Water, and Hygiene

Unsafe disposal of human waste, unsafe water, and poor hygiene are associated with 3.2% of the total deaths in low- and middle-income countries and 3.7% of the DALYs.[3] Studies that have been done suggest that within the African region, about 85% of the DALYs from these risk factors are related to the oral-fecal route of disease transmission and to diarrheal disease, primarily among young children. These studies also suggest that schistosomiasis, in the water-based

group, has the second largest loss of DALYs related to these risk factors in Africa.

We should expect globally that the burden of disease related to these risk factors will fall disproportionately on children, who suffer such a large share of the global burden of disease from diarrhea. The burden of these risk factors will also fall overwhelmingly on poor and less well-educated people in the poorer countries of South Asia and of Sub-Saharan Africa. They have less access than others to improved water supply and sanitation and to the knowledge of good hygiene they need to avoid illness in the face of unsafe water and sanitation.

It is very complicated to try to assess individually the relative contribution of unsafe sanitation, unsafe water, and poor hygienic practices to the burden of diarrheal disease, partly because they are all so closely linked with each other. Nonetheless, both historical experiences in what are now the developed countries and a number of studies in developing countries suggest that improving water supply alone will not reduce diarrheal disease as needed. This seems to stem from the large amount of diarrhea that is associated with food that is unsafe and the way in which people use water if they are not knowledgeable about and do not practice good personal hygiene. More will be said about this later.

Separate from any impact on the reduction of diarrheal disease, improvements in water supply are associated with important reductions in the burden of disease from dracunculiasis, schistosomiasis, and trachoma, as shown in Table 7-5.[23]

THE COSTS AND CONSEQUENCES OF KEY ENVIRONMENTAL HEALTH PROBLEMS

The social and economic consequences of the environmental health issues that have been discussed are enormous. First, they constitute 8.4% of the total deaths in low- and middle-income countries and 7.2% of their total burden of disease. Taken together, the burden of disease from these causes is about 25% more than unsafe sex and about twice as much as tobacco use.[3] The magnitude of their burden itself suggests substantial social and economic costs related to these issues.

Second, as indicated earlier, the burden of these causes falls disproportionately on relatively poorer people. It is the poorer people who cook with biomass fuels and coal, not the better-off people. These burdens also fall on low- and middle-income countries more than on high-income countries. People in high-income countries do not customarily cook with biomass fuel or coal and they do not have to contend with the problems of unsafe water and sanitation that people in the lower- and middle-income countries face. Their knowledge of good hygiene practices is also superior to the level of knowledge of most people in the developing world.

Third, these environmental health burdens have very negative consequences on productivity. It is women who suffer the ill effects of indoor air pollution the most. The results of this are very costly to women in terms of morbidity and disability and days of reduced productivity from both acute and chronic illnesses. In addition, the economic and social consequences of ill health for women in many low- and middle-income countries go considerably beyond the poor health of the women. Rather, they spillover onto the health of the rest of her family, especially young children, whose own health and survival depend in important ways on the health of the mother.

Young children are especially at risk to all three forms of the environmental issues discussed in this chapter. They are especially vulnerable to unsafe water and diarrheal disease can put them into a cycle of infection and malnutrition, ultimately retard their growth and development, or be deadly. Indoor air pollution can also lead to a cycle of illness and respiratory infection, death from pneumonia, or disability from asthma. To a lesser extent, outdoor air pollution can do the same. The elderly face particular risks from outdoor air pollution. This can exacerbate chronic health problems they already have, leading to additional disability and its attendant reduction in productivity.

REDUCING THE BURDEN OF DISEASE

Important progress has been made in some settings in addressing the environmental health issues discussed here. The next section examines some of the lessons learned to date and some of the most cost-effective measures that can be taken to enhance health in low- and middle-income countries by addressing selected environmental health issues.

Outdoor Air Pollution

Outdoor air pollution is a very broad topic, and there is very little published data on the cost-effectiveness of approaches to addressing outdoor air pollution in developing countries. The studies that have been done on developed countries, however, suggest that developing countries could take a number of cost-effective steps to reduce the health burden of outdoor air pollution.[24]

A number of cities, including Jakarta, Manila, Kathmandu, and Mumbai, participated in a World Bank assisted effort to assess their outdoor air pollution and take measures to reduce it. They examined:

- the amount and type of pollution
- how it was being dispersed
- the health impacts of reductions in particulate matter
- time and cost to implement reductions

TABLE 7-5 Selected Waterborne Pathogens

Waterborne Pathogens
Enteric protozoal parasites
- *Entamoeba histolytica*
- *Giardia intestinalis*
- *Cryptosporidium parvum*
- *Cryptosporidium cayetanensis*

Bacterial enteropathogens
- *Salmonella*
- *Shigella*
- *Escherichia coli*
- *Vibrio cholerae*
- *Campylobactor*

Viral Pathogens
- Enteroviruses
- Adenoviruses
- Noroviruses

Source: Adapted with permission from Friis RH. "Water Quality." *Essentials of Environmental Health.* Sudbury, MA: Jones and Bartlett Publishers, Inc.; 2007:211.

- health benefits
- the value of those health benefits
- how the benefits compared to the costs of the intervention[24]

Some of the first measures that these cities and some other large cities in the developing world have taken to reduce outdoor air pollution have included:

- the introduction of unleaded gasoline
- low smoke lubricant for two stroke engines
- the banning of two stroke engines
- shifting to natural gas to fuel public vehicles
- tightening emissions inspections on vehicles
- reducing the burning of garbage[24]

It would also be reasonable to ensure that governments use their regulatory authority to incorporate information about outdoor air pollution in their policies on transportation and industrial development.[24] In line with this, many of the low-income countries do not yet have a significant problem of outdoor air pollution. It will be much more cost-effective for those countries to put in place cost-effective approaches now to minimizing outdoor air pollution and its health effects than it will be to try later to mitigate those effects. In doing so, they should take account of vehicular and industrial pollution.

Indoor Air Pollution

There are a number of areas in which actions could be taken to reduce indoor air pollution from the burning of solid fuels for cooking and heating. In terms of the source of pollution, cooking devices can be improved, less polluting fuels can be used, and families can reduce their need for these fuels by using solar cooking and heating. Some changes can also be made to the living environment. Mechanisms for venting smoke can be built into the house, for example, or the kitchen can be moved away from the main part of the house. People can also change their behaviors to reduce pollution or exposure to it by using dried fuels, properly maintaining their stoves and chimneys, and keeping children away from the cooking area.[25]

Public policy can also play a helpful or hurtful role in trying to reduce indoor air pollution. The public sector, for example, can promote information and education about indoor air pollution and how to reduce it in schools, in the media, and in communities. The government can also use tax policy to reduce the cost of cooking appliances and fuels that will reduce pollution. If necessary, it could subsidize the cost of improved fuels and appliances for those below a certain income level. Governments could also undertake surveillance of the problem and if possible, set standards for indoor air pollution, although this will certainly be beyond the capacity of most low-income countries.[25]

Calculating the cost-effectiveness of different approaches to reducing the health effects of indoor air pollution is a very complicated matter and requires many assumptions. Nonetheless, the conclusions of the analyses that have been done are instructive. The main findings are that the most cost-effective approach to reducing indoor air pollution in Sub-Saharan Africa and South Asia, where the needs are greatest, would be to promote the use of improved stoves. The most cost-effective approach in East Asia would be to promote the use of better fuels, such as kerosene and gas. Of course, these conclusions presume that the stoves get maintained and the fuels are of good quality, which may not always be the case and which would detract from the effectiveness of these approaches.[26]

In addition, a number of lessons have been learned about how to encourage the uptake of better stoves and better fuels, some drawn from extensive experiences in China and India. These include:

- Involve end users, especially women, in helping to assess needs and design approaches
- Promote demand for better stoves and fuels to encourage the development of competitive suppliers and market choice

- Consider subsidies and microcredit for selected interventions to help defray the cost of improvements for the poor
- Establish national and local policies that encourage the needed changes in stoves and fuels[27]

Sanitation

There are a number of different levels of technology associated with excreta disposal, many different forms of toilets, and a wide array of costs associated with them. Sanitation could range from the simple technology of bucket latrines to modern urban sewage systems. Table 7-6 lists the different approaches to excreta disposal. Although we usually think of toilets as owned by individuals, they can also be public and shared by many individuals and families.

The cost per person for methods of sanitary removal of human waste varies considerably. At the bottom levels of service, it appears that pour-flush latrines, ventilation improved latrines, and simple pit latrines can be constructed in low- and middle-income settings for about US$60. Assuming that these last approximately 5 years, the annual cost per capita would be about US$12. The construction cost of conventional sewage systems in some countries is more than 10 times that amount. In addition, they need water to function properly and water is often in short supply.[28] Work is ongoing to develop more cost-effective toilets, and in Bangladesh a simple pour-flush pan has been developed that only costs about US$0.27 per household to construct.[28]

Contrary to what we might normally believe, all of these systems can be operated in a hygienic manner that addresses health concerns. A very important review that was done in the early 1980s, for example, concluded that from the point of view of health, pit latrines would be just as hygienic as modern sewage systems, even if they were considerably less convenient.[29]

Given the relatively low cost of simple methods of sanitation and their relative effectiveness, it might be surprising that such a small share of households in low- and middle-income countries have a sanitary means of excreta disposal. Yet, besides the cultural constraints to their use, there are some other important constraints, as well:

- Lack of knowledge of options—especially the poor may not understand the options available to them and may believe that toilets cost more to install than they do
- Cost—even at relatively low prices, the poor may not have the money to pay for the up-front costs of the toilet

- Construction—there may be a lack of skills to help install the toilets
- Local laws—particularly in urban areas, local laws may forbid low-cost sanitation, even if the area has no modern sewage system[30]

There are some countries in which the public sector leads the effort to build low-cost sanitation systems. In some places, the public sector also subsidizes the cost of toilets for the poorest families, given what can be seen as the benefits to society as a whole of toilets being used by individual families. In addition, the public sector can try to enforce regulations to require the use of toilets. Although such regulatory authority is weak in most low-income and many middle-income countries, one of the main cities in Burkina Faso was able to promote toilet construction by taking away the title of homes if their owners did not install a toilet within a specific period of time.[31]

It is also possible, if the private sector believes that there is a market for low-cost sanitation, for such efforts to be handled in the private sector. In this case, the public sector may confine its role to areas needed to encourage private sector involvement and public demand for the toilets. This would include, for example, promoting the use of toilets, encouraging private sector involvement, setting standards, and helping to train people in installation and maintenance techniques.[31]

Promotion of improved sanitation can also be done with a public and private partnership and led by NGOs. Two of the most successful cases of improving low-cost sanitation were led by NGOs in Zimbabwe and Bangladesh. In Zimbabwe, an NGO was able to help communities construct 3400 latrines for about $13 per unit, or only about $2.25 per person served.[32] In Bangladesh, an NGO has helped to make 100 villages free of open defecation for a cost of only about $1.50 per person served.[33] In both of these cases, the families in the communities served paid for the latrines themselves.

The largest impact of improved sanitation is in the reduction of diarrhea and studies that have been done suggest that this impact may be on the order of about 35% overall. Some studies, such as one in Brazil suggested that children living in slum homes with a toilet suffered only one third the number of cases of diarrhea as children in homes without a toilet. It is very important to note that having a toilet seems to also increase the hand washing habits of families, which itself brings benefits, as discussed later.

Finally, the benefits of sanitary excreta removal go beyond diarrhea. Improving sanitation should reduce the prevalence of several worms, including Ascaris, Trichuris, and

---

TABLE 7-6 Selected Sanitation Technologies

- Simple pit latrine
- Small bore sewer
- Ventilation-improved latrine
- Pour-flush
- Septic tank
- Sewer connection

Source: Data with permission from The World Bank. Cairncross S, Valdmanis V. Water supply, sanitation, and hygiene promotion. In: Jamison DT, Breman JG, Measham AR, et al., eds. *Disease Control Priorities in Developing Countries.* 2nd ed. New York: Oxford University Press; 2006:780.

---

hookworm.[34] Given the low-cost of some forms of latrines, they would be cost-effective approaches to reducing the prevalence of these worms. As noted earlier, the same would be true in terms of the positive impact and low costs of reducing trachoma through improved sanitation.[35]

Water Supply

There are many analogies between water supply and sanitation. For water, as well as for sanitation, there are many different levels of technology and the costs vary considerably according to the level of technology employed. One could get water, for example from the following types of improved water sources:

- House connection
- Standpost
- Borehole
- Dug well
- Rainwater collection

The section below examines the relative cost-effectiveness of different approaches to achieving health benefits from improved water supply. In considering these costs and benefits, reasonable access to water was considered to be access to at least 20 liters per day from one of these sources from not more than 1 kilometer distance.[36]

Improving water supply can lead to a variety of health benefits. The most important studies that have been done have shown that providing a continuous supply of water with good bacteriological quality can reduce the morbidity of a number of diseases, as shown in Table 7-7 for the Africa region. Studies showed a median reduction in trachoma, for example, of 27%, schistosomiasis of 77%, and dracunculiasis of 78%.[23]

Other studies have looked at the health benefits from different combinations of investments in water quantity, water quality, sanitation, and the promotion of hygiene. The results of these studies are somewhat surprising to those not involved in the environmental field. They suggest that the largest reductions in diarrhea morbidity—approximately 30%—come from investing in sanitation only, water and sanitation, or hygiene only. The lowest reductions, between 15% and 20%, came from investing in water quantity only, or a combination of water quality and quantity, all without complementary investments in hygiene or in sanitation.

As noted earlier, many of the pathogens that are waterborne are also carried on food. Thus, sanitation has a large potential impact on reducing those pathogens. However, water alone may not yield the results that sanitation would. For this, among other reasons, complementary investments for the promotion of hygiene are critical to realizing gains from water and sanitation.[37]

Another important lesson is that the greatest effect of investments in water on health are realized when people have water connections in their homes. Unfortunately, community standpipes, for example, do not produce the level of health gains of individual household water connections.[37] A review in New Guinea, for example, showed that there was 56% less diarrhea in homes with an individual connection than in homes that got their water from standpipes.[37] This may partly be the case because people with individual connections use considerably more water than those without such connections and much of the additional water may be used to engage in better hygiene.

TABLE 7-7 Potential Morbidity Reduction from Excellent Water Supply

Condition	Percentage Reduction
Scabies	80
Typhoid fever	80
Trachoma	60
Most diarrheas and dysentery	50
Skin and subcutaneous infections	50
Paratyphoid, other Salmonella	40

Source: Adapted with permission from The World Bank. Cairncross S, Valdmanis V. Water supply, sanitation, and hygiene promotion. In: Jamison DT, Breman JG, Measham AR, et al., eds. *Disease Control Priorities in Developing Countries*. 2nd ed. New York: Oxford University Press;2006:776.

Hygiene

Unfortunately, there have been relatively few studies of the impact of hygiene promotion on actual health behaviors and on related reductions in the burden of disease. The studies that have been done showed that investing in hygiene promotion led to a 33% reduction in diarrhea. They also found that to be successful and sustainable, hygiene promotion efforts need to focus on simple messages about hand washing and avoid trying to promote too many messages at once. It appears that the messages that families acquire through hygiene promotion do stay with them and that retraining is necessary only once every five years.[38] Studies have also been done on the impact of hand washing on respiratory infections. Hand washing was associated in these studies with a significant reduction in acute respiratory infections.[38]

Integrating Investment Choices about Water, Sanitation, and Hygiene

When the information from the studies previously discussed is reviewed together, it appears that the promotion of hygiene, the promotion of sanitation, and the construction of standposts are all likely to be cost-effective in low- and middle-income countries. Using public funds to provide individual household connections to water supply systems is likely to be above the cut-off for cost-effective investments. This is shown in Table 7-8.

The costs of hygiene and sanitation promotion compare favorably, for example, with the costs per DALY averted of oral rehydration. In addition, such investments might help to reduce the burden of diarrhea and decrease the need for oral rehydration. (See Table 7-10.)

On that basis, what would be a sensible approach to improving health through investments in water supply, sanitation, and hygiene in low- and middle-income countries? First would be to promote hygiene. This is necessary both for its own sake and to maximize the value that will accrue from investments in water supply and sanitation. Second, governments should promote low-cost sanitation schemes. In doing this, they should encourage the private sector to invest in this business, encourage demand from consumers, try to ensure that there are skills to install the latrines, and try to set and enforce standards to which they have to be built. Third, low-cost water supply schemes should also be developed. This can often be done best in conjunction with communities and with community-based approaches. Finally, the government should use its regulatory and other authority to be sure that it helps consumers meet the costs of these schemes and also encourages investment in water supply schemes with household connections that families pay for. Much has been written about approaches to water and sanitation. Those interested in how such schemes get designed, built, operated, and financed are encouraged to review some of the literature on those topics, which is beyond the scope of this book.

FUTURE CHALLENGES

There will be many challenges to reducing the burden of disease that is related to hygiene, water supply, and sanitation; indoor air pollution; and outdoor air pollution. One important challenge has to do with population growth. The population is continuing to grow in many developing countries and will do so for some time. As the population grows, and as increasing numbers of people move to cities, for example, will low- and middle-income countries be able to provide the infrastructure needed for improved water supply and sanitation when they already face such substantial gaps in this provision?

At the same time, as the economies of low- and middle-income countries hopefully grow at a relatively rapid and sustained pace, how will they manage the pollution that is related, for example, to increased use of energy and greater use by better-off people of automobiles? In addition, will relatively poorly governed societies be able to manage and regulate industrial forms of pollution that could further harm air and water quality?

Many of the more difficult problems of indoor air pollution and health impacts of unsafe water and sanitation exact a larger tool on rural people than urban people, on the poor rather than the better-off, and on women and children. In this light, many countries will need to explore ways to reduce indoor air pollution and improve the safety of the water supply through community-based approaches that will often have to link the public, private, and NGO sectors with communities and that will have to explicitly focus on women and children.

Reducing the burden of environmentally-related health problems will also require that people be better informed about that burden. At the societal level, people and communities will need to understand more about the links between their health and the environment. At national, regional, local, and family levels, people will also need to be more aware of the solutions to these problems that might be available to them. The need for better and more information about issues and options for addressing them will be especially important among the poor, poorly educated, the rural, and women.

Another challenge of addressing environmental health issues is that efforts to address them generally require action outside the health sector. Urban water supply systems are

TABLE 7-8 Cost per DALY of Selected Investments in Water, Sanitation, and Hygiene

Investment	US$/DALY
Hygiene promotion	3.35
Sanitation promotion only	11.15
Water sector regulation and advocacy	47.00
Hand pump or standpost	94.00
House connection	223.00
Construction and promotion	≤ 270.00

Source: Adapted with permission from The World Bank. Cairncross S, Valdmanis V. Water supply, sanitation, and hygiene promotion. In: Jamison DT, Breman JG, Measham AR, et al., eds. *Disease Control Priorities in Developing Countries.* 2nd ed. New York: Oxford University Press; 2006:791.

usually under the control of public or private companies. Urban sanitation is usually managed by individual cities. In rural areas, water supply and sanitation are most likely to be controlled by communities and individuals. Indoor air pollution is an issue that can best be addressed by working with families and communities to change the way they cook and the fuel that they use for cooking. Outdoor air pollution comes, among other things, from industrial plants and vehicles, the control of which depends on an array of economic and policy matters beyond the scope of the health ministry.

MAIN MESSAGES

Environmental health issues have a large impact on the global burden of disease. These impacts occur at the individual, household, community, and global level. Broadly speaking, about one third of the total global burden of disease is related to environmental factors.[39] About 8% of the global burden of disease is associated with the environmental factors discussed in this chapter, including outdoor air pollution, indoor air pollution from the use of sold fuels, and water, sanitation, and hygiene.[3]

The risks of these environmental factors are greatest for poor women and their children due to their exposure to indoor air pollution from the burning of solid fuel and to poor quality water. The risks of environmental impacts on health are greatest in the low-income countries of Africa and Asia. Environmental risk factors are especially important causes of illness and death from diarrhea and acute respiratory infections among young children. They also have a large impact on the burden of disease from certain parasitic infections, such as worms. Given the prominence of these risk factors, it is essential that improvements be made in water, sanitation, and hygiene if the MDGs are to be met.

The burden of indoor air pollution stems largely from cooking on unventilated stoves with solid biomass fuels or coal, as done by a large share of poor people in the world. The sources of outdoor air pollution are many and vehicle emission is among the most important in most cities. Poor sanitation allows pathogens in human waste to spread but only about 40% of the people in the world have access to improved sanitation. Unsafe water carries pathogens. The lack of water prevents people from engaging in appropriate hygiene practices. Poor hygiene practices, including open defecation and the failure to engage in hand washing, are common in the developing world, especially among people who lack education.

Data are weak on cost-effective approaches to reducing outdoor air pollution in the developing countries. However, it appears that there are a number of measures that could be taken to reduce pollution and enhance health including eliminating leaded gasoline, eliminating two stroke engines, strengthening emissions standards, and shifting vehicle fuel to natural gas. In Africa and South Asia, the most cost-effective approach to reducing indoor air pollution will be to promote the use of improved stoves. In Asia, the most cost-effective approach would be to encourage a shift from biomass fuels and coal to kerosene or gas.

The most cost-effective approach to reducing the burden of water-related diseases, especially diarrhea, is to invest in low-cost sanitation and standposts for water and to promote hand washing. Investments in water can have numerous benefits, including saving the time of women who are usually charged with getting water and often have to expend large amounts of energy to do so. The provision of water can also contribute to reduction in certain parasitic diseases. However, in the absence of improved hygiene, the provision of improved access to water alone still fails to address an important share of the burden of diarrheal disease.

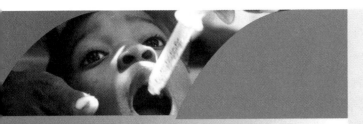

Study Questions

1. Why are environmental health issues important in global health? Which of them are the most important and why?

2. Why would the burden of disease from indoor air pollution in low- and middle-income countries be larger than that from outdoor air pollution?

3. In what regions of the world would the burden from indoor air pollution be the greatest? Why?

4. What are the different ways in which unsafe water is related to the spread of disease? Give some examples of specific diseases that are spread in various water-related ways.

5. What are some of the health problems associated with outdoor air pollution?

6. Why is it important to promote hand washing?

7. What approach would you take in a low-income African country to enhancing the access of the poor to better water supplies? Why?

8. How would you try to expand access to low-cost sanitation in Nepal? Why?

9. What would constrain poor people in Nepal from investing their own resources in improved low-cost sanitation? How could those constraints be overcome?

10. How would you help people in Guatemala to adopt the use of better stoves?

REFERENCES

1. Lopez AD, Mathers CD, Murray CJL. *Global Burden of Disease and Risk Factors*. New York: Oxford University Press; 2006.

2. Smith KR, Corvalan CF, Kjellstrom T. How much global ill health is attributable to environmental factors? *Epidemiology*. 1999;10(5):573.

3. Lopez AD, Mathers CD, Ezzati M, Jamison DT, Murray CJL. Measuring the global burden of disease and risk factors 1990–2001. In: Lopez AD, Mathers CD, Ezzati M, Jamison DT, Murray CJL, eds. *Global Burden of Disease and Risk Factors*. New York: Oxford University Press; 2006:10.

4. Friis RH. *Essentials on Environmental Health*. Sudbury, MA: Jones and Bartlett Publishers, Inc.; 2007.

5. Yassi A, Kjellstrom T, de Kok T, Guidotti TL. *Basic Environmental Health*. New York: Oxford University Press; 2001.

6. McMichael AJ, Kjellstrom T, Smith KR. Environmental health. In: Merson MH, Black RE, Mills A, eds. *International Public Health: Diseases, Programs, Systems, and Policies*. Gaithersburg, MD: Aspen Publishers; 2001:379.

7. The World Bank. Environmental Health. Available at: http://web.worldbank.org/WBSITE/EXTERNAL/TOPICS/EXTHEALTHNUTRITIONANDPOPULATION/EXTPHAAG/0,,contentMDK:20656146~menuPK:2175463~pagePK:64229817~piPK:64229743~theSitePK:672263,00.html. Accessed October 27, 2006.

8. World Health Organization. Protection of the Human Environment. Available at: http://www.who.int/phe/en/. Accessed May 19, 2005.

9. World Health Organization. Indoor Air Pollution and Health: Fact Sheet No. 292. Available at: http://www.who.int/mediacentre/factsheets/fs292/en/index.html. Accessed October 29, 2006.

10. Yassi A, Kjellstrom T, de Kok T, Guidotti TL. Health and energy use. *Basic Environmental Health*. New York: Oxford University Press; 2001:315.

11. Yassi A, Kjellstrom T, de Kok T, Guidotti TL. Health and energy use. *Basic Environmental Health*. New York: Oxford University Press; 2001:317.

12. Yassi A, Kjellstrom T, de Kok T, Guidotti TL. Air. *Basic Environmental Health*. New York: Oxford University Press; 2001:188.

13. Yassi A, Kjellstrom T, de Kok T, Guidotti TL. Air. *Basic Environmental Health*. New York: Oxford University Press; 2001:193–194.

14. Yassi A, Kjellstrom T, de Kok T, Guidotti TL. Water and sanitation. *Basic Environmental Health*. New York: Oxford University Press; 2001:233.

15. Cairncross S, Valdmanis V. Water supply, sanitation, and hygiene promotion. In: Jamison DT, Breman JG, Measham AR, et al., eds. *Disease Control Priorities in Developing Countries*. 2nd ed. New York: Oxford University Press; 2006:776.

16. Cairncross S, Valdmanis V. Water supply, sanitation, and hygiene promotion. In: Jamison DT, Breman JG, Measham AR, et al., eds. *Disease Control Priorities in Developing Countries*. 2nd ed. New York: Oxford University Press; 2006:784.

17. World Bank. Access to Safe Water. Available at: http://www.worldbank.org/depweb/english/modules/environm/water/. Accessed November 3, 2006.

18. United Nations. The Millennium Development Goals Report 2005. Available at: www.un.org/Docs/summit2005/MDGBook.pdf. Accessed November 3, 2006.

19. UNICEF. Press Release: 400 Million Children Deprived of Safe Water. Available at: http://www.unicef.org/media/media_31772.html. Accessed November 3, 2006.

20. Ostro B. Outdoor Air Pollution: Assessing the Environmental Burden of Disease at National and Local Levels. Available at: http://www.who.int/quantifying_ehimpacts/publications/ebd5.pdf. Accessed November 3, 2006.

21. Kjellstrom T, Lodh M, McMichael AJ, Ranmuthugala G, Shrestha R, Kingsland S. Air and water pollution: burden and strategies for control. In: Jamison DT, Breman JG, Measham AR, et al., eds. *Disease Control Priorities in Developing Countries*. 2nd ed. New York: Oxford University Press; 2006:820.

22. Cohen AJ, Ross Anderson H, Ostro B, et al. The global burden of disease due to outdoor air pollution. *J Toxicol Environ Health A*. 2005;68(13-14):1301–1307.

23. Cairncross S, Valdmanis V. Water supply, sanitation, and hygiene promotion. In: Jamison DT, Breman JG, Measham AR, et al., eds. *Disease Control Priorities in Developing Countries*. 2nd ed. New York: Oxford University Press; 2006:778.

24. Kjellstrom T, Lodh M, McMichael AJ, Ranmuthugala G, Shrestha R, Kingsland S. Air and water pollution: burden and strategies for control. In: Jamison DT, Breman JG, Measham AR, et al., eds. *Disease Control Priorities in Developing Countries*. 2nd ed. New York: Oxford University Press; 2006:825–826.

25. Bruce N, Rehfuess E, Mehta S, Hutton G, Smith K. Indoor air pollution. In: Jamison DT, Breman JG, Measham AR, et al., eds. *Disease Control Priorities in Developing Countries*. 2nd ed. New York: Oxford University Press; 2006:800.

26. Bruce N, Rehfuess E, Mehta S, Hutton G, Smith K. Indoor air pollution. In: Jamison DT, Breman JG, Measham AR, et al., eds. *Disease Control Priorities in Developing Countries*. 2nd ed. New York: Oxford University Press; 2006:802–808.

27. Bruce N, Rehfuess E, Mehta S, Hutton G, Smith K. Indoor air pollution. In: Jamison DT, Breman JG, Measham AR, et al., eds. *Disease Control Priorities in Developing Countries*. 2nd ed. New York: Oxford University Press; 2006:808–811.

28. Cairncross S, Valdmanis V. Water supply, sanitation, and hygiene promotion. In: Jamison DT, Breman JG, Measham AR, et al., eds. *Disease Control Priorities in Developing Countries*. 2nd ed. New York: Oxford University Press; 2006:780.

29. Feachem R, Bradley D, Garelick H, Mara D. *Sanitation and Disease: Health Aspects of Excreta and Wastewater Management*. Chichester, U.K.: John Wiley & Sons; 1983.

30. Cairncross S, Valdmanis V. Water supply, sanitation, and hygiene promotion. In: Jamison DT, Breman JG, Measham AR, et al., eds. *Disease Control Priorities in Developing Countries*. 2nd ed. New York: Oxford University Press; 2006:780–182.

31. Cairncross S, Valdmanis V. Water supply, sanitation, and hygiene promotion. In: Jamison DT, Breman JG, Measham AR, et al., eds. *Disease Control Priorities in Developing Countries*. 2nd ed. New York: Oxford University Press; 2006:781.

32. Waterkeyn J. Cost-Effective Health Promotion: Community Health Clubs. Abuja, Nigeria: Paper presented at the 29th WEDC Conference; 2003.

33. Allan S. The WaterAid Bangladesh/VERC 100% Sanitation Approach; Cost, Motivation and Subsidy. *M.Sc. dissertation, London School of Hygiene and Tropical Medicine*; 2003.

34. Cairncross S, Valdmanis V. Water supply, sanitation, and hygiene promotion. In: Jamison DT, Breman JG, Measham AR, et al., eds. *Disease Control Priorities in Developing Countries*. 2nd ed. New York: Oxford University Press; 2006:783–784.

35. Emerson PM, Lindsay SW, Alexander N, et al. Role of flies and provision of latrines in trachoma control: cluster-randomised controlled trial. *Lancet*. 2004;363(9415):1093–1098.

36. Cairncross S, Valdmanis V. Water supply, sanitation, and hygiene promotion. In: Jamison DT, Breman JG, Measham AR, et al., eds. *Disease Control Priorities in Developing Countries*. 2nd ed. New York: Oxford University Press; 2006:772.

37. Cairncross S, Valdmanis V. Water supply, sanitation, and hygiene promotion. In: Jamison DT, Breman JG, Measham AR, et al., eds. *Disease Control Priorities in Developing Countries*. 2nd ed. New York: Oxford University Press; 2006:777.

38. Cairncross S, Valdmanis V. Water supply, sanitation, and hygiene promotion. In: Jamison DT, Breman JG, Measham AR, et al., eds. *Disease Control Priorities in Developing Countries*. 2nd ed. New York: Oxford University Press; 2006:784–785.

39. Smith KR, Corvalan CF, Kjellstrom T. How much global ill health is attributable to environmental factors? *Epidemiology*. 1999;10(5):573–584.

Nutrition and Global Health

By the end of this chapter, the reader will be able to:

- Define key terms related to nutrition
- Describe the determinants of nutritional status
- Discuss nutrition needs at different stages of the life cycle
- Discuss the burden of nutrition problems globally
- Review the costs and consequences of the burden of nutrition problems
- Discuss measures that can be taken to address key nutrition problems
- Discuss important successes that countries have had in dealing with nutrition issues

VIGNETTES

Shireen was 1 year old and lived in Dhaka, the capital of Bangladesh. Shireen was born with low birthweight. In addition, her family lacked the income needed to provide her with adequate food after she was no longer breastfeeding. Shireen had also repeatedly been ill with respiratory infections and diarrhea and she was now hospitalized with pneumonia. Despite the best efforts of the hospital, Shireen died after 2 days there.

Ruth lived in Liberia and was pregnant with her first child. Ruth had been anemic for all of her adult life, partly from hookworm infection and partly from not having enough iron rich foods in her diet. She also had no access during pregnancy to iron and folic acid tablets or to foods that were fortified with vitamins and minerals. Ruth went into labor one evening and delivered the baby with the help of a traditional birth attendant. After the baby was born, however, Ruth began to bleed severely.

Her family was not able to get her to a hospital and Ruth died.

Dorji was 15 years old and lived in the mountains of northern India. Dorji was very short and was also severely mentally retarded. Dorji was not the only one in his village with these problems. Dorji lived in an area in which the soils had little iodine. Although the government of India was encouraging the fortification of salt with iodine, such salt was not sold in Dorji's region of the country.

Rachel and her mother lived in Mombassa, a port city in Kenya. Rachel had already received her first polio vaccine and she was soon to get another. When the children participated in "polio days" not only did they get polio vaccine, but they also got a dose of vitamin A. Until recently, there were many young children who were blind due to the lack of vitamin A. Since the polio campaign started and children got extra vitamin A as part of that campaign, almost no children had become blind.

THE IMPORTANCE OF NUTRITION

Some things really are more important than others, and the role of nutrition in health is one of them. As noted in Table 8-1, nutritional status has a profound impact on and relationship to health status, as elaborated upon in the section that follows.

Nutritional status is fundamental to the growth of young children, their proper mental and physical development, and their health as adults. In addition, because of the impact of nutrition on health, nutritional status is intimately linked with whether or not children enroll in school, perform effectively while there, or complete their schooling. Nutritional

TABLE 8-1 Selected Links Between Nutrition and the Health of Mothers and Children

Good maternal nutrition is essential for good outcomes of pregnancy for the mother

Exclusive breastfeeding for 6 months promotes better health for infants than mixing breastfeeding with other foods during that period

Nutritional deficits in fetuses and in children under 2 years of age may produce growth and development deficits in infants and young children that can never be overcome

About half of all deaths in children under five years worldwide are associated with nutritional deficits

Underweight and micronutrient deficiencies in children make those children more susceptible to illness, cause illnesses to last longer, and can lead to deaths from diarrhea, pneumonia, and malaria that might have been preventable

Source: The Author

status, therefore, has a profound effect on labor productivity and people's prospects for earning income.

Despite the importance of nutrition to health, an exceptional number of people in the world are malnourished, especially poor women and children in low-income countries. In fact, more than 30% of all children in the world are underweight or stunted in growth.[1,2] In addition, about 50% of the young children who die in the world every year die of causes related to being underweight.[3] This means that about 5.5 million children in the world die every year of malnutrition. Remarkably, this is equal to 15,000 children dying of nutrition-related causes every day.[3] In addition, undernutrition is the single largest risk factor for the loss of health in low- and middle-income countries.[4]

These nutritional gaps are even more difficult to accept because there are a number of low cost, but highly effective, nutrition interventions that can dramatically improve nutrition status, which are not being implemented sufficiently. Many improvements in nutrition can be enabled largely by communication efforts, such as the promotion of breastfeeding, the introduction of appropriate complementary foods, and the eating of foods that are rich in certain micronutrients. Such communication efforts, however, are not put in place frequently enough. The fortification of salt with iodine has been carried out in high-income countries for more than 50 years but un-iodized salt is still sold in many countries. The importance of iron and folic acid to successful outcomes

of pregnancy has also been well-known for decades,[5] yet most women in low-income countries, like Ruth in the vignette, do not get supplements of iron and folic acid or eat food that is fortified with iron and folate.

In fact, there is enormous scope to improve nutrition status globally simply by implementing a number of these interventions. Indeed, the Copenhagen Consensus, about which you read in Chapter 3, concluded that some of the highest yielding investments that could be made in developing countries include measures to improve nutritional status, such as the provision of micronutrients, the development of new agricultural technologies, improvements in infant and child nutrition, and reductions in the prevalence of low birthweight.[6]

Nutrition is also central to the achievement of the MDGs. Directly or indirectly, nutrition is related to almost all of these goals, as noted in Table 8-2.

In fact, this table makes clear that there are *no* prospects for meeting the MDGs without substantial improvements in nutrition. The hunger goal is completely linked with nutrition, and nutrition deficits are intimately connected to whether or not people are poor. The large number of children who are poorly nourished will challenge the realization of the education goal. In addition, if about 50% of all child deaths are related to nutrition, then how can the child mortality goal be met unless nutrition problems are tackled more effectively? The nutritional concerns that are particular to women will constrain their productivity, limit improvements in their economic and social status, and preclude gains in the reduction of maternal mortality.

In light of the exceptional importance of nutrition to human health, this chapter will provide an overview of the most critical matters concerning nutrition globally. First, it will introduce you to the most important terms used in discussing nutrition. It will then examine the determinants of nutritional status. After that, the chapter will explore the most important nutritional needs of people at different stages in their life cycle. It will then review the nutritional state of the world and the costs and consequences of key nutrition problems. The chapter will then examine what can be done to address nutrition problems in effective and efficient ways. The chapter will conclude by examining some of the challenges of trying to further improve nutritional status worldwide.

This chapter will deal almost exclusively with undernutrition. It is true that there is a growing epidemic of overweight and obesity in the world, often side by side with underweight. It is also increasingly true that this is occurring in low- and middle-income countries, as well as in high-income countries.[7] However, the focus of this book is on low-income people in low- and middle-income countries and for them undernutrition will remain for many years the most important nutrition concern. It should be noted, however, that Chapter 12 discusses the relationship between diet and non-communicable diseases, examines obesity, and reviews measures to reduce the burden of disease associated with being overweight and obese. Nutritional problems related to famine, drought, and civil conflict are touched on in Chapter 14.

DEFINITIONS AND KEY TERMS

There are a number of terms related to nutrition that will be used throughout this chapter and in other sections of the book, as well. These terms are noted and defined in Table 8-3.

The term "malnutrition" should be used to refer to those who do not get proper nutrition, whether too little, too much, or of the wrong kind. This is the way that this book will use "malnutrition." In addition, people who lack sufficient nutrients will be referred to as "undernourished." People who have low weight for their age will be called "underweight." People who are nourished to the point of being too heavy for their height will be called "overweight" or "obese," depending on how overweight they are.

THE DETERMINANTS OF NUTRITIONAL STATUS

Nutritional status depends on a number of factors, as shown in Figure 8-1, which follows the UNICEF framework.[8]

In line with that, we can consider first the "immediate causes" of malnutrition. The two most important are inadequate dietary intake and illness. People may get an insufficient amount of food or not enough of some of the nutrients they need. These factors weaken the body, open the person to illness and infection, and lead to longer and more frequent illness than would otherwise be the case. Inadequate dietary intake becomes part of a vicious cycle with illness and infection, because they make it harder for people to eat, more difficult for them to absorb what they do take in, and actually raise the need for some nutrients. The relationship between infection and nutritional status is very important to keep in mind, especially when considering how to improve the nutritional status of poor children in low- and middle-income countries.

The UNICEF framework also includes a set of "underlying causes" to inadequate dietary intake and infectious disease that include "inadequate access to food in a household; insufficient health services and an unhealthful environment; and, inadequate care for children and women."[8] Whether or not people get enough food within a household depends on a

TABLE 8-2 Nutrition and the MDGs

Goal 1—Eradicate Poverty and Hunger
Link—Poor nutritional status is both a cause and a consequence of poverty. Improving income and nutritional status will improve health status.

Goal 2—Achieve Universal Primary Education
Link—Children who are properly nourished enroll in school at higher rates than undernourished children, attend school for more years, and perform better while they are there than undernourished children.

Goal 3—Promote Gender Equality and Empower Women
Link—Women suffer very high rates of some nutritional deficiencies, such as iron deficiency anemia, that constrain their health and their productivity. Improving the nutritional status of women will enhance their income earning potential and ability to be more productive in all of their work.

Goal 4—Reduce Child Mortality
Link—About half of all child deaths worldwide are associated with malnutrition. It will not be possible to make major strides in reducing child mortality without significant improvements in the nutritional status of young children.

Goal 5—Improve Maternal Health
Link—Maternal health and pregnancy outcomes are intimately connected to the nutritional status of the pregnant women.

Goal 6—Combat HIV/AIDS, malaria, and other diseases
Link—Poor nutritional status makes people more susceptible to illness and to being sick for longer periods of time. Good nutrition is especially important for people suffering some health conditions, such as TB and HIV/AIDS. Supplementation with some micronutrients, even in the absence of anti-retroviral therapy, can lengthen the time that HIV positive people can go without progressing to full-blown AIDS.

Source: Author commentary on the UN Millennium Goals. Available at: www.un.org/millennium goals. Accessed July 11, 2006.

number of factors. These include access to land and the ability to produce food for those living in rural areas. They also include having access to food and the money to purchase it. In addition, the amount and type of food one gets depends in many families on social position, with girls and women sometimes getting less food or less nutritious food than men and boys get. It is also important to note that in rural areas in low-income countries, there may be a "hungry season," in which families have exhausted the food from their last harvest, have

TABLE 8-3 Key Terms and Definitions

Anemia—Low level of hemoglobin in the blood, as evidenced by a reduced quality or quantity of red blood cells

Body mass index (BMI)—Body weight in kilograms divided by height in meters squared (kg/m2)

Iodine deficiency disorders (IDDs)—The spectrum of IDD includes goiter, hypothyroidism, impaired mental function, stillbirths, abortions, congenital anomalies, and neurological cretinism

Low birthweight—Birthweight less than 2500 grams

Malnutrition—Various forms of poor nutrition. Underweight or stunting and overweight, as well as micronutrient deficiencies, are forms of malnutrition.

Obesity—Excessive body fat content; commonly measured by BMI. The international reference for classifying an individual as obese is a BMI greater than 30.

Overweight—Excess weight relative to height; commonly measured by BMI among adults. The international reference for adults is as follows:

- 25–29.99 for grade I (overweight)
- 30–39.99 for grade II (obese)
- > 40 for grade III

For children, overweight is measured as weight-for-height 2 z-scores above the international reference.

Stunting—Failure to reach linear growth potential because of inadequate nutrition or poor health. Stunting is measured as height-for-age 2 z-scores below the international reference.

Undernutrition—Poor nutrition. The three most commonly used indexes for child undernutrition are height-for-age, weight-for-age, and weight-for-height. For adults, undernutrition is measured by a BMI less than 18.5.

Underweight—Low weight-for-age; that is, 2 z-scores below the international reference for weight-for-age. It implies stunting or wasting and is an indicator of undernutrition.

Vitamin A deficiency—Tissue concentrations of vitamin A low enough to have adverse health consequences such as increased morbidity and mortality, poor reproductive health, and slowed growth and development, even if there is no clinical deficiency.

Wasting—Weight, measured in kilograms, divided by height in meters squared, that is 2 z-scores below the international reference.

Z-score—A statistical term, meaning the deviation of an individual's value from the median value of a reference population, divided by the standard deviation of the reference population.

Source: Adapted with permission from The World Bank. *Repositioning Nutrition as Central to Development.* Washington, DC: The World Bank; 2006:xvii.

not yet produced the food for this year and do not have the income to buy food, even if a market is accessible to them.

As discussed in Chapter 7, the lack of safe water and sanitation are extremely important causes of diarrheal disease and, therefore, greatly contribute to the cycle of infection and malnutrition. This is made worse when people live in generally unhygienic circumstances, in which food is often handled in unhygienic ways. These are also the circumstances under which people, especially children, are likely to get parasitic infections, such as worms, about which you will read in Chapters 10 and 11. These parasites sap the energy of children and make it harder for them to absorb what they do eat.

Child caring practices affect the nutritional status of children in similar ways to the manner in which they impact children's health status. If a child is exclusively breastfed for 6 months, if complementary foods are intro-duced that are of sufficient quality and quantity, and if food and water are handled in hygienic ways, then the nutritional status of young children will be enhanced. In addition, as discussed earlier, the nutrition and health status of the mother is an exceptionally important determinant of whether or not the child will be born with low birthweight and will thrive thereafter.

Access to appropriate health services is also very important to nutritional status, in a manner similar to its importance for health status. Receiving basic childhood immunizations is an important way to avoid illness and infection. The same is true for vitamin A supplements that are provided by many health services. Medicines to rid children of worms can also be very important to their nutritional status. Unfortunately, as noted in Chapter 5, there are still too many health systems that are not capable of effectively providing even these basic services.

FIGURE 8-1 Determinants of Nutritional Status—the UNICEF Framework

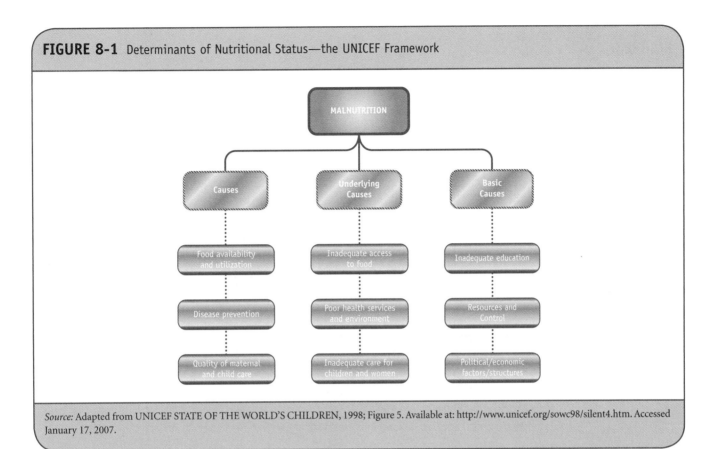

Source: Adapted from UNICEF STATE OF THE WORLD'S CHILDREN, 1998; Figure 5. Available at: http://www.unicef.org/sowc98/silent4.htm. Accessed January 17, 2007.

Of course, at the root of nutritional status are the factors that UNICEF calls "basic causes." In a manner similar to the factors that determine health, the root causes of nutritional status also have to do with socioeconomic status, family income, the level of knowledge people have of appropriate health and nutritional practices, and the amount of control that people have over their lives. Governmental and global policies that affect agricultural production, marketing, and distribution, and that impact education, health, and nutrition programs can also have a profound effect on the nutritional status of individuals, communities, and societies.

GAUGING NUTRITION STATUS

The nutritional status of infants and children is largely gauged by measuring and weighing these children and then plotting their weight and height on growth charts, like the one shown in Figure 8-2.

These growth charts have been standardized. The place of the child on the growth curves indicates whether the child is growing normally or not. The nutrition status of adults is generally determined on the basis of the person's weight in relation to the person's height, while also taking account of his or her age.

We usually think of deficits in nutrition as being large and evident. However, it is extremely important to note that this is not necessarily the case. Rather, a very large share of the nutritional deficits that exist globally are "mild" or "moderate" and may not be very obvious. Nonetheless, even mild and moderate malnutrition can have very negative consequences on the biological development of people, on their health, and on their productivity, and some of these negative effects will be irreversible.

KEY NUTRITIONAL NEEDS

Many nutrients are important; however, from the point of view of global health, several are of paramount importance. These include protein, energy, and the four micronutrients: vitamin A, iron, iodine, and zinc. The next section examines each of these topics in greater detail and Table 8-4 summarizes the sources of these nutrients and their key impacts.

Undernutrition

It is also extremely important to note that the failure of children to grow properly often begins around their 6th month, as they move away from exclusive breastfeeding. At this time, they begin to eat complementary foods that may not be suf-

FIGURE 8-2 Model Growth Chart

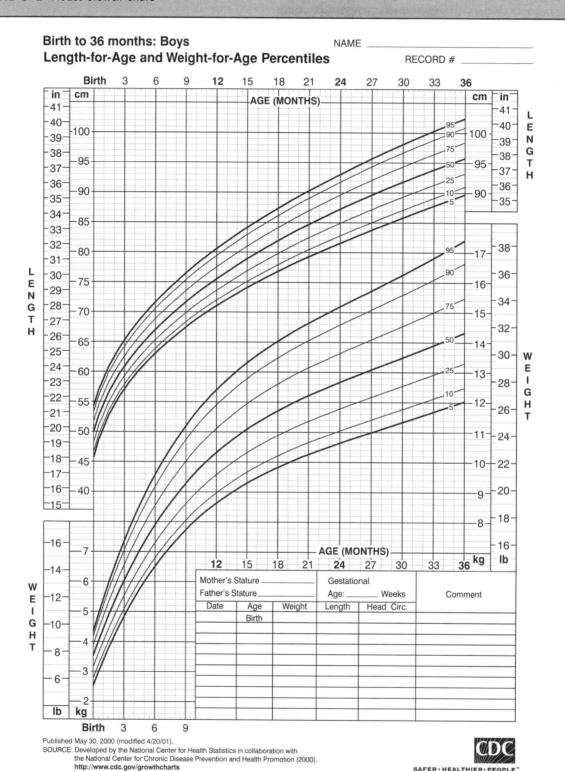

Birth to 36 months: Boys
Length-for-Age and Weight-for-Age Percentiles

NAME _____

RECORD # _____

Published May 30, 2000 (modified 4/20/01).
SOURCE: Developed by the National Center for Health Statistics in collaboration with
the National Center for Chronic Disease Prevention and Health Promotion (2000).
http://www.cdc.gov/growthcharts

Source: CDC. Available at: http://www.cdc.gov/nchs/data/nhanes/growthcharts/set1clinical/cj41l017.pdf. Accessed January 31, 2007.

TABLE 8-4 Key Nutritional Needs, Sources, and Selected Functions

Key Nutritional Needs	Sources	Selected Functions
Protein	Milk, eggs, chicken, and beans	Proper growth of children and immune functions
Vitamin A	Liver, eggs, green leafy vegetables, orange and red fruits and vegetables	Proper immune function and prevention of xerophthalmia
Iodine	Selected seafoods and plants grown in iodine containing soil	Growth and neurological development
Iron	Fish, meat, poultry, grains, vegetables, and legumes	Prevent iron deficiency anemia, prevent low birthweight and premature babies
Zinc	Red and white meat and shellfish	Promote growth, immune function, and cognitive development

Source: Data from *The Journal of Nutrition.* Nutrient Information. Available at: http://jn.nutrition.org/nutinfo/. Accessed February 8, 2007.

ficient in quality or quantity, and they are also increasingly exposed to the risks of infection and illness. A continuous lack of sufficient protein and energy at young ages would be chronic undernutrition and would produce children who are stunted.[9]

Undernutrition has a number of other deleterious effects. Being malnourished in childhood, for example, is associated with diminished intellectual capacity and undernutrition also greatly raises the risk of illness for a child. In addition, there is a hypothesis that early malnutrition is associated with later hypertension, diabetes, and cardiovascular disease.[9]

Furthermore, malnourished women have a greatly increased risk of delivering premature or low birth weight babies. Such babies are, in turn, at much greater risk than full-term babies or babies with a birthweight of over 5.5 pounds of growing poorly, not developing properly, or dying.[9]

Vitamin A

Vitamin A is found in a variety of plants but mostly in green leafy vegetables, yellow and orange fruits that are not citrus, and carrots. It is also found in some animal products, including liver, milk, and eggs.[9] The lack of vitamin A is associated with the development of a condition known as xeropthalmia. The person with this condition first gets "night blindness." Later, the eye dries out, which can lead to permanent blindness.[10]

What is less well known, however, is that vitamin A is extremely important to the proper functioning of the immune system and to a child's growth. Deficiency in vitamin A has a profound impact on whether a child will survive a bout of pneumonia, malaria, measles, or diarrhea.[9] Vitamin A deficiency also increases the risk of maternal mortality.[11]

Iodine

Iodine is generally found in some types of seafood and in plants that are grown in soil that naturally contains iodine.[12] People who live in mountainous areas often do not get enough iodine in their diets, because they do not consume much seafood and mountainous soils often lack iodine. This was the case, for example, for Dorji, in the vignette at the start of this chapter. The lack of iodine is most often associated with a growth on the thyroid, called a goiter, and the failure to develop full intellectual potential.[12] However, iodine deficiency disorders "can also include fetal loss, stillbirth, congenital anomalies, and hearing impairment."[13] In fact, iodine deficiency most often manifests itself in mild mental retardation[13] and people with cretinism have an IQ that is on average 10 to 15 points below that of people who do not suffer this deficit.[14] In extreme forms, iodine deficiency may also lead to severe mental retardation and being both deaf and mute. Iodine deficiency "is the most common form of preventable mental illness in the world."[15]

Iron

The most easily absorbable form of iron is found in fish, meat, and poultry. Less absorbable forms can be found in fruits, grains, vegetables, nuts, and dried beans. The lack of iron is most often associated with iron deficiency anemia, which we usually associate with weakness and fatigue. This is especially a problem for adolescent women and pregnant women, because women who are iron deficient have an increased risk of giving birth to a premature or low birthweight baby or of hemorrhaging in childbirth.[16] Iron deficiency is also associated with poor mental development and reduced immune function.[13] In addition, iron is a critical requirement for children in the 6 to 24 month age group to ensure optimal development of their cognitive and motor skills.

Zinc

The importance of zinc to good health has only recently become better understood. The best sources of zinc are red and white meat and shellfish.[17] Severe deficiency in zinc is associated with "growth retardation, impaired immune function, skin disorders, hypogonadism, and cognitive dysfuncion."[13] Mild to moderate deficiency increases susceptibility to infecion.[13] Indeed, children who receive zinc supplementation when they have diarrhea recover more rapidly than those who do not,[18] and zinc deficiency is a major risk factor for morbidity and mortality from diarrhea, pneumonia, and malaria, as discussed later.[13]

NUTRITIONAL NEEDS THROUGHOUT THE LIFE CYCLE

Nutritional needs vary with one's place in the life cycle. Having outlined the most important nutritional needs that concern global health issues, therefore, it will now be valuable to examine how those needs change from pregnancy, through infancy, childhood, adolescence, adulthood, and old age. This will assist us in getting a better understanding of the nature of the nutrition problems globally, the burden of disease related to nutrition, and how this burden might be addressed.

Pregnancy and Birth Weight

The nutritional status of a pregnant woman is especially important to the outcome that she will have in pregnancy, both for herself and for her newborn. It is critical that a pregnant woman stay well-nourished and healthy. During pregnancy, the woman will need to get a sufficient amount of protein and energy from the food she eats, and it is generally recommended that she consume 300 calories more per day than when she is not pregnant. In addition, iron, iodine, folate, zinc, and calcium will be very important to the health of the woman and her newborn.[19]

The birthweight of a baby is an extremely important determinant of the extent to which a child will thrive and become a healthy adult. Fetuses that do not get sufficient and appropriate nutrition from the mother may suffer a number of problems, including stillbirth, mental impairment, or a variety of severe birth defects. They could also undergo a general failure to grow properly, referred to as intrauterine growth retardation. Babies who are low birthweight have a much greater risk of getting diarrhea and pneumonia and more than a 10 times greater risk of dying then babies born between about 6.5 pounds and about 8 pounds.[20] The most important nutritional needs in pregnancy and the consequences of deficits in them are outlined in Table 8-5.

Infancy and Young Childhood

An important share of a child's biological development takes place between conception and 2 years of age. It is essential to understand that nutritional gaps that arise during that period may produce problems in stature or mental development that can never be overcome. They may also lead to more frequent infection and infections that last longer than would be the case in a better-nourished child. Thus, it is extraordinarily important that infants and young children get a sufficient amount of protein, energy, and fat from their foods. They also need sufficient amounts of iodine, iron, vitamin A, and zinc.

There is very strong evidence worldwide that infants will grow best and stay healthiest if they are exclusively breastfed for the first 6 months of their lives. They will also thrive best if foods other than breast milk or infant formula begin to be introduced around 6 months of age, while breastfeeding continues.[3] Especially in low-income countries in which nutritional deficits are likely to be considerable, such foods will be especially valuable if they are fortified with key vitamins and minerals.

The nutrition needs of the infant continue into young childhood, but the nutritional status of many children faces risks as the child stops breastfeeding, as noted earlier. At this stage, the child's nutritional status depends on the ability of the family to provide an adequate diet and to help the child avoid illnesses and infections. Among the most critical issues concerning childhood nutrition is that stunted children have very little chance to catch up in their growth and that most of the damage done to their development, both physical and mental, can not be changed.[20]

This fact has enormous implications for public policy aimed at enhancing nutrition status. It means that the focus of attention in addressing undernutrition and its consequences must be on children under 2 years of age, and it must start by trying to ensure that pregnant women are well nourished and healthy enough to give birth to healthy babies of acceptable birthweight. As some have said, there is a "window of opportunity" for ensuring that children grow properly and reach their biological potential. This window opens at conception and closes, at least most of the way, around the time the child is 2 years of age.[21]

Adolescence

Adolescent girls who are well nourished grow faster than adolescent girls who are not well nourished. Adolescent girls who are poorly nourished, but still growing, are much more likely than well-nourished girls to give birth to an underweight baby. This may stem from the fact that the fetus and the girl are competing for nutrients in the adolescent who is still growing.[20] Poorly nourished and very small adolescent girls also have more complications of pregnancy than do older girls who are taller. This relates partly to the difficulties of very small women giving birth, because of their size. In addition, all adolescents go through a growth spurt, although children who are stunted are unable to make up in adolescence for their retarded growth. For adolescents to grow properly and become healthy adults, they need appropriate protein and energy. They also have particular needs for iodine, iron, and folic acid. Because of their growth during this period, calcium is also especially important for adolescents.[20]

Adulthood and Old Age

Adults need appropriate, well-balanced nutrition to stay healthy and productive. Adults also need to pay particular attention in their diets to foods that can be harmful to their health, such as foods that contain too much fat, cholesterol, sugar, or salt. Older adults have special nutritional needs that are very important, but often forgotten. The ability of older people to live on their own and to function effectively depends in many ways on their nutritional status; however, many older people lack the income or the support needed to eat properly. Like other adults, they need to get enough protein, energy, and iron and avoid obesity. They also have to pay particular attention to getting enough calcium to reduce the risk of osteoporosis, which is a condition in which bones become fragile and can break.[22]

THE NUTRITION TRANSITION

In high-income countries, people tend to eat more manufactured foods. These foods are likely to be higher in calories, higher in fat, and contain more sugar than locally produced foods. As people in low- and middle-income countries have more disposable income, they also tend to change their eating habits and move from locally produced foods to more processed foods. This transition, often referred to as "the nutrition transition"[23] has already occurred in better-off countries and among better-off people in poor countries. It is now spreading to other people in developing countries.[23] It is linked with a growing trend toward diet related non-communicable diseases, which is discussed in Chapter 12.[23]

TABLE 8-5 Selected Nutritional Needs in Pregnancy

Protein is needed for muscles, uterus, breasts, blood supply, and baby's tissues. Low protein intake is related to smaller-than-average weight babies who may have health problems.

Folate is required to build protein tissues. Low folate levels are linked to birth defects, such as spina bifida.

Calcium is needed by the baby for strong bones. If calcium is not supplied by the mother's diet, calcium is taken from the mother's bones for the baby.

Low **Zinc** levels during pregnancy can cause long labor and small babies who may have health problems.

Iron deficiency is common in pregnant women. Both mother and baby need iron for their developing blood supplies.

Source: Data with permission from the Ohio State University Extension, Fact Sheet, Nutritional Needs of Pregnancy. Available at: http://ohioline.osu.edu/mob-fact/0001.html. Accessed November 1, 2006.

THE NUTRITIONAL STATE OF THE WORLD

There has been some important progress in reducing the burden of malnutrition over the last decade. The rate of children younger than five years in developing countries who are underweight, for example, fell from 32% to 28%.[24] In addition, there were a number of countries that were able to reduce levels of malnutrition in their under-five children by 25% or more, including Bangladesh, China, Indonesia, Mexico, and Vietnam.[24] Important progress has been made in addressing micronutrient deficiency, as well. The number of households using iodized salt has increased from about 20% in 1990 to about 70% today.[24] There has also been a dramatic increase in the share of the world's children who receive Vitamin A supplements, which now stands at about 50%. As importantly, this supplementation is associated with saving the lives of about 300,000 young children a year.[24]

Despite this progress, however, the nutritional state of the world is, in many respects, deplorable. About 800 million people worldwide are malnourished to at least some degree.[25] More than 25% of the under-five children in developing countries are moderately or severely underweight and about 30% are moderately or severely stunted.[26] Many poor women in the world are also underweight. A large share of the poor women and children in the world also suffer from deficiencies in important micronutrients. Nutritional problems remain a fundamental cause of ill health and of premature death for infants, children, and pregnant women. The economic costs of undernutrition are great.

The section that follows examines the burden of nutrition disorders that relate to undernutrition and reviews undernutrition as a risk factor for ill health. For undernutrition and for deficiencies in vitamin A, iodine, iron, and zinc, it looks first at the prevalence of deficiencies and then examines the contribution of each issue to the global burden of disease. Table 8-6 summarizes the deaths that are directly attributable to these nutritional concerns. The much larger number of deaths and DALYs that are precipitated by these problems are addressed in the text that follows.

Undernutrition

Undernutrition is still disturbingly prevalent. Almost 150 million children, or about 27% of the children younger than five years in low- and middle-income countries are stunted.[21] Almost 130 million children, or about 23% of the children younger than five years in those countries are underweight.[21]

The rates of wasting and stunting vary considerably, both across countries and within countries. However, South Asia and Sub-Saharan Africa have the highest rates of undernourished children younger than five years. About 46% of the under-five children in South Asia are moderately or severely underweight and about 44% of the under-five children in that region are moderately or severely stunted.[26] In fact, it is estimated that in South Asia there are almost 90 million children who are younger than five years who are underweight and just over 90 million children younger than five years who are stunted.[1] In Sub-Saharan Africa, almost 40% of the under-five children are severely or moderately

stunted and about 30% are moderately or severely underweight.[2,21] Table 8-7 shows the prevalence of underweight children by region.

Only about 0.5% of the total deaths in low- and middle-income countries are directly due to undernutrition, referred to as "protein-energy malnutrition" in the studies on the global burden of disease.[27] About 1% of the DALYs lost are directly due to undernutrition.[28] However, undernutrition, as discussed earlier, is an exceptionally important risk factor for illness, disability, and death from other causes. It has been estimated, for example, that 5–16% of the illness from pneumonia, diarrhea, and malaria is directly attributable to undernutrition and the extent to which it increases the susceptibility to illness.[9] Moreover, it has also been estimated that 44–60% of the deaths due to measles, malaria, pneumonia, and diarrhea are also attributable to undernutrition, and 53% of these deaths could be eliminated if these children were not undernourished.[9]

Low Birthweight

Given the extent of undernutrition in South Asia, it should not be a surprise that about 30% of the babies born in South Asia are born with low birth weight. The Middle East, North Africa, and Sub-Saharan Africa have the next highest prevalence of low birth weight, at about 15%.[29] More than 20 million low birthweight babies are born each year in the developing countries.[29] Table 8-8 shows the prevalence of low birth weight by region.

About 2.5% of the total deaths that occur in low- and middle-income countries are attributable to low birth weight.[27] About 3% of the DALYs lost in low- and middle-income countries are attributable to low birth weight.[28] The

---

TABLE 8-6 Nutrition-Related Deaths in Children Under Five Years, by Region, 2001, in Thousands

Region	Undernutrition	Vitamin A	Iron Deficiency Anemia	Zinc Deficiency
East Asia & Pacific	125	11	18	15
Europe & Central Asia	14	0	3	4
Latin America & the Caribbean	22	5	10	15
Middle East & No. Africa	305	70	10	94
South Asia	870	157	66	252
Sub-Saharan Africa	1334	383	21	400

Note: Underweight is weight for age less than 1 standard deviation

Source: Adapted with permission from The World Bank. Caulfield LE, Richard SA, Rivera JA, Musgrove P, Black RE. Stunting, wasting, and micronutrient disorders. In: Jamison DT, Breman JG, Measham AR, et al., eds. *Disease Control Priorities in Developing Countries.* New York: Oxford University Press; 2006:552.

difference between the two figures stems from the illness and disability that many low birth weight children will face, if they do survive.

Vitamin A

More than 250 million children worldwide suffer from vitamin A deficiency.[3] The prevalence of vitamin A deficiency among children younger than 72 months of age in the developing world varies from a low of about 20% in Central America and the Caribbean to more than 50% in South Asia. In India alone, more than 60% of the children younger than 72 months of age are vitamin A deficient.[30] As shown in Table 8-9, more than 40% of the children of this age in Sub-Saharan Africa are also vitamin A deficient.

Vitamin A deficiency has an enormous impact on morbidity, disability, and deaths in young children. It has been estimated that 20–24% of the deaths from measles, diarrhea, and malaria, or 630,000 deaths each year, are attributable to vitamin A deficiency.[31] In addition, it is estimated that between 250,000 and 500,000 children each year are blinded due to vitamin A deficiency.[31]

Iodine

Iodine deficiency disorders are estimated to affect more than 70 million people worldwide.[32] The highest rates of such disorders are found in the Eastern Mediterranean region and in Africa, where about 30% of the population suffers from goiter. This is followed by South Asia, where more than 20% of the population has goiter.[33]

Iodine deficiency is associated with only a small number of deaths. However, such deficiencies are associated with substantial DALYs lost in low- and middle-income countries, equal to about the same amount as chlamydia, syphilis, or intestinal worms.[34] The DALYs lost from iodine deficiency disorder are about 30% as many DALYs as are lost from iron deficiency anemia in low- and middle-income countries.[34]

Iron

About 500 million women of childbearing age worldwide, equal to about 40% of all women aged 15–49 in the developing world, are anemic.[35] This includes about 60% of all pregnant women.[36] The highest prevalence among women appears to be in the Middle East, North Africa, and South Asia.[36] It is estimated that as many as 80% of the pregnant women in South Asia are anemic.[37] It is also estimated that about 45% of all children younger than five years in the developing world are iron deficient.[38] Twenty countries have prevalence rates of iron deficiency among their children who are younger than 5 of more than 70%. This includes a num-

TABLE 8-7 Prevalence of Underweight in Low- and Middle-Income Countries, by Region, Children Under Five Years

Region	Prevalence Rate of Underweight
East Asia & Pacific	18
Europe & Central Asia	6
Latin America & the Caribbean	6
Middle East & No. Africa	21
South Asia	48
Sub-Saharan Africa	32

Note: Underweight is weight for age less than 2 standard deviations

Source: Adapted with permission from The World Bank. Caulfield LE, Richard SA, Rivera JA, Musgrove P, Black RE. Stunting, wasting, and micronutrient disorders. In: Jamison DT, Breman JG, Measham AR, et al., eds. *Disease Control Priorities in Developing Countries.* New York: Oxford University Press; 2006:552.

TABLE 8-8 Prevalence of Low Birth Weight, Low- and Middle-Income Countries, 2001

Region	Percent of Babies Born with Low Birth Weight
East Asia & Pacific	7
Europe & Central Asia	6
Latin America & the Caribbean	8
Middle East & No. Africa	14
South Asia	28
Sub-Saharan Africa	13

Source: Adapted with permission from The World Bank. *Repositioning Nutrition as Central to Development.* Washington, DC: World Bank; 2006:47.

ber of countries in Sub-Saharan Africa in which more than 80% of such children are iron deficient.[38]

Iron deficiency anemia is thought to be the underlying factor related to about 840,000 maternal and perinatal deaths per year.[13] It is also estimated that this anemia is the direct cause of 134,000 deaths a year of young children.[13] The number of deaths directly relating to iron deficiency anemia in low- and middle-income countries is about the same as the total number of deaths caused by a group of six tropical diseases. It is also similar to the deaths caused individually

TABLE 8-9 Prevalence of Vitamin A, Iron, and Zinc Deficiency in Children Under Five Years, Low- and Middle-Income Countries, 2001, by Region

Region	Vitamin A	Iron	Zinc
East Asia & Pacific	11	40	7
Europe & Central Asia	<1	22	10
Latin America & the Caribbean	15	46	33
Middle East & No. Africa	18	63	46
South Asia	40	75	79
Sub-Saharan Africa	32	60	50

Source: Adapted with permission from The World Bank. Caulfield LE, Richard SA, Rivera JA, Musgrove P, Black RE. Stunting, wasting, and micronutrient disorders. In: Jamison DT, Breman JG, Measham AR, et al., eds. *Disease Control Priorities in Developing Countries.* New York: Oxford University Press; 2006:552.

by prostate, bladder, and pancreatic cancer.[27] About 0.7% of the total DALYs lost in low- and middle-income countries is related to iron deficiency anemia. This is similar to the DALYs lost in these countries due to sexually transmitted diseases (not including HIV), stomach cancer, schizophrenia, or asthma.[34]

Zinc

The data on zinc deficiency are not as well established as that on the other micronutrient deficiencies noted earlier; however, a study has estimated the prevalence rate of zinc deficiency by region for children younger than five years. Prevalence in low- and middle-income regions ranges from a low of 7% in the East Asia and the Pacific Region to almost 80% of the children younger than five years in South Asia. In high-income countries, it is estimated that only about 5% of the children younger than 5 are zinc deficient.[9] The information available on deaths and DALYs for zinc deficiency has not been calculated as part of recent studies of the burden of disease. However, other studies have suggested that as many as 800,000 deaths occur every year in children younger than 5 from diarrhea, pneumonia, and malaria as a result of deficiencies in zinc.[13]

NUTRITION, HEALTH, AND ECONOMIC DEVELOPMENT

Nutrition has an important bearing on the economic development prospects of people, communities, and countries. In some of the early thinking about economic development, many economists saw nutrition as something that people consumed, but they did not see it as a "productive" investment. However, as we will see later, nutrition is an extremely important contributor to human health, the development of human intellectual and biological potential, and therefore, has an extremely important link with what people learn, their strength and ability to use their own labor, and other factors relating to their potential productivity. The following comments follow the life cycle.

First, nutritional deficits can take an enormous toll on maternal health, with important economic consequences. Women are responsible for child care in most low- and middle-income countries. In addition, they often contribute to household income. The death of a woman in the prime of her life, in childbirth, due to undernutrition or deficiencies in iron or vitamin A, can leave poor families with needs for child care they can not meet and with reduced income. It is common, in fact, in poor families in low-income countries for very young children to die not long after their mothers die.

In addition, we have seen that low birthweight is a powerful predictor of the future productivity of a child and that a number of forms of malnutrition contribute to the failure of infants and children to grow or to achieve their full mental potential. Children who are malnourished and small in stature enroll in schools at lower rates or later in age than students who are perceived by their parents to be normal in size. Children who are malnourished have IQs that are lower than students who are properly nourished. These malnourished students are less attentive in class and less able to learn than other students. Children who are malnourished fall ill more than well-nourished children. Thus, they miss more school, learn less from school, and are much more likely than well-nourished children to drop out of school, with its attendant economic consequences.

Nutritional status also plays an important part in the productivity of adults. Numerous studies have shown that improvements in nutritional status, such as eliminating iron deficiency anemia, can improve worker productivity by 5–15%.[39] The contribution of nutrition to maintaining good health also has important economic returns. It helps people to avoid disease and the costs associated with treating disease.

Moreover, through its impact on health, nutritional status also has an important bearing on life expectancy. Infants and children who are better nourished live longer than those who are poorly nourished, and they also can contribute to the economy for longer. Adults who are properly nourished get sick less and for shorter periods, live longer, and work more years than adults who are not well nourished. Thus, they, too, can make more contributions to the economy than people who are not well nourished.

A look at social and economic history also speaks to the importance of nutrition to economic development. Studies that have been done of the economic development of England showed that improvements in nutritional status of adults in England in the late 19th century were important to improving the stature and strength of workers, their health, and their economic outputs.[40] Other studies have shown that there is a correlation between height and wages. Rubber tappers in Indonesia significantly improved the amount of rubber they could tap when their anemia was treated with iron supplements, and road construction workers in Kenya were 4–12.5% more productive after getting calorie supplements.[41] Female mill workers in China increased their production efficiency by 17% after being given iron supplements for 12 weeks.[42]

CASE STUDIES

In fact, there are a number of investments in improving nutrition status on a large scale that have made a significant difference to the communities in which they took place. One of the best known is the Tamil Nadu Nutrition Project in India. The CHILD Project in Uganda also appears promising. China has also made considerable progress in the last 10 years in controlling iodine deficiency.

Tamil Nadu State, India[43]

Background

The Tamil Nadu Integrated Nutrition Project in India is one of the most important efforts ever undertaken to improve nutritional status on a large scale. This project began in 1980 in the South Indian state of Tamil Nadu. It aimed at improving the nutritional status of poor women and children in the rural areas of the state through a set of well-focused interventions.

These specific goals were set for several reasons. First, the levels of malnutrition in poor women and children in Tamil Nadu were very high at the time the project was conceived. Second, malnutrition persisted despite considerable investments that had already been undertaken to improve nutrition status. Third, studies that had been done on those investments showed that they were not working as planned and were not cost-effective. Rather, the children who needed assistance most were not getting it. In addition, food that was given to children at feeding centers that was meant to supplement other food often replaced that food or was taken home and consumed by family members other than the intended children. The form of the food supplement was also difficult for children to eat. Moreover, little attention had been paid to

nutrition education for families or to health investments that could complement the investments made in nutrition.

The project design was based on the idea that much of the malnutrition present in Tamil Nadu was because of inappropriate child care practices, rather than just a lack of money to buy food. Thus, the project focused considerable attention on nutrition education and efforts to improve care and feeding practices for young children. In addition, because deficits at an early age often produce irreversible damage to children's physical and mental development, project interventions focused on pregnant and lactating women and on children younger than 3 years of age.

The Intervention

In line with this approach, the project included a package of services that were delivered by health and nutrition workers that consisted of nutrition education, primary health care, supplementary on-site feeding for children who were not growing properly, vitamin A supplementation, periodic de-worming, education of mothers for managing childhood diarrhea, and the supplementary feeding of a small number of women.

An important innovation of the project was that it used growth monitoring of the children as a device for mobilizing community action. Groups of mothers met regularly to weigh their young children. They then plotted their weight- for-age on a growth chart. Together with the community nutrition worker, they identified which children were not growing properly. A related innovation of great importance was that supplementary feeding was targeted only to the children identified as faltering. In addition, children received food supplements only while they were not growing well. This was done in conjunction with nutrition education for mothers. The intent of this approach was that short-term feeding, combined with better child care practices, could return the child to normal growth. This was a major change compared with previous practice in which supplementary feeding was more universal and longer term.

Impact

The nutrition interventions of the project were largely implemented as planned, but the health efforts were not fully implemented. Nonetheless, through careful evaluation the project was shown to have reduced significantly the levels of malnutrition of the targeted children. These improvements also continued over a substantial time, suggesting that the gains of the project were sustainable. The project was also more cost-effective than other investments that had tried to achieve similar aims in India.

Lessons Learned

This project was pioneering and revealed some very important lessons, including:

- Growth monitoring, coupled with short term supplementary feeding of children who are faltering, can be a cost effective way of improving nutritional status
- More universal and longer term feeding of children is not necessary to achieve improvements in nutrition
- Women can be organized to participate actively in growth monitoring efforts
- Nutrition education can have a permanent and sustainable impact on child care and child feeding practices, even in the absence of other interventions

Uganda CHILD Project[45]

Background

The Community Home Initiative for Long Term Development (CHILD Project) began in Uganda in 2001. This project focused on early childhood development. It sought to reduce the prevalence of underweight children a third, address children's psychosocial needs, empower women, and help to raise their income. To achieve these aims, the project supported health and nutrition education, extensive outreach on child rearing and child feeding practices, and growth monitoring and immunization for infants and young children. It also supported credit and savings programs for women.

The Intervention

This project contained a number of innovative features. First, it supported the establishment and operation of "Child's Days." These were events held every 6 months that would be like a "festival for child health." On Child's Days, families could bring their children to selected locations where the children would receive in one place, at one time, an integrated package of health and nutrition services. In many developing countries, such services would normally not be available in an integrated way. Second, the project included a grant fund to support creative ideas that communities would propose to improve child development in their area. Third, the project included another fund that could support investments by women in activities that could generate income. The aim of this was to help women to earn more income, become more empowered, and in conjunction with their improved knowledge of child care practices, use some of their new income to improve the health and nutrition of their children.

Impact

The project has been associated with reductions in severe and moderate malnutrition in all four of the regions in which it was implemented among children from birth to 3 years of age. These fell from 24.4% to 17.1% and from 10.3% to 5.1%, respectively. The project was also associated in three of the four regions with significant reductions in severe and moderate malnutrition among children aged 3 to 6 years. The project also increased the knowledge of adults of appropriate child care and child feeding practices and the knowledge of adults of the need to exclusively breastfeed children for the first 6 months by almost 14%. There was also an increase in the awareness of children's dietary needs and the importance of enriching foods for infants and young children. Other positive benefits that can be attributed to the project include an 18% increase in improved sanitation and hygiene practices, a rise in immunization rates by 23%, increased participation by men in child rearing, and an increase of 13.6% and 38.7% for vitamin A supplementation and de-worming practices.

Lessons Learned

Although it is too early in the life of the project to draw definitive lessons from it, the efforts to date suggest that a number of possible lessons may emerge from this project, most of which are consistent with the lessons from the Tamil Nadu Integrated Nutrition Project. These include:

- the importance of embedding projects in the community
- the centrality of having events around which one could mobilize the community, in this case, Child's Days
- the importance of effective mass communication to support significant behavior change about child rearing and feeding practices
- the value of integrating health and nutrition efforts in a single program
- the value of having good monitoring and evaluation of the project, so that it can be better managed and so that lessons can emerge from it

The Challenge of Iodine Deficiency Disease in China

Background

China bears the heaviest burden of iodine deficiency in the world. In 1995, 20% of children aged 8 to 10 showed signs of goiter. Overall, some 400 million people in China were estimated to be at risk of iodine deficiency disorders, constituting 40% of the global total. Fortunately, iodine deficiency can be simply remedied by adding iodine to salt, a cheap and universally consumed food. Implementing this in a relatively poor and vast country like China, however, is far from simple.

The Intervention

Scientific evidence linking iodine deficiency to mental impairment was seen by the Chinese government as a threat to its one-child-per-family policy, and so the government strengthened its resolve to tackle this widespread health risk. In 1993, China launched the National Iodine Deficiency Disorders Elimination Program, with technical and financial assistance from the donor-funded Iodine Deficiency Disorders Control Project. The public needed to be made aware of the risk of iodine deficiency, especially in regions where goiter was so common that it was regarded as normal. A nationwide public education campaign was launched, using posters on buses, newspaper editorials, and television documentaries to inform consumers and persuade them to switch to iodized salt. Provincial governors ensured that government education efforts reached even the most remote villages. The supply of iodized salt was increased by building 112 new salt iodation factories and enhancing capacity at 55 existing ones. Bulk packaging systems were installed to complement 147 new retail packaging centers, with packaging designed to help consumers easily recognize iodized salt. The sale of non-iodized salt was banned, and technological assistance was provided to salt producers to adopt iodation. Salt quality was monitored, both at production, where the amount of iodine added needs to be just right, and in distribution and sales, because iodine in salt dissipates easily, reducing the shelf life of iodized salt. China's nationally controlled network of production and distribution made licensing and enforcement of legislation easier.

The Impact

By 1999, iodized salt was reaching 94% of the country, compared to 80% in 1995. The quality of iodized salt also improved markedly. As a result, iodine deficiency was reduced dramatically, and goiter rates for children aged 8 to 10 fell from 20.4% in 1995 to 8.8% in 1999.[44]

Costs and Benefits

Fortifying salt with iodine costs about 2 to 7 cents per kilogram, or less than 5% of the retail price of salt in most countries. The Chinese government invested approximately $152 million in the program, recovering some of this cost by rais-

ing the price of iodized salt. The World Bank, one of several donors, deemed the project extremely cost-effective.

Lessons Learned

China's success in reducing iodine deficiency offers valuable lessons for future efforts to reduce through fortification other micronutrient deficiencies such as iron and vitamin A. The government made a firm and long-standing commitment to tackle the problem and brought about administrative, legal, technical, and socio-cultural changes that were needed to do so. Donor coordination was strong and effective and was managed by the Chinese government and the donors themselves, and the major players offered mutual support across all activities. The financing strategy was clearly defined from the start. The salt industry seized the opportunity of the investment in eliminating iodine deficiency to restructure and modernize the industry, gaining a firmer commercial footing and positioning itself to compete in the international market, given its cost advantages.

China's iodation program continues, with special targeting of resources on areas where the consumption of iodized salt is particularly low, usually in poor and remote mountainous regions where residents see iodized salt as too costly, especially when salt can be obtained cheaply from local salt hills, dried lakes, or the sea. Research will be needed to determine the best way to ensure iodine intake in these areas—through price subsidies, iodation of well or irrigation water, or even iodine capsules or injections, in the case of nomadic peoples. Through a variety of approaches, China is fast approaching the day when iodine deficiency will be unknown throughout its population. A more detailed review of this case is available in *Case Studies in Global Health: Millions Saved.*

ADDRESSING FUTURE NUTRITION CHALLENGES

The world has made some progress in the last several decades in addressing key nutrition problems, as reflected in the case studies and as noted earlier. Nonetheless, as we have seen, the overall state of the world's nutrition still faces numerous and serious gaps. This is especially so in South Asia and Sub-Saharan Africa. At the present rate of progress in addressing those gaps, the world will not meet the MDGs that relate to nutrition. What steps will have to be taken to speed the world's progress on nutrition? These are discussed briefly below.

It has already been noted that knowledge and behaviors are important determinants of what foods people eat, how they cook them, and how they consume them. Studies have shown that people can improve what they eat, how they cook, and how they eat their food by improvements in knowledge, even in the absence of improvements in income.[46] Nutrition education needs to be spread much more widely and in more appropriate ways to promote appropriate breastfeeding and complementary feeding and to help people eat better and more nutritious foods.

The two-way relationship between infection, disease, and nutrition status has been noted. Many infections and diseases reduce one's ability to eat or ability to absorb food. At the same time, poor nutritional status reduces immunity to disease. To set the foundation for improvements in the nutritional status of poor people in the developing world, especially poor infants, children, and women, it is very important to improve the control of parasitic infections such as hookworm, and to also control diarrheal diseases, malaria, and measles. Of course, doing this will also demand renewed efforts at health education and improvements in water supply and sanitation.

There will be some people who will simply not eat enough food or enough of the right foods, largely because of income gaps. These problems are also the result of, or are compounded by, natural disaster and conflict. Under these circumstances, it may be necessary that people receive food supplements. Alternatively, they may receive vouchers for food, such as "food stamps," which are cash transfers that can be used only to buy certain health and nutrition services, or the right to buy certain foods at reduced prices.

Vitamin and mineral supplementation is widespread in the world, is not expensive, and is often used as a way of improving the micronutrient status of large numbers of people, especially infants, children, and pregnant and lactating mothers. These can be given in capsules or syrups. Vitamin A should be given twice per year and should be integrated with child survival and other health services to minimize the cost of distribution.[47] In the last decade, vitamin A has been given orally to infants and children during national polio immunization days in many countries. These efforts can be expanded. At the same time, additional and carefully monitored efforts can be made to provide iron and folate to pregnant women. Unfortunately, these efforts have not worked as well as planned and need to be carefully reviewed and refined to enhance both coverage of supplementation and the extent to which women take the pills they do get.

Food fortification is practiced in many countries for a number of micronutrients. In fact, fortification in the industrialized countries has contributed greatly to the disappearance of several deficiencies. The fortification of salt with iodine is a very widespread practice and is very inexpensive,

as we have seen in the China case noted earlier. Nearly two thirds of the world now consumes iodized salt and the impact of fortification of salt could be further expanded through its double fortification with iron, as well as iodine. In addition, many different food products can be fortified. The key to effective fortification is to find a food product that is very widely consumed, for which there are no technical impediments to fortification, and for which fortification is inexpensive.[48] Thus, increasingly one can see flour, cooking oil, margarine, and other products fortified, as well as salt. Fortification can cost as little as three to five cents per person reached per year.[49] Clearly, fortification is a good way to harness the resources of commercial marketing networks to enhance the health of the population. Given the difficulties of iron supplementation, it may be that the most effective way of reducing iron deficiency in women is to operate an effective program of fortification for iron and folic acid.

If the world is to do better in nutrition, it will also have to take a number of policy steps. First, policy makers who work both globally and on individual countries need to understand the exceptional importance of nutrition to good health and human productivity and act accordingly. More than 50% of the child deaths globally are associated with nutritional causes. In addition, low cost, highly effective solutions are available to deal with a number of critical nutrition issues, but they are not being implemented sufficiently. Thus, much greater attention needs to be paid by all concerned parties to nutrition as an underlying health issue. Nutrition does not fit neatly into governmental bureaucracies because it touches many government units, such as agriculture, health, and education. Thus, governments will also need to think creatively about how to ensure that there are government units accountable and responsible for promoting enhanced approaches to nutrition.

Improving government policy and action on nutrition will also require a good understanding of the nature of the nutrition problem in different settings. Nutritional concerns will vary considerably by income group, gender, and ethnicity, and solutions to these problems will need to be carefully crafted to local circumstances. In addition, governments need to work more effectively with the food industry to improve the way in which foods are fortified. Legal and financial arrangements need to be made in many countries so that more fortification can take place and the demand for fortified foods will be increased. We have also seen the power in TINP, for example, of focusing efforts on community-based action, in which affected people are involved in the design, implementation, and oversight of nutrition activities.

Although there is much knowledge of "what works" in nutrition, there are also other areas in which additional knowledge could fill important gaps. The world needs to continue gathering scientific knowledge about the causes and consequences of malnutrition and different ways in which it can be addressed. It would be very valuable to the world's nutrition status and health if more easy to make, nutritious, and inexpensive food supplements were available; if better formulas were available for some of the vitamin and mineral supplements that could be given less frequently, very cheaply and without side effects; and, if additional cost-effective ways were found for fortifying foods.

Lastly, it is important for all societies to make the health and nutritional well-being of their citizens a national priority. One way to do this would be to create partnerships of civil society, government, and the private sector that can work together to identify nutrition issues, plan on how they can best be addressed, and then collaborate with each other and with communities to implement solutions to these problems.

MAIN MESSAGES

Nutritional status is a major determinant of health status. It has an important bearing on the health of pregnant women and of pregnancy outcomes. It is a major determinant of the birthweight of children, how children grow, and the extent to which their cognitive functions develop properly. Nutrition status is also closely linked with the strength of one's immune system and one's ability to stay healthy.

In addition, nutritional status has an important bearing on people's capacity to learn and on their productivity. Nutritional deficits can seriously hamper the ability of children to attend school, concentrate while they are there, and learn effectively. Numerous studies have shown that workers who are anemic produce less than workers who do not suffer from iron deficiency anemia.

From the global health perspective, the most important nutritional concerns are whether or not people get enough of the right foods to have sufficient energy and protein and the extent to which people have a sufficient intake of vitamin A, iodine, iron, and zinc. The importance of these nutrients and micronutrients varies with the place of people in their life cycle, with needs differing for adolescents, pregnant and lactating women, infants, children, adults, and older adults.

About 800 million people in the world today suffer from energy and protein malnutrition and deficiencies in key micronutrients. These problems often stem from people's lack of income to purchase enough food or food of appropriate quality. However, these problems also relate to culture, customs, and eating behaviors. Malnutrition disproportionately affects poor people, marginalized people, and females.

Energy and protein malnutrition is associated with being underweight, failing to grow properly, and a weakening of immunity. Vitamin A deficiency is well known for its impact on vision, but is also closely associated with general immunity and child growth. The lack of iron is the primary cause of iron deficiency anemia, which leads to weakness and fatigue; however, it is also associated with maternal morbidity and mortality, poor and stunted growth in children, and poor mental development in children, as well. The lack of iodine causes thyroid problems, goiter, and important deficits in mental abilities. Iodine is also essential for proper child growth. The lack of zinc is associated with general immunity, the growth of children, and the development of children's cognitive and motor abilities. About 50% of the child deaths in the world today are associated with malnutrition.

There are cost-effective solutions to the most important nutritional concerns. People can wash their hands more frequently with soap to reduce the rate of infections and diarrhea that take such terrible tolls on nutritional status. Efforts can be enhanced to promote exclusive breastfeeding for 6 months, followed by the appropriate complementary feeding. Food supplements can be given to those people who are not getting enough protein and energy. Nutritional supplements can be provided for vitamin A and iron. Salt can be fortified with iodine. Families can also learn, even in the absence of income gains, to improve what they eat. These actions will be most successful if they are tied to approaches that are taken by communities.

Finally, it is critical to remember that the "window of opportunity" for ensuring that children are well-nourished and develop properly is a small one. It begins at conception and lasts until the children are about 2 years of age. Damage done to the child's development in this period is largely irreversible. The most critical interventions, therefore, are to:

- ensure that pregnant women are well-nourished and have sufficient amounts of needed micronutrients
- promote exclusive breastfeeding for all children until they are 6 months of age
- encourage the provision of appropriate complementary foods for infants beginning at 6 months of age
- fight infection and illness through better hygiene, improved water and sanitation, and appropriate food and health behaviors
- support effective programs in supplementation and fortification, based on nutritional needs at the local level and embed them in community-based approaches
- focus on South Asia and Sub-Saharan Africa

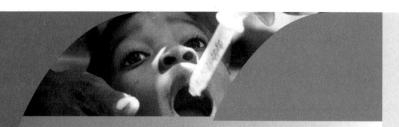

Study Questions

1. What is the importance of nutrition to the MDGs?

2. What are "stunting" and "wasting?"

3. What are some of the direct and indirect causes of undernutrition?

4. What are the links between nutrition and health?

5. How are growth charts used to gauge nutrition status?

6. What are the most important micronutrient deficiencies and what health problems do they cause?

7. Why is anemia a special risk in pregnancy?

8. Why is exclusive breastfeeding for the first 6 months so important?

9. What parts of the world have the worst nutritional problems?

10. What are the links between nutrition and economic development?

REFERENCES

1. DeOnis M, Blossner M, Borghi E, Frongillo E, Morris R. Methodology for estimating regional and global trends of child malnutrition. *Int J Epidemiol.* 2004;33:1260–1270.

2. DeOnis M, Blossner M, Borghi E, Frongillo E, Morris R. Estimates of global prevalence of childhood underweight in 1990 and 2015. *JAMA.* 2004;291(21):2600–2606.

3. Black RE, Morris SS, Bryce J. Where and why are 10 million children dying every year? *Lancet.* 2003;361(9376):2226–2234.

4. Ezzati M, Vander Hoorn S, Lopez AD, et al. Comparative quantification of mortality and burden of disease attributable to selected risk factors. In: Lopez AD, Mathers CD, Ezzati M, Jamison DT, Murray CJL, eds. *Global Burden of Disease and Risk Factors.* New York: Oxford University Press; 2006:251.

5. UNICEF and The Micronutrient Initiative. *Vitamin and Mineral Deficiency: A Global Progress Report.* Ottawa.

6. Copenhagen Consensus Center. Outcome and Results of Copenhagen Consensus 2006—A United Nations Perspective. Available at: http://www.copenhagenconsensus.com/Default.aspx?ID=675. Accessed July 14, 2006.

7. ACC/SCN. *Fifth Report on the World Nutrition Situation.* Geneva: United Nations Administrative Committee on Coordination/Sub-Committee on Nutrition; 2004.

8. UNICEF. *State of the World's Children: Focus of Nutrition.* New York City: Oxford University Press; 1998:23–25.

9. Caulfield LE, Richard SA, Rivera JA, Musgrove P, Black RE. Stunting, wasting, and micronutrient disorders. In: Jamison DT, Breman JG, Measham AR, et al., eds. *Disease Control Priorities in Developing Countries.* 2nd ed. New York: Oxford University Press and The World Bank; 2006:552.

10. GP Notebook: Xerophthalmia. Available at: www.gpnotebook.co.uk/cache/664403984.htm. Accessed July 5, 2006.

11. West Jr. KP, Vitamin A deficiency as a preventable cause of maternal mortality in undernourished societies: plausibility and next steps. *Int J Gynaecol Obstet.* 2004;85(Suppl 1):S24–27.

12. Government of Australia. Iodine Explained. Available at: http://www.betterhealth.vic.gov.au/BHCV2/bhcarticles.nsf/pages/Iodine_explained?open. Accessed June 27, 2006.

13. Caulfield LE, Richard SA, Rivera JA, Musgrove P, Black RE. Stunting, wasting, and micronutrient disorders. In: Jamison DT, Breman JG, Measham AR, et al., eds. *Disease Control Priorities in Developing Countries.* 2nd ed. New York: Oxford University Press; 2006:554.

14. World Bank. *Repositioning Nutrition as Central to Development.* Washington, DC: The World Bank; 2006:23.

15. Mercer LP, Wests Jr. KP. Nutrient Information: Iodine. Available at: http://nutrition.org/nutinfo/content/iodi.shtml. Accessed July 14, 2004.

16. Hunt J. Nutrient Information: Iron. Available at: http://nutrition.org/nutinfo/content/iron2.shtml. Accessed July 14, 2004.

17. Cousins RJ. Nutrient Information: Zinc. Available at: http://jn.nutrition.org/nutinfo/. Accessed July 29, 2006.

18. Brown KH, Wuehler SE. The Micronutrient Initiative. Ottawa: The Micronutrient Initiative; 2000:7.

19. Ohio State University. Ohio State University Extension Fact Sheet: Nutritional Needs of Pregnancy. Available at: http://ohioline.osu.edu/mobfact/0001.html. Accessed June 28, 2006.

20. International Food Policy Research Institute. The Life Cycle of Malnutrition. Available at: http://www.ifpri.org/pubs/books/ar1999/08-13LC.pdf. Accessed July 4, 2006.

21. The World Bank. *Repositioning Nutrition as Central to Development.* Washington, DC: The World Bank; 2006.

22. National Osteoporosis Foundation. Fast Facts. Available at: http://www.nof.org/osteoporosis/diseasefacts.htm. Accessed June 28, 2006.

23. Popkin BM. The nutrition transition in low-income countries: an emerging crisis. *Nutr Rev.* 1994;52(9):285–298.

24. UNICEF. Nutrition: What are the Challenges? Available at: http://www.unicef.org/nutrition/index_challenges.html. Accessed June 28, 2006.

25. Food and Agriculture Organization. *The State of Food Insecurity in the World.* Rome: Food and Agriculture Organization; 2004:5.

26. UNICEF. *State of the World's Children: Focus of Nutrition.* New York: Oxford University Press; 1998:109.

27. Lopez AD, Mathers CD, Murray CJL. The burden of disease and mortality by condition: data, methods, and results for 2001. In: Lopez AD, Mathers CD, Ezzati M, Jamison DT, Murray CJL, eds. *Global Burden of Disease and Risk Factors.* New York: Oxford University Press; 2006:126.

28. Lopez AD, Mathers CD, Murray CJL. The burden of disease and mortality by condition: data, methods, and results for 2001. In: Lopez AD, Mathers CD, Ezzati M, Jamison DT, Murray CJL, eds. *Global Burden of Disease and Risk Factors.* New York: Oxford University Press and The World Bank; 2006:180.

29. UNICEF and WHO (World Health Organization). *Low Birth Weight: Country, Regional, and Global Estimates.* New York: UNICEF; 2004.

30. UNICEF and MI (Micronutrient Initiative). *Vitamin and Mineral Deficiency: A Global Progress Report.* Ottawa.

31. Caulfield LE, Richard SA, Rivera JA, Musgrove P, Black RE. Stunting, wasting, and micronutrient disorders. In: Jamison DT, Breman JG, Measham AR, et al., eds. *Disease Control Priorities in Developing Countries.* 2nd ed. New York: Oxford University Press; 2006:553.

32. World Health Organization. World Health Organization Sets Out to Eliminate Iodine Deficiency Disorder. Available at: http://www.who.int/inf-pr-1999/en/pr99-wha17.html. Accessed July 15, 2006.

33. Mason JB, Lofti M, Dalmiya N, Sethuraman K, Deitchler M. *The Micronutrient Report.* Ottawa: Micronutrient Initiative; 2001.

34. Lopez AD, Mathers CD, Murray CJL. The burden of disease and mortality by condition: data, methods, and results for 2001. In: Lopez AD, Mathers CD, Ezzati M, Jamison DT, Murray CJL, eds. *Global Burden of Disease and Risk Factors.* New York: Oxford University Press; 2006:180–184.

35. UNICEF and MI (Micronutrient Initiative). *Vitamin and Mineral Deficiency: A Global Progress Report.* Ottawa.

36. Mason JB, Lofti M, Dalmiya N, Sethuraman K, Deitchler M. *The Micronutrient Report.* Ottawa: Micronutrient Initiative; 2001.

37. Mason JB, Lofti M, Dalmiya N, Sethuraman K, Deitchler M. *The Micronutrient Report.* Ottawa: Micronutrient Initiative; 2001.

38. UNICEF and MI (Micronutrient Initiative). *Vitamin and Mineral Deficiency: A Global Progress Report.* Ottawa.

39. Hunt JM. Reversing productivity losses from iron deficiency: the economic case. *J Nutr.* 2002;132(Suppl 4):794S–801S.

40. Fogel R. *New Sources and New Techniques for the Study of Secular Trends in Nutritional Status, Health, Mortality, and the Process of Aging.* National Board of Economic Research; 1991.

41. Wolgemuth JC, Latham MC, Hall A, Chesher A, Crompton DW. Worker productivity and the nutritional status of Kenyan road construction laborers. *Am J Clin Nutr.* 1982;36(1):68–78.

42. Li R, Chen X, Yan H, Deurenberg P, Garby L, Hautvast JG. Functional consequences of iron supplementation in iron-deficient female cotton mill workers in Beijing, China. *Am J Clin Nutr.* 1994;59(4):908–913.

43. The World Bank. *Impact Evaluation Report: Tamil Nadu Integrated Nutrition Project.* Washington, DC: The World Bank; 1994.

44. Goh, CC. Combating Iodine Deficiency: Lessons from China, Indonesia, and Madagascar. Food and Nutrition Bulletin 23, No. 3:280–290.

45. Skolnik R. Evaluation of the CHILD Project: Unpublished Paper for the World Bank; 2003.

46. Griffiths M, Dicken K, Favin M. *Promoting the Growth of Children: What Works: Rationale and Guidance for Programs.* Washington, DC: Human Development Department and The World Bank; 1996.

47. The World Bank. *Repositioning Nutrition as Central to Development.* Washington, DC: World Bank; 2006:72.

48. Lofti M, Merx R, Naber P, Van der Heuvel P. *Micronutrient Fortification of Foods: Current Prospectus, Research and Opportunities.* Ottawa: International Agriculture Centre; 1996.

49. The World Bank. *Repositioning Nutrition as Central to Development.* Washington, DC: The World Bank; 2006:132–135.

CHAPTER 9

Women's Health

By the end of this chapter the reader will be able to:

- Describe the importance of women's health to individuals, families, and communities
- Describe the determinants of women's health and how they vary in different settings
- Discuss the burden of disease for women worldwide, with a focus on women in low- and middle-income countries
- Describe critical challenges in improving women's health in low- and middle-income countries
- Describe some success stories in improving women's health and the lessons they suggest for other women's health efforts

VIGNETTES

Suneeta was pregnant with her first child. She lived in northern India where many families prefer to have sons rather than daughters, especially for their first-born child. Eager to have a son, Suneeta's husband took her to get a sonogram to determine the sex of the baby. When they learned the baby would be a girl, they decided that Suneeta should abort the fetus and try again to get pregnant, in hopes of having a boy.

Sarah lived in rural Pakistan and was pregnant with her second child. When she went into labor, Sarah called for the traditional birth attendant, as most women did in her town. As Sarah's labor continued, she and the birth attendant realized that the labor was complicated. Sarah needed to go to a hospital to deliver the baby. In this part of Pakistan, however, women could not be taken to hospitals without their husband's permission. Sarah's husband was working in another

city and was not available to give such permission. Several hours later, Sarah and the baby died at Sarah's home.

Carmen lived in a slum in Guatemala City, Guatemala. She was not married but became pregnant after relations with a man she had met several months before. In her culture, to become pregnant without being married was a source of great shame to a woman's family. Fearing the reaction of her family to her pregnancy, Carmen decided to get an abortion. Although abortions are illegal in Guatemala, except to save the life of the mother,[1] they are performed there by both licensed physicians and by unlicensed medical practitioners. Sarah could not afford the fee charged by a physician and went instead to an unlicensed abortionist. Carmen's abortion was not performed properly; she bled profusely as a result of the procedure, and she died before she could be taken to a hospital.

Elizabeth was a 15-year-old girl in Capetown, South Africa. She was a good student but came from a poor family and was always short of the money she needed to pay for school supplies, uniforms, and books. John had been eyeing Elizabeth for some time. He was 25 years old, had a good job, and was always interested in spending time with the young ladies at Elizabeth's school. At the start of the second semester, when Elizabeth was trying to get together the money for school, John convinced her to sleep with him in exchange for a small amount of money. Elizabeth had heard about HIV, but John convinced her that he was healthy and there was no need to use a condom. About a year later, Elizabeth fell ill, was given an HIV test, and turned out to be HIV positive.

THE IMPORTANCE OF WOMEN'S HEALTH

The vignettes above suggest several reasons why women's health issues must be given a prominent place in this book and in the global health agenda. First, women in many countries face a number of specific and serious health problems. Second, there are important and often unacceptable differences in the health of men and women in a large number of countries. Third, women play especially important roles in

---

TABLE 9-1 Key Linkages between the Millennium Development Goals and Women's Health

Goal 1—Eradicate Poverty and Hunger
Link—Poor health and nutritional status of women is both a cause and an effect of poverty. Enhancing the nutritional status of women will improve both their health and the health of their babies, with many attendant beneficial consequences for both.

Goal 2—Achieve Universal Primary Education
Link—Improving the health of females will enhance their enrollment in, attendance at, and performance in schools. Improving the educational attainments of females will lead to improvements in their health and the health of their children.

Goal 3—Promote Gender Equality and Empower Women
Link—Improvements in equity and empowerment will lead to better education for females, more income earning opportunities for them, and less violence against them, all of which will improve their health status.

Goal 4—Reduce Child Mortality
Link—An important share of child mortality is linked with poor health and nutritional status of the mother. Improving the health and nutritional status of the mother is the starting point for reducing the share of children born with low birth weight, a major contributor to child morbidity and mortality.

Goal 5—Improve Maternal Health
Link—This is directly connected to the health of women.

Goal 6—Combat HIV/AIDS, Malaria, and Other Diseases
Link—The share of the total number of HIV-affected people who are women is growing worldwide and HIV/AIDS is a major cause of illness, disability, and death for women. Combating HIV/AIDS would have a major impact on the health of females and, as a result, on their families as well.

Source: Author commentary on the UN Millennium Development Goals. Available at: http://www.un.org/millenniumgoals. Accessed July 10, 2006.

---

their families, and when they are in poor health it has important negative consequences on their families and especially on their children. Finally, many investments in improving the health of women would result, at relatively low cost, in a substantial number of deaths and DALYs averted.

In addition, the health of women is intimately linked with the MDGs.[2] Table 9-1 indicates how six of the eight goals have a powerful relationship to women's health.

The aim of this chapter is to give readers a sense of the health challenges that women face in the world today, with a particular focus on the health of poor women in low- and middle-income countries. First it will look at the determinants of women's health and then it will examine selected causes of women's illness, disability, and death and the risk factors related to them. The chapter will then review the costs and consequences of key women's health issues for both women and for society more generally. The chapter will also look at some success stories in improving women's health. The chapter will conclude by looking at the challenges that must be tackled in the future if the health of women is to be improved significantly and by recommending ways to address those challenges.

KEY DEFINITIONS

As one reviews the most important health issues that affect women worldwide, a number of terms will be used repeatedly. The most important of these are shown in Table 9-2.

THE DETERMINANTS OF WOMEN'S HEALTH

The determinants of a woman's health relate to both sex and gender. "Sex is biological."[3] It has to do with being born a female. "Gender is cultural."[3] Gender has to do with societal norms about the roles of women and their social position relative to men.[4] Some health issues are primarily determined by biology, such as the fact that women alone get ovarian cancer. Other women's health issues are determined mostly by social factors, such as sex selective abortion of female fetuses. Most women's health issues, however, are determined by a combination of biological and social determinants, such as the case of Sarah in the opening vignettes, who died in childbirth for a number of biological and social reasons that interacted. Further comments are given now on the biological and social determinants of women's health.

Biological Determinants

Women face a number of unique biological risks. One is iron deficiency anemia related to menstruation. Other risks are associated with pregnancy, including complications of

TABLE 9-2 Selected Definitions on Women's Health

Abortion—The premature expulsion or loss of embryo, which may be induced or spontaneous.

Cesarian Delivery (Section)—The surgical delivery of a fetus through abdominal incision.

Eclampsia—A serious, life-threatening condition in late pregnancy in which very high blood pressure can cause a woman to have seizures.

Family Planning—The conscious effort of couples to regulate the number and spacing of births through artificial and natural methods of contraception.

Female Genital Cutting—Traditional practices which are all related to the cutting of the female genital organs.

Gestational Diabetes—Diabetes that develops during pregnancy because of improper regulation of blood sugar.

Hemorrhage (related to pregnancy)—Significant and uncontrolled loss of blood, either internally or externally from the body. Antepartum (prenatal) hemorrhage after the 20th week of gestation but before delivery of the baby. Postpartum hemorrhage is the loss of 500ml or more of blood from the genital tract after delivery of the baby. Primary postpartum hemorrhage occurs in the first 24 hours after delivery.

Maternal Death—The death of a woman while pregnant, during delivery, or within 42 days of delivery.

Obstetric Fistula—An injury in the birth canal that allows leakage from the bladder or rectum into the vagina, leaving a woman permanently incontinent.

Preeclampsia (previously called toxemia)—A condition characterized by pregnancy-induced high blood pressure, protein in the urine, and swelling (edema) due to fluid retention.

Sepsis—A serious medical condition caused by a severe infection, leading to a systemic inflammatory response.

Sex Selective Abortion—The practice of aborting a fetus after a determination that the fetus is an undesired sex, typically female.

Source: Author created with data from: The University of New South Wales; WordNet: a lexical database; UKHealthCare; The White Ribbon Alliance [for Safe Motherhood]; Federal Ministry for Economic Cooperation and Development (BMZ); MayoClinic.com; The United Nations Population Fund; Wikipedia; The Queensland Government Health Professionals Resource.

the pregnancy itself, diseases that may be aggravated by pregnancy, and the effects of some unhealthy lifestyles, such as smoking, on pregnancy.[5] During pregnancy, there are a number of conditions, for example, that can cause women to become ill or to die, including hypertensive disorders of pregnancy. In addition, a woman can be left with a number of permanent disabilities related to pregnancy, including uterine prolapse and obstetric fistulas. Women can also die of preeclampsia or eclampsia. It is hemorrhage, however, that is the leading cause of maternal mortality. The conditions that can exacerbate pregnancy-related health risks could include malaria, hepatitis, tuberculosis, malnutrition, and obesity, as well as certain mental health issues, such as depression. Unsafe abortions lead to significant morbidity and mortality for women. In terms of the effects of lifestyles on pregnancy, it is clear that certain occupations and the use of alcohol, tobacco, and drugs are especially important to avoid during pregnancy.

Women are also biologically more susceptible to some sexually transmitted infections than men are, including to the HIV virus.[6] This relates to the fact that women have a greater mucosal area that is exposed during sexual relations than men have. There are also certain health conditions specific to women for biological reasons, such as uterine cancer or ovarian cancer, as mentioned above. There are other health conditions in which women have a disproportionate share of the burden of disease, such as breast cancer. As women age, they also have a higher rate of heart disease than men have, although it is diagnosed far less frequently.[4]

Social Determinants

The social determinants of a woman's health are also very important, especially in societies that favor males. These social determinants relate predominantly to gender norms, which assign different roles and values to males and females, usually to the disadvantage of females. In many societies, women's inferior status leads to social, health, and economic problems for women that men do not face.

The social determinants of health begin even before young women are born. In some societies where male preference is very strong, such as in India and in China, some families are determining the sex of their unborn children with the use of sonograms and then aborting females, especially for the birth of their first child.[7–9] This was the case for Suneeta in one of the opening vignettes.

Female infants are often breastfed less than boys of the same age and then fed less complementary food when they become toddlers.[10] In addition, young girls in many societies are also fed less than their male siblings. Older women in some cultures feed men first and then eat only the portions that are remaining. Others eat less nutritious food than the men in their family eat. Poor nutrition, often stemming partly from social causes, makes women more susceptible to illness. It also contributes to stunting and small pelvic size, which are hazards to the health of pregnant women.

There are a number of critical social issues that relate to women's sexual experiences. The low social status of women in many societies is linked to the physical and sexual abuse of women. Furthermore, male dominance means that women often have only a limited choice about when to have sexual relations, with whom, how to have them, and whether or not to use protection. As a result, women are often forced to have sex, often at young ages, and often without a condom or other contraceptives. For these social reasons, women face heightened risks of becoming pregnant, of having repeated pregnancies at close intervals, and of getting sexually transmitted diseases, including HIV/AIDS.

A dowry is the gifts that a bride's family gives to the family of a groom, and among the worst forms of violence against women is "dowry death." The data on mortality for young women in India suggest that there are a disproportionate number of young married women who suffer burns, which are often alleged to occur when women are cooking. It appears, however, that some of these deaths are not accidental. Rather, the husband's family sometimes perpetrates the burning of the young women when they are not satisfied with the dowry that she has brought to her marriage.[11]

High levels of depression also appear to be related to the low status position of women in different societies and the expectations that those societies have of them. There is also widespread reporting in many societies of general gynecologic discomfort without physical explanation, which may be related to the stresses on the lives of many women.[12]

Especially in low-income populations, there are many households that are headed by females who are divorced, separated, or widowed, or by women whose husbands are working elsewhere. These households tend to be among the poorest people. These women also tend to be among the least well-educated people in a community and low income and education mitigate severely against the health of such women.

The roles that women play in different cultures can also pose important hazards to their health. In many societies, for example, women cook indoors on open fires without adequate ventilation, as discussed in Chapter 7. This is strongly associated with respiratory problems and asthma for such women and for their children.

Poverty, lack of or low levels of education, and low social status of women in many societies seriously constrain the access of women to health services. In addition, girls and women who need health services often do not take advantage of such services in a timely way. There are also numerous instances in which women can not use health services without the permission of a husband or male relative or without having a male relative take them to the health services, which also constrains their attendance. In some settings, even when women need emergency care, such as during complications of pregnancy, social constraints sometimes prevent them from seeking such care and inhibit their husbands from taking them for treatment, as well, as reflected in the vignette about Sarah.

THE BURDEN OF HEALTH CONDITIONS FOR FEMALES

Having looked at the biological and social determinants of health for women, we can now look at some of the key health issues that females face, their prevalence, and the critical risk factors for those health conditions. This part of the chapter will examine selected women's health issues through their life cycle. In particular, it will focus on sex-selective abortion, female genital cutting, sexually transmitted infections, violence against women, and complications of pregnancy. It will comment on nutrition only briefly, because nutrition is largely covered in Chapter 8.

Sex-Selective Abortion

How common is sex-selective abortion worldwide? How many unborn children are affected? Sex-selective abortion appears to be a phenomenon that is more prevalent in India and China than in any other countries in the world.[13] A number of studies have been done of this phenomenon and "one study suggested that close to one million female fetuses were aborted in India in the last 20 years."[14]

An important consequence of sex-selective abortion is the skewed ratios of males to females in a number of countries. Naturally, one would expect that there would be about 105 females born for every 100 males. However, in China today, there are about 120 males born for every 100 females, with similar male to female ratios in Taiwan, Singapore, and parts of India. South Korea also has 10% more male births than female births.[15]

There is considerable evidence worldwide that both family size and preferences for males go down as income and education rise. In the case of the countries cited above, however, this has not been the case. Rather, as incomes and education have risen, and as technology has become more available, some families have used their income, knowledge, and access to technology—ultrasound in this case—to express their preference for males by engaging in sex-selective abortion. Punjab State, for example, is the wealthiest state in India. Yet, it has the most skewed ratio in India of males to females. The one-child policy in China has exacerbated male preference in that country.

Deaths of Young Girls

Females are born with biological advantages over males. If they received the same child care as boys, the same nutrition, and the same access to health care, then they would be less affected than boys by certain childhood illnesses, and boys would die at higher rates than do girls. However, in many countries, girls receive less parental attention, poorer nutrition, and less access to health care than do boys. Thus, girls younger than five years have higher rates of mortality than boys younger than five years.[10]

Female Genital Cutting

Female genital cutting (FGC) is also known as "female genital mutilation" and "female circumcision." The WHO has grouped FGC into four types, generally varying from excision of the prepuce, the fold of skin surrounding the clitoris, to excision of part or all of the external genitalia and the stitching and narrowing of the vaginal opening. There are also a variety of related practices, including pricking of the genitalia or using chemicals to narrow the vaginal opening.[16]

Female genital cutting is generally carried out on girls 4 to 14 years of age by traditional practitioners, although it is sometimes carried out on infants. The cutting is done with razor blades, knives, or glass. It is estimated that between 100 million and 140 million women worldwide have had female genital cutting performed on them. Estimates also suggest that as many as 3 million girls in Sub-Saharan Africa and in Egypt have such cutting performed on them each year.[16] In some countries, such as Egypt, FGC is practically universal among women who are 15 to 49 years old. However, there are other countries in Africa in which only a small share of the women have had FGC, such as Niger.[16] The practice appears to be diminishing almost everywhere, with fewer younger girls being cut than their mothers. FGC is very closely related to ethnicity. It also varies inversely with education; the higher the level of education of the mother, the lower the level of FGC.

When FGC is done initially, it can result in terrible pain or shock. It is also associated with infection and blood poisoning, because the instruments used for FGC are not always clean. Over the longer term, it can lead to the retention of urine, infertility, and obstructed labor. If infection and hemorrhage linked to the act of FGC are not addressed in a timely and appropriate manner, FGC can also lead to death.[16]

Sexually Transmitted Infections

Chapter 11, which is on infectious diseases, discusses HIV/AIDS and its relationship with other sexually transmitted infections (STIs). This chapter highlights the facts that women are more biologically susceptible to sexually transmitted infections because of more exposed mucosal surfaces, because they often show no symptoms of those diseases, and because of their roles in society they are less likely to get treated for sexually transmitted infections than are men.

Sexually transmitted infections that are not treated in a timely and appropriate manner can have a number of long-lasting effects on the health of women. These include pelvic inflammatory disease, chronic pain, ovarian abscesses, ectopic pregnancies, and infertility.[17] When pregnant women can not get STIs treated in appropriate and timely ways can lead to fetal wastage, stillbirths, low birth weight babies, eye and lung damage in their babies, and congenital abnormalities.[17] Human papiloma virus is associated with cervical cancer,[17] and the complications of syphilis can lead to death.[18] Chlamydia bears special mention because it is nine times more prevalent in women than in men.[19] Chlamydia is very prevalent in low-income countries and is associated with chronic conjunctivitis, reproductive tract infections, genital ulcer disease, and infertility.[19]

The data on the burden of STIs, other than HIV, is incomplete. However, based on the best available studies about chlamydia, gonorrhea, and syphilis, it appears that about 176,000 people worldwide died in 2001 from STIs in low- and middle-income countries[20] and about 0.6% of the global burden of disease in those countries in 2001 was from STIs.[21] Sub-Saharan Africa faces a disproportionately high share of morbidity and mortality from STIs. In fact, about half of all the DALYs lost from STIs were in that region.[21]

From the limited studies available, the prevalence of chlamydia, gonorrhea, and syphilis appears to vary widely. Studies done in China showed that rates of chlamydia ranged from 1–24%.[22] Studies done in other parts of Asia indicated that the prevalence of syphilis ranged from almost negligible to about 15%.[22] Studies done in Sub-Saharan Africa have shown ranges for chlamydia from 2–30%, for gonorrhea from 2–32%, and for syphilis from almost negligible to 23%.[23]

Worldwide, it is the group aged 15 to 44 in whom we find the largest burden of STIs, and within that group, women have a larger share of disease than men have. About 1.9% of the total DALYs lost in this group to women were lost to STIs.[21] About 0.5% of the total DALYs lost to men in this age group were lost to these infections.[21]

The risk factors for a woman getting an STI are well known and include young age when engaging in sexual relations, often because of child marriage, especially in Asia and Sub-Saharan Africa; multiple sexual partners; sex with high risk partners, including partners considerably older than the woman; and inability to use a condom. The use of alcohol and drugs is also associated with unprotected sex, as is unequal power between the woman and the man who are engaging in sexual relations.

Violence and Sexual Abuse Against Women

Violence and sexual abuse against women occur with remarkable frequency throughout the world. Violence is usually episodic, it is often not reported, and it is often associated with sexual abuse.[24] "Sexual abuse, which can include rape, sexual assault, sexual molestation, sexual harassment, and incest."[25] It is very hard to get reliable data on violence and sexual abuse against women. However, UNAIDS suggests that 10–50% of women worldwide have been abused physically by an intimate partner at least once in their lives.[26] Another study on intimate partner violence indicated that "one third of women have been beaten, coerced into sex, or subjected to extreme emotional abuse."[27] Other data suggest that between 20–60% of women report having been beaten by their partners.[28] A study about forced sex done in a number of countries concluded that "between 20–50% of adolescent girls aged 10–25 report their first sexual encounter was forced."[26] In addition, there have been a number of conflicts in which rape has been used systematically, as a "tool of war."[29]

Violence and abuse against women have a number of negative consequences for the health of women. These include injuries, unwanted pregnancies, STIs, depression, and sometimes permanent disability or death.[30] The risk factors for whether or not a woman will suffer violence can be complicated, are often a result of many factors, and are not well documented. However, it appears that such violence is associated with factors such as young age of the male partner, a history of violence of the male partner, low socioeconomic status of the male and female involved, proximity to drugs or alcohol, social isolation, and gender inequality. The likelihood of violence is heightened in conflict and post-conflict situations.[31]

Maternal Morbidity and Mortality

There are about 530,000 maternal deaths per year in the world, meaning deaths that occur during pregnancy, during childbirth, or until 42 days after the baby is born.[32] This is equal to about 400 maternal deaths for every 100,000 live births.[33] It is estimated that between 11–17% of maternal deaths happen during childbirth.[30] Between 50–71% of maternal deaths occur in the postpartum period, with most of those occurring in the first week after birth.[30] Of the estimated 530,000 annual maternal deaths, it is thought that about 70,000, or 13%, were due to unsafe abortions.[34]

There are both indirect and direct causes of maternal death. About 20% of maternal deaths are from indirect causes, meaning diseases that complicate pregnancy or that are complicated by pregnancy. These include malaria, anemia, HIV/AIDS, and cardiovascular disease.[33] The importance of these problems depends on the presence of these diseases in different communities and how effective the health system is in responding to them. About 80% of maternal deaths stem from direct causes, including hemorrhage, infection, eclampsia, and obstructed labor. Figure 9-1 indicates the major causes of maternal death and the share of maternal deaths worldwide that are associated with them.

The ratio of maternal deaths to the number of live births varies considerably across regions. The highest maternal mortality ratios are in Sub-Saharan Africa, where there are 940 maternal deaths per 100,000 live births.[35] The lowest maternal mortality ratios are in Western Europe, where only about 5 women die of maternal causes per 100,000 live births.[36] Table 9-3 shows the maternal mortality ratio by region and the lifetime chance of maternal death.

The risk of maternal death is a stark reflection of the disparities in the health status between different countries and within those countries. A woman in Western Europe has only a 1 in 10,000 chance of dying a maternal death. In some of the poorest countries of Sub-Saharan Africa, however, a woman has a 1 in 20 lifetime chance of dying a maternal death. This means that a woman in some countries in Sub-Saharan Africa faces 500 times the risk of dying a maternal death as does a woman in Western Europe.

There are a number of risk factors for maternal death. Among the first are the nutritional status and general health status of the mother. There is also a very strong correlation between maternal death and the level of education and income of the mother. Clearly, well-educated women with comfortable incomes do not suffer many maternal deaths; uneducated and poor women do. Maternal death also var-

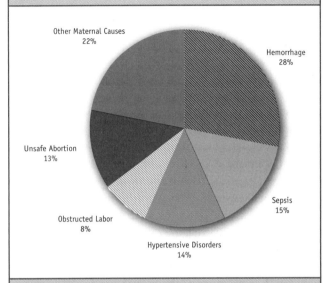

FIGURE 9-1 Maternal Death by Cause, Low- and Middle Income Countries, Percentage Distribution, 2000

Source: Data from Maternal Mortality in 2000, Estimates Developed by WHO, UNICEF, UNFPA. Geneva: WHO; 2000:Annex 2.

ies with ethnicity and location, with rural women being at greater risk than urban dwellers. The risk of maternal death is also associated, among other things, with childbirth by adolescents,[37] women having their first child,[38] women having more than five children,[38] and childbirth at ages older than 35 years.[39] Short intervals between the births of subsequent children are also a risk factor for maternal death. Having a birth attended by a skilled healthcare provider and having

TABLE 9-3 Maternal Mortality Ratio and Lifetime Risk of Dying a Maternal Death, by Region, 2000

Region	Maternal Mortality Ratio	Lifetime Risk of Dying a Maternal Death (1 in X)
Central & E. Europe and Central Asia	64	770
East Asia & Pacific	110	360
Latin America & the Caribbean	190	160
Middle East & No. Africa	220	100
South Asia	560	43
Sub-Saharan Africa	940	16
High-Income Countries	13	4000

Source: Adapted with permission from The World Bank. Graham WJ, Cairns J, Bhattacharya S, Bullough CHW, Quayyum Z, Rogo K. Maternal and perinatal conditions. In: Jamison DT, Breman JG, Measham AR, et al., eds. *Disease Control Priorities in Developing Countries.* 2nd ed. New York: Oxford University Press; 2006.

access to emergency obstetric care are important to successful outcomes of pregnancy. In addition, consumption of alcohol, tobacco, and drugs during pregnancy can also be harmful to both mother and child.

Unsafe Abortion

Many pregnancies are not wanted. It is estimated that there are 211 million pregnancies worldwide each year, of which about 46 million end in induced abortion.[30]

One critical issue concerning abortion is whether they are "safe" or "unsafe." WHO defines "safe" abortion as those abortions that are performed "by trained healthcare providers, with proper equipment, correct technique, and sanitary standards." "Unsafe" abortions are essentially the opposite of that definition—performed by an untrained provider, with inappropriate equipment, poor technique, and unhygienic conditions.[30] It is thought that only about 60% of the abortions that are carried out every year worldwide are safe.[30]

Fewer than 1 woman per 100,000 who have a safe abortion will die as a result of the abortion. The mortality rate for unsafe abortions, however, is at least 100 times greater, although it varies by country, from about 100 per 100,000

such abortions to about 600 per 100,000. It is estimated that about 70,000 women in the world die every year from unsafe abortions. This would be equal to about 13% of the total maternal deaths that occur annually worldwide.[40,41]

Figure 9-2 shows the extent to which unsafe abortions take place in different regions of the world. The age of those having an unsafe abortion also varies by region. About 60% of the unsafe abortions in Africa take place among women younger than 25 years of age, compared to about 30% for women this age in Asia. In Latin America and the Caribbean, about half of the unsafe abortions are carried out on women 20 to 29 years of age.[42]

Obstetric Fistula

It is difficult to get good estimates of the number of women who suffer from obstetric fistula every year. Studies suggest that for every 100,000 births, between 50 and 80 women in Sub-Saharan Africa, North Africa, West and South Asia, and about 30 women in Latin America and China suffer a fistula.[43] At these rates, about 50,000 to 100,000 women each year will suffer a fistula.[44] It is thought that about 2 million women worldwide are living with fistula.[44]

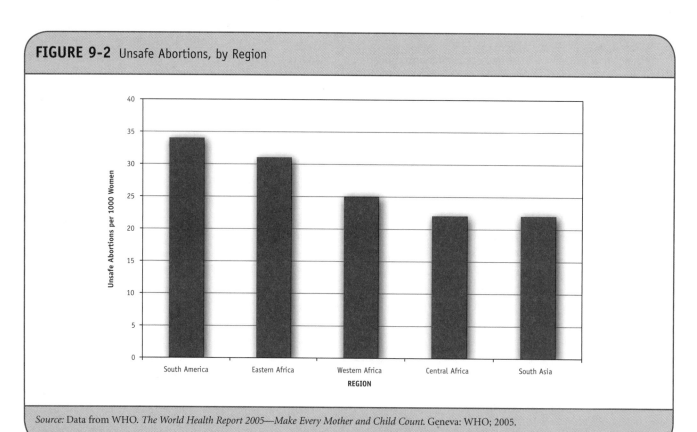

FIGURE 9-2 Unsafe Abortions, by Region

Source: Data from WHO. *The World Health Report 2005—Make Every Mother and Child Count.* Geneva: WHO; 2005.

The risk factors for fistula are those that are linked with an obstructed delivery, which is the precipitating factor for a fistula. These include undernutrition, young age at first birth, and having had multiple births. In addition, female genital cutting and some traditional practices that damage the birth canal can also cause prolonged labor and lead to fistula. The lack of access to emergency obstetric care and the failure to make use of such care, if available, also contribute to the prevalence of fistula.[44]

Cardiovascular Disease

Cardiovascular disease is the leading cause of death world-wide, as discussed earlier, and it affects people in both low- and high-income countries. There is a strong correlation between lifestyle and cardiovascular disease. As women around the world begin to eat more processed foods, become more obese, and take up smoking, their rates of cardiovascular disease will increase.

DIFFERENCES BETWEEN THE HEALTH OF MEN AND WOMEN

Much of the attention paid to the health of women over the last several decades has focused on reproductive health and on "women as child bearers." More recently, however, greater focus has been put on females in all of their roles and on the extent to which gender discrimination negatively impacts their overall health. Although still somewhat limited, increasing amounts of information are available on the health of females compared to the health of males.[45] Overall, women have a higher life expectancy at birth than men. On average, women in low-income countries live 1 year longer than men and women in high-income countries live on average 7 years longer than men.[45]

However, an analysis of the extent to which females suffer a burden of disease greater than males identified 19 conditions that disproportionately affect females. Some of these relate to conditions that are specific to women, such as maternal conditions and cancers that overwhelmingly affect females. Some of these conditions are associated with the fact that females live longer than males, such as Alzheimer's disease, osteoarthritis, cerebrovascular and cardiovascular disease, and age related vision disorders. In fact, it has been estimated that females lose 80% more DALYs from Alzheimer's disease, more than 60% more DALYs from osteoarthritis and age related vision disorders, and more than 40% more DALYs from cerebrovascular and cardiovascular disease than men. Females also lose more than 50% more DALYs than males from depression and almost three times more DALYs than men from migraine headaches. As

noted earlier, a condition affecting females that appears to be driven solely by discrimination is the excess burden of disease that women in South Asia suffer from fires and burns. In South Asia, females lose more than 250% more DALYs from fire and burns than males lose.[46] In fact, South Asia is the region of the world in which females are the least healthy compared to males.

THE COSTS AND CONSEQUENCES OF WOMEN'S HEALTH PROBLEMS

The costs and consequences of women's health problems have not been examined carefully, and there are insufficient data on the social and economic costs related to them. Nonetheless, it is possible to make a number of comments on the economic and social costs of the health problems that women face in low- and middle-income countries.

First, there are a number of important social costs that relate to women's health issues. Violence against girls and women tends to isolate them socially. When a woman dies in childbirth, the social impacts are enormous. In most societies, women are the primary caregivers for children; therefore, when a mother dies, the death usually has a profound impact on the health of her children, with young children often dying thereafter. The social costs of some problems are particularly high. For example, women who have obstetric fistula are often socially isolated from their community.

Second, there are exceptional economic costs related to women's health conditions, and these are not often given the attention they deserve. The economic costs of nutritional issues have already been examined. The costs of violence against women, especially in low-income countries, have not been studied carefully. However, it is clear that these would include the direct costs of caring for women against whom violence has been perpetrated, as well as the indirect costs of earnings lost due to the impact of violence on their health and ability to work. A study in Chile, for example, suggested that the costs of domestic violence in Chile were equal to 2% of Chile's GDP. A similar study in Nicaragua indicated that such violence cost 1.6% of GDP. A review of intimate partner violence in the United States indicated that it led to 2 million injuries in a year and costs of about $6 billion.[47]

The economic costs of maternal health conditions are substantial but not well documented. As noted earlier, women play important economic roles both inside and outside the home. If a woman can not attend to her home chores because of ill health following a delivery, then families often have to search for help in doing those activities. This is essential because in low-income societies, many women are responsible, among other things, for gathering water and fuel, cooking, doing the laundry, and caring for the children. In addition, many women in low- and middle-income settings do work outside their home chores. Illness associated with maternal conditions seriously constrains women's productivity and reduces the income they can contribute to their family. Similarly, women's higher proportion of depression is also likely to have high economic costs.

CASE STUDIES

There has been some progress in a number of countries in dealing with the critical health issues discussed previously. The next section of this chapter examines three cases about efforts to address health conditions among women and to promote family planning. The first deals with the reduction of maternal deaths in Sri Lanka, the second concerns efforts to encourage family planning in Bangladesh, and the third is about a program to deal with obstetric fistula in Tanzania. The Sri Lanka and Bangladesh cases are well-documented success stories. The case about Tanzania concerns a promising new effort to help women with fistula.

Maternal Mortality in Sri Lanka

Background

Sri Lanka has had an impressive history of public-sector commitment to education and health, even when its income per capita was low. Today, the female literacy rate in Sri Lanka is more than double the South Asian average, and free health services have been available in rural areas since the 1930s.[48] Another unusual strength of Sri Lanka is that it has a good civil registration system that has recorded maternal deaths since about 1900.

Interventions

Sri Lanka has taken a number of steps to reduce maternal deaths. First, Sri Lanka improved access to health services. Starting in the 1930s, Sri Lanka established health facilities throughout the country that were staffed by medical officers. In addition, Sri Lanka expanded secondary and tertiary facilities in the 1950s and around the same time established a working ambulance service.

Second, as early as the 1940s, Sri Lanka introduced policies to expand the number of midwives, who were the front line workers dealing with pregnant women and childbirth. The focus on midwifery and on promoting easy access to higher-level health services in Sri Lanka has contributed to a wide acceptance by women and their families of giving birth with the assistance of a trained midwife at home or in the hospital. Midwives in Sri Lanka today serve a population of 3000 to 5000 people and they provide an invaluable link between the local community and the health system.

Another step that Sri Lanka took to reduce maternal deaths was to make use of its civil registration data to identify what areas of the country had the most significant problems with maternal mortality. On this basis, the government was able to target its efforts to especially vulnerable groups, including women who were isolated both physically and socially, such as on distant tea estates. The government coupled these efforts with continuous activities, starting in the 1960s, to ensure that the quality of maternal health services was always appropriate. The lessons learned from individual maternal deaths, for example, were disseminated throughout the health system so that the quality of services could be improved and errors in dealing with obstetric problems could be reduced.

At the same time, the government made considerable progress in other health areas. This included efforts to improve health by improving sanitation and by measures to combat malaria and hookworm. These actions also contributed to improved health and lowered maternal mortality rates.[49]

Impact

As a result of these efforts, Sri Lanka has halved maternal deaths every 6 to 12 years since 1935. This has meant a decline in the maternal mortality ratio from between 500 and 600 maternal deaths per 100,000 live births in 1950 to 60 per 100,000 today. Skilled medical practitioners now attend 97% of the births in Sri Lanka, compared with 30% in 1940.

One very important point to note about Sri Lanka is that it has achieved better health outcomes than many countries that have higher per capita incomes and spend more on health than Sri Lanka. In India, for example, the maternal mortality ratio is more than 400 per 100,000 live births, and spending on health constitutes over 5% of the GNP. In Sri Lanka, however, the ratio of maternal deaths to live births is less than one-quarter of that for India, even though the country spends only 3% of its GNP on health. Low-cost, but dedicated and well-trained health personnel, including midwives, helped make the expansion of access to health care in Sri Lanka affordable.

Lessons

Sri Lanka's success in reducing maternal deaths can be attributed to widespread access to maternal health care, including emergency obstetric care, built upon a strong health system that provides free services to the entire population. The professionalism and broad use of midwives, the systematic use of health information to identify problems and guide decision making, and targeted quality improvements for vulnerable groups were also ingredients for success. Sri Lanka's tradition of public-sector commitment to human development created conditions where gains were reinforced by good education, an emphasis on gender equity, the promotion of family planning, and a coordinated network of health services. Although factors such as the introduction of antibiotics and national efforts against malaria helped lower maternal mortality rates, it was the step-by-step actions of the government rather than better living conditions alone that led to most of the improvements in maternal health. Sri Lanka's success offers important lessons for other low- and middle-income countries that have unacceptably high levels of maternal deaths. Detailed information on this case is available in *Case Studies in Global Health: Millions Saved.*

Reducing Fertility in Bangladesh

Background

Despite the existence of several family planning methods, more than 150 million women in developing countries who wish to limit or space childbearing do not use contraception. In Bangladesh, where more than half the women are illiterate and cultural traditions favor large families, each woman had, on average, almost seven children in the mid-1970s, thereby jeopardizing her health and that of her children. For a country with the world's highest population density[50,51] where almost 80% of the people live in poverty, it became clear that lowering population growth would be very important.

The Intervention

In 1975 the government of Bangladesh launched a program to reduce the national birth rate. The program had four components. First, young, married women were trained as outreach workers to visit women at home and offer information and contraceptive services. The number of these family welfare assistants (FWAs) eventually exceeded 40,000. Their outreach surpassed all expectations, with virtually all Bangladeshi women having been contacted at least once by an FWA, including many women isolated by cultural practices, geographical location, or poor transportation. The second element of the program was the provision of a wide range of family planning methods through a well-managed distribution system. The third component was the establishment of thousands of family planning clinics in rural areas to which outreach workers could refer clients for long-term family planning methods such as sterilization. The fourth

element was the information, education, and communication (IEC) campaign. The IEC program successfully tailored its message to achieve different aims, such as persuading men to talk to their wives about contraception, and winning social acceptance for FWAs by creating a story about a compelling soap opera heroine who eventually becomes an FWA. In fact, the IEC campaign's remarkable success has inspired similar mass media initiatives in other countries such as Kenya, Tanzania, and Brazil.[52]

The government's program evolved substantially over time, benefiting greatly from the existence of the Matlab Health Research Center that has operated for over 35 years as a site for large-scale research on the operation of health, nutrition, and family planning programs. Within villages in the Matlab area, researchers have tested various approaches to the delivery of health services. Matlab evaluations have shaped maternal and child health programs both in Bangladesh and throughout the developing world.

The Impact

The program resulted in virtually all women in Bangladesh becoming aware of family planning options. Contraceptive use increased from 8% in the mid-1970s to its current level of about 50%, and fertility declined from 6.3 births per woman in the early 1970s to about 3.3 in the mid-1990s.[53] Although other factors such as increased education and employment opportunities for women also increased demand for contraception, the family planning program has been shown to have had an independent effect on attitudes and behaviors.[54]

Costs and Benefits

The program is estimated to have cost about $100 million to $150 million per year, with more than half the funding coming from the United States Agency for International Development (USAID), the United Nations Development Program (UNDP), the World Bank, and other agencies. Efforts are under way to increase program efficiency. The most expensive program component is that of FWAs, who were once critical to program success but are now valued by clients more as a convenience than as an essential source of information.[55] Research suggests that the most cost-effective strategy for the continued promotion of family planning is a fixed site approach that provides health and family planning services from clinics, complemented with targeted outreach to hard-to-reach clients.[56] However, some of those involved in women's health believe that "doorstep delivery" by FWAs would continue to be cost-effective if the FWAs delivered not only family planning, but also other messages on sexual and reproductive health, such as safe motherhood, STIs, and

HIV/AIDS. They also note the benefits of the FWAs as role models for women's status in rural areas. [25]

Lessons Learned

The success of the program can be attributed to four factors. The first was political commitment on the part of Bangladesh and the international agencies involved. The second was the broad use of FWAs who carried the program's message into almost every home, however isolated. The third was the excellent use of mass media strategies to target audiences and change behavior. The fourth was the research and data provided by the Matlab center that helped to constantly identify problems and improve the program. Although the program is far from perfect and the optimal outreach strategy is yet to be identified, Bangladesh is one of the few low-income countries to have reduced fertility rapidly without resorting to coercive measures. More detailed information on this case is available in *Case Studies in Global Health: Millions Saved*.

Fistula in Tanzania

Background

The emotional and physical side effects of obstetric fistulas stem largely from the fact that urine or feces leak from the fistula of affected women and cause them to be shunned by others. As a result of a fistula, women lose their babies, suffer constant pain or discomfort created by the unrelenting moisture from the leak, and are often deserted by their husbands and communities. Moreover, the women become socially isolated, lose the ability to sustain normal lives, and become economically dependent on others. To make matters worse, many communities view fistulas as a curse and hide the women away, rather than realizing that it is a medical condition. Decreasing the prevalence of obstetric fistulas is challenging, because it requires altering cultural practices on the one hand and strengthening very weak healthcare systems on the other.[57]

To assist in addressing the problem of fistula, the Bill & Melinda Gates Foundation[58] provided funding in 2002 to the United Nations Population Fund (UNFPA) and two NGOs, EngenderHealth and the Women's Dignity Project, to create The Obstetric Fistula Partnership. In conjunction with this funding, UNFPA initiated in 2003 The Global Campaign to End Fistula. The aim of the partnership and campaign, among other things, was to prevent obstetric fistulas by strengthening emergency obstetric care, to enhance the capacity of the health system to deal with the large number of women who already have a fistula, and to help through advocacy to promote greater attention to and resources for dealing with maternal health.[57]

Surgery for uncomplicated cases of fistula is about 90% effective. Surgery for complicated cases of fistula is about 60% effective.[13] Most women with a fistula are unaware of any opportunities for repairing their fistula or of getting support to help them return to normal lives.

The Intervention

The Women's Dignity Project (WDP), called *Utu Mwanamke* in Swahili, is a program operated by a Tanzanian NGO that is dedicated to "addressing fistula and advocating for the health rights of the poor, within a human rights framework."[59] The WDP is a partner of the UNFPA's Campaign to End Fistula. It is estimated that more than 1000 new cases of fistula occur every year in Tanzania.[60]

The WDP carries out activities in four areas: participatory research, organizational strengthening, policy and advocacy work, and the funding of fistula repairs. The research work of the WDP began in 2001, with a survey of the magnitude of the fistula problem in Tanzania and of the resources available to help address the problem. This has been followed by other community-based surveys. In addition, the WDP has worked with the Ministry of Health in Tanzania to establish a national referral system for fistulas and to train healthcare workers how to deal with fistula. The WDP has also advocated to help make the community, the government, and Tanzania's development partners more aware of the fistula problem and to allocate additional resources to address it. Moreover, the WDP has provided funds to five hospitals to support the health services needed to deal with fistulas more effectively.[61]

In carrying out those efforts, the WDP has:

- Identified women with fistula through community-based efforts and arranged transport for them to a hospital at which they could have surgery.[62]
- Published a booklet to raise awareness about fistulas that is based on the life stories of seven women who are affected by this condition.[63]
- Worked with a number of other NGOs, such as the African Medical and Relief Foundation (AMREF),[64] to raise additional money for fistula efforts. AMREF, for example, now contributes $100 to hospitals for each fistula repair they carry out.
- Collaborated with some NGOs, such as Engender Health, to identify and address the risk factors for fistula.[57]

The Impact

The impact of the WDP efforts has not been studied scientifically or documented extensively and independently.

However, it does appear that the activities described have led to an increase in the number of women who are getting fistulas repaired and who can, therefore, return to productive and healthy lives. The work of the WDP is also strengthening the capacity within Tanzania to continue dealing with fistulas more effectively in the future, through work at the community level in identifying the problem, training health providers, and helping to increase financial resources.

Costs and Benefits

According to the UNFPA, the average cost of treating fistula is $300.[65] This includes the reconstructive surgery, post-operation stay at the hospital or clinic, and rehabilitation. There are no data on the economic returns to fistula repair in Tanzania. However, one should expect that a woman with a successful fistula repair could return to a productive life that she could not have without that surgery. In addition, of course, there would be large social benefits to the surgery, because the woman whose fistula is repaired can also overcome the social ostracism that she faced earlier and can return to a more normal social life with her family and community.

Lessons Learned

The WDP's program in Tanzania suggests some promising approaches to dealing with difficult global health issues. First, it appears that combining a global effort such as The Campaign to End Fistula, with a local effort, such as the work of the WDP, can set a valuable foundation for addressing some global health problems. Second, careful advocacy efforts with the right stakeholders in a country, such as local communities, key government agencies, and selected development partners can help to build both awareness and support for trying to address health problems. Third, the initial successes of the WDP seem to stem from its efforts to embed its work at the level of the community and to involve the community in helping to identify problems and then act on them. Finally, carefully trying to build capacity through training and financial support can provide both immediate benefits and set the basis for programs to be sustained in the longer run.

ADDRESSING FUTURE CHALLENGES

The health of females in low-income countries is a powerful reflection of biological susceptibility and gender norms that assign certain roles, restrictions, and values to females, compared to males. They also reflect the fact that the health systems in many countries have profound gender gaps and can not or do not serve effectively the health needs of females. In this light, making major improvements in the future in the health of females in low- and middle-income countries will require attention to an array of social and public health measures.

One future challenge will be to improve the nutritional status of females, because it is poor nutrition in utero and from infancy that later can lead to women becoming stunted, not reaching their full biological potential, and experiencing a variety of health conditions. Measures to address nutritional concerns more effectively are discussed in Chapter 8.

Another challenge that is central to the long-term improvement in the health of females is access to education. The empowerment of females socially is strongly associated with their level of education. Empowerment will improve the status of females and reduce the extent to which discrimination against them hurts their health. In addition, education improves access to important health information that can make a difference in women's and children's health.

Major changes must also be made in the perception that communities have of female roles and the health of females. This will require significant efforts at the level of communities and populations as a whole to put greater value on women's health. This will help to reduce the abortion of female fetuses and to ensure that women in obstructed labor do not die because they lack appropriate and timely medical attention.

A continuing challenge will also be to put greater emphasis on the health of females as people, rather than as just "women who give birth." This would encourage policy makers to take a number of steps that are essential to improving the health of females globally, including gaining a better understanding of the health conditions affecting females and what can be done about them and making the health of females central to all health efforts. In addition, in many cultures, females are constrained in dealing with male medical workers and it is also very important to train more female health workers.

The next section comments on further measures that can be taken to deal with some of the particular health problems discussed previously, such as female genital cutting, sexually transmitted infections, violence against women, and other reproductive health issues, including maternal mortality, unsafe abortion, and fistula.

Female Genital Cutting

Although fewer families appear to be practicing FGC, there is little evidence so far about cost-effective interventions to reduce harmful FGC practices. It is clear, however, that efforts to achieve this aim will have to be based on good data about who is practicing FGC and how they practice it, which will require additional research on this topic. In addition, advocacy efforts that promote change need to be specifically tailored to local practices and to local beliefs. Linking these efforts with other measures that promote female empowerment, female education, and female control over economic resources will also be needed. FGC is intimately linked with deep-seated local beliefs and traditions that vary with location, ethnicity, education, and income. Only by taking account of these underlying issues will one be able to address FGC.[66]

Violence Against Women

We have already discussed the extent to which violence against women is usually a result of a complex set of factors and the interactions among them. Although there is increasing evidence on the factors linked to violence against women, there is little evidence about what works to reduce such violence and what are the most cost-effective approaches to doing so.

Some studies have shown that protecting women against violence through legislation, as has been done in the United States and some other high-income countries, can have important positive effects in some settings. Shelters for abused women can also be used to reduce violence against them. Ensuring that the police, judges, and healthcare personnel are trained to deal with violence against women in more sensitive and more effective ways has also been useful. It also appears that many non-governmental organizations can deal with violence against women as effectively and at lower cost than some government services can do.[67]

In the end, however, it is a combination of measures adapted to local circumstances that can best address the combination of factors that put women at risk of violence. Some of the most important of these measures are noted in Table 9-4.

TABLE 9-4 Selected Measures to Reduce Intimate Partner Violence

Prevention and education campaigns to increase awareness of intimate partner violence and change cultural norms about violence against women
Treatment for those who engage in intimate partner violence
Programs to strengthen ties to family and jobs
Couples counseling
Shelters and crisis centers for battered women
Mandatory arrest for offenders

Source: Adapted with permission from The World Bank. Rosenberg ML, Butchart A, Mercy J, Narasimhan V, Waters H, Marshall MS. Interpersonal Violence. In: Jamison DT, Breman JG, Measham AR, et al., eds. *Disease Control Priorities in Developing Countries.* 2nd ed. New York: Oxford University Press; 2006:755–770.

Sexually Transmitted Infections

Sexually transmitted infections are important not only because of the morbidity and mortality associated with them, particularly among women in Sub-Saharan Africa, but also because they increase the chance of getting HIV/AIDS. It is critical, therefore, that the burden of these diseases be addressed. Some comments follow about addressing three of the most common STIs among women: syphilis, gonorrhea, and chlamydia.

The goals of any program for reducing these sexually transmitted infections have to be to reduce infection, reduce the complications of infections, and reduce the spread of STIs to infants when they are born.[68] It is much more cost-effective to prevent these diseases and to treat them before they lead to complications. Achieving these goals requires that young women initiate their first sexual relations at later ages; be able to refuse unwanted sex, even from their husbands; have relations with fewer partners; use condoms; and have any STIs diagnosed early and treated properly.

Meeting these aims will also require that young people get "the information and skills for making good decisions;" have access to "a range of health services that help them to act on those decisions;" and "live within a social, legal, and regulatory framework that supports health behaviors and protects young people from harm . . ."[69]

The successes in reducing STIs to date have focused on a common set of health system interventions and capacities. First, the health system must have an ability to carry out surveillance of STIs. Second, there needs to be a program of health education, targeted to those people most at risk of infection. Third, appropriately trained health workers need to be able to provide proper treatment of infection. Fourth, a system of partner notification must be in place so that the partners of the infected people can also be tested and treated, if necessary. Finally, there must be an effective program for access to health services, including condom use, generally referred to as "condom promotion."[70]

Sweden made important strides in reducing chlamydia. Sweden offered free diagnosis, coupled with a major health education campaign in schools, partner notification, and condom promotion. Linked to this, Sweden was able to reduce the prevalence of gonorrhea by 15 times and cut the prevalence of chlamydia by one half over a 15 year period. Zambia also made good progress in reducing the burden of sexually transmitted infections by expanding the number of STI clinics, improving the training of health educators and clinicians, and expanding health education.[70] South Africa's "Love Life" initiative focuses on improving the sexual health of adolescents aged 12 to 17 years. Some reviews of this program suggest that is associated with "better understanding of health risks, delayed debut of sexual relations, fewer partners, more assertive behavior regarding condom use, and better communication with parents about sex."[71]

Maternal Mortality

We have already seen that more than 500,000 women die a year of maternal causes, and that 70,000 die as a result of unsafe abortion. There is also considerable morbidity related to pregnancy. The fact that childbirth itself is such a risk in some settings is usually a result of the "three delays:" a delay in identifying complications and seeking care, a delay in transporting the woman to a hospital, and a delay in providing appropriate emergency obstetric care in the hospital.[70] There is also considerable disability, illness, and death related to unsafe abortion.

Unsafe Abortion

Most of the disability, morbidity, and mortality associated with abortion is the result of "unsafe abortion," mostly in low-income and middle-income countries in which abortion is legally restricted. To address the effects of unsafe abortion, it is essential that the health system in these settings be able to provide hygienic and appropriate post-abortion care at the lowest level of the health system possible. This means that they must be able to deal effectively with sepsis, hemorrhage, and shock. This may require a hospital stay, antibiotics, the ability to perform anesthesia, and the ability to transfuse blood. The most cost-effective manner in which to deal with incomplete abortion will be to perform vacuum aspiration, rather than to depend on the more surgical dilation and curettage approach. Prevention of unsafe abortion is also important, including universal access to family planning and services, including after abortion.[72]

In countries in which abortion laws are more liberal, it is essential that services be widely available so that women do not turn to unsafe abortion providers. In addition, it is critical that legal abortions be safe and hygienic and that services also be available to deal with any post-abortion complications. In these cases, including countries in eastern Europe and Japan in which abortion is a common method of family planning, it is also important that counseling be available about choices of family planning methods.[73]

Family Planning

Because pregnancy and abortion are such important risks for disability, illness, and death, one way to avoid these problems is to reduce unwanted pregnancy through the promotion and widespread availability of family planning. In fact, it has been suggested that in countries with high rates of maternal mortality, as much as one third of the maternal deaths could be avoided through an effective family planning program.[72] The importance of family planning is highlighted by the fact that many women in the world today would like to avoid pregnancy or space their births, but they do not have the access to family planning needed to do this. Indeed, studies done in Sub-Saharan Africa suggest that 20% of the women in the region who would like to avoid pregnancy do not have access to family planning.

There are permanent methods of family planning that include sterilization of either males or females, although only about 8% of the total number of sterilizations worldwide are among men.[74] There are also long-term methods of family planning, including intrauterine devices and implants. Short-term methods include contraceptive pills, injectables, and barrier methods, including condoms or diaphragms. In addition, exclusive breastfeeding for at least 6 months—before the mother's menstrual period returns—acts as a natural contraception. There are also methods for natural family planning that focus on periodic abstinence.

A number of countries have made important progress in promoting the use of family planning, including Bangladesh, Brazil, Colombia, Korea, and Vietnam. The experience from these countries suggests that an effective family planning program has to include information, education, and communication to promote informed choices by families about family planning; the need for a good selection of family planning technologies; the use of many points of service in both the public and private sector; services that are free or inexpensive enough for the poor to afford them; and health workers who are trained to work on family planning with knowledge and sensitivity, especially female health workers for women who are reluctant to see male health workers.[75] There is considerable evidence that "social marketing" is an effective tool for promoting family planning, as well. Social marketing refers to the use of commercial marketing techniques to sell health related measures, such as family planning or prevention of malaria.

Family planning is a cost-effective investment in reducing maternal death, but it is not clear which approach to family planning programs is more cost-effective than other approaches. The high rate of maternal death in Sub-Saharan Africa and South Asia suggest that these are the two regions in which family planning would be most cost-effective to reduce maternal morbidity, disability, and mortality.[41]

Complications of Pregnancy

The risks of complications of pregnancy increase when the general health of the mother is not good. Thus, the nutritional status of the mother is very important. In addition, malaria is very dangerous for pregnant women, especially in Sub-Saharan Africa.

Some of the conditions that affect pregnancy outcomes can be identified during prenatal care. However, although it is important for pregnant women to get regular medical exams during their pregnancy—and WHO recommends four such visits—some complications of pregnancy can not be foreseen during those checks-ups. Thus, it is also critical to ensure that births are attended by a skilled healthcare provider who can handle the complications of pregnancy and who can refer the pregnant woman to a facility where these complications can be handled. In addition, it is important that communities have transportation to get women to emergency obstetric care urgently when they have complications of pregnancy and that health services be able to address the most important complications appropriately.

TABLE 9-5 Basic Care Packages for Pregnancy at the Primary Level

Routine Prenatal Care
Clinical examination
Obstetric and gynecological examination
Urine test
Laboratory tests: hemoglobin, blood type and rhesus status, syphilis and other symptomatic testing for sexually transmitted diseases
Advice on emergencies, delivery, lactation, and contraception
Education
Iron and folic acid supplementation
Tentanus toxoid immunization
Screening and treatment for syphilis

Delivery Care
Clean delivery technique, clean cord cutting, clean delivery of baby and placenta
Active management of the third stage of labor
Episiotomy in appropriate cases
Recognition and first-line management of delivery complications
Intravenous fluid
Intravenous uterotonics, if bleeding occurs
Partograph
Essential newborn care
Intravenous antibiotics

Source: Adapted with permission from The World Bank. Graham WJ, Cairns J, Bhattacharya S, Bullough CHW, Quayyum Z, Rogo K. Maternal and Perinatal Conditions. In: Jamison DT, Breman JG, Measham AR, et al., eds. *Disease control priorities in developing countries.* 2nd ed. New York: Oxford University Press; 2006:515.

Studies show that there are several cost-effective packages of services that can reduce maternal death due to complications of pregnancy. The basic package of essential obstetric services that all countries should have is shown in Table 9-5. Countries that have more financial resources may wish to also provide some additional services that can address food, multivitamin supplements and malaria prophylaxis, the ability to deal with complicated deliveries of an HIV positive mother, and arrangements for caring for a high risk infant,[76] which are also shown on Table 9-5.

MAIN MESSAGES

As discussed by one women's health advocate, "being born female is dangerous to your health."[12] Some of the health conditions that women face are biologically determined. Others are socially determined. Some result from the interplay between biological and social determinants of health. The inferior social status of women in many cultures, however, is reflected in certain health conditions that women face and in some of the differentials that favor men between the health of men and the health of women.

As one looks globally at the health of women, especially poor women in low- and middle-income countries, one notes the importance of several key health issues. One is nutrition. Another is sex-selective abortion. A third is discriminatory healthcare practices toward young girls that cause these girls to suffer higher rates of mortality before age 5 than boys. Sexually transmitted infections are an important cause of DALYs lost for women in the reproductive age group, especially in Sub-Saharan Africa. Female genital cutting is also a practice that is widespread, especially in parts of Africa, and it is associated with important morbidity and disability for women. Violence against women is also an important cause of ill health for women.

Illness, disability, and death from maternal causes are also unnecessarily high. More than 500,000 women die each year of maternal causes, of which about 70,000 are due to unsafe abortions. Complicated labor that is not properly attended can also lead to problems, such as fistula, which an estimated 2 million women suffer worldwide.

The costs of women's health problems are very substantial. In many societies, women are the primary caregivers to children, and when the health of the mother suffers, there is often a negative effect on the health of the children, as well. In addition, women play important economic roles in many families and the morbidity, disability, and mortality associated with particular problems of women's health have substantial economic implications.

There are countries, such as Sri Lanka, that have been able to improve the health of women at relatively low levels of expenditure by making wise choices about investments in health and education. These included increasing female education, providing widespread access to midwives, and ensuring adequate back up for the midwives at hospitals.

Improving the health of women in the future will require that health systems provide a cost-effective package of services, including nutrition, family planning, prenatal care, deliveries attended by skilled healthcare providers, emergency transportation of women who are having complicated labors, and emergency obstetric services at a hospital. In the long run, it will be important to change the gender roles that favor males, promote the education and empowerment of females, promote their prospects for employment, and educate communities to better understand the health conditions that females face and the measures that can be taken to address them. These measures could help to reduce sex-selective abortion, female infanticide, violence against women, and avoid the "three delays" that are associated with maternal morbidity, disability, and mortality.

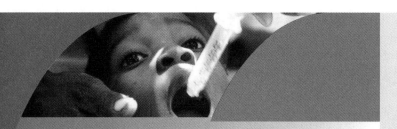

Study Questions

1. Why can it be said that "being born female is dangerous to your health?"

2. Why should we pay particular attention to the health of females?

3. In what ways do gender issues affect the health of females?

4. What are some of the key differences in the burden of disease between males and females?

5. What are the sources of those differences?

6. What are the "three delays" and why are they important?

7. What steps do countries need to take to deal with the complications of unsafe abortions?

8. What measures might be taken to reduce intimate partner violence?

9. How could one reduce the risk to women of sexually transmitted infections?

10. What are some of the most cost-effective investments that should be made to improve the health of women in low-income countries?

REFERENCES

1. Prada E, Restler E, Sten C, et al. *Abortion and Postabortion Care in Guatemala: A Report from Health Care Professionals and Health Facilities.* Occasional Report. New York: Guttmacher Institute; 2005:No. 18. Available at: http://www.alanguttmacher.org/pubs/2005/12/30/or18.pdf. Accessed June 24, 2006.

2. UN Millenium Development Goals. Available at: http://www.un.org/millenniumgoals/. Accessed March 15, 2006.

3. Murphy EM. Being born female is dangerous for your health. *The American Psychologist.* 2003;58(3):1.

4. Buvinic M, Medici A, Fernandez E, Torres AC. Gender differentials in health. In: Jamison DT, Breman JG, Measham AR, et al., eds. *Disease Control Priorities in Developing Countries.* 2nd ed. New York: Oxford University Press; 2006:195–210.

5. WHO. *The World Health Report 2005: Make Every Mother and Child Count.* Geneva: World Health Organization; 2005.

6. Quinn TC, Overbaugh J. HIV/AIDS in women: an expanding epidemic. *Science Mag.* 2005;308(5728):1582–1583.

7. Sex-selective Abortion and Infanticide. Available at: http://en.wikipedia.org/wiki/Sex-selective_abortion. Accessed June 10, 2006.

8. Abeykoon ATPL. Sex Preference in South Asia: Sri Lanka an outlier. *Asia-Pacific Popu J.* 1995;10(3):5–16.

9. Gu B, Roy K. Sex ratio at birth in China, with reference to other areas in East Asia: what we know. *Asia-Pacific Popu J.* 1995;10(3):17–42.

10. Tinker A. *A New Agenda for Women's Health and Nutrition.* The World Bank; 1994:15–17.

11. Rov K. *Encyclopaedia Against Women & Dowry Death in India.* New Delhi: Anmol Publications Pvt Ltd; 1999.

12. Murphy EM. Being born female is dangerous for your health. *Am Psychol.* 2003;58(3):205.

13. Case Study: Female Infanticide. Available at: http://www.gendercide.org/case_infanticide.html. Accessed June 10, 2006.

14. Jha P, Kumar R, Vasa P, Dhingra N, Thiruchelvam D, Moineddin R. Low female-to-male sex ratio of children born in India: national survey of 1.1 million households. *Lancet.* 2006;367(9506):211–218.

15. Walker M. The geopolitics of sexual frustration. *Foreign Policy.* 2006;(153):60.

16. UNICEF. *Female Genital Mutilation/Cutting, A Statistical Exploration 2005.* New York: UNICEF; 2005.

17. Rowley J, Berkley S. Sexually transmitted diseases. In: Murray CJL, Lopez AD, eds. *Health Dimensions of Sex and Reproduction.* Geneva: World Health Organization; 1998:21.

18. Rowley J, Berkley S. Sexually transmitted diseases. In: Murray CJL, Lopez AD, eds. *Health Dimensions of Sex and Reproduction.* Geneva: World Health Organization; 1998:68-72.

19. Buvinic M, Medici A, Fernandez E, Torres AC. Gender differentials in health. In: Jamison DT, Breman JG, Measham AR, et al., eds. *Disease Control Priorities in Developing Countries.* 2nd ed. New York: Oxford University Press; 2006:203.

20. Lopez AD, Mathers CD, Murray CJL. The burden of disease and mortality by condition: data, methods, and results for 2001. In: Lopez AD, Mathers CD, Ezzati M, Jamison DT, Murray CJL, eds. *Global Burden of Disease and Risk Factors.* New York: Oxford University Press; 2006:174.

21. Lopez AD, Mathers CD, Murray CJL. The burden of disease and mortality by condition: data, methods, and results for 2001. In: Lopez AD, Mathers CD, Ezzati M, Jamison DT, Murray CJL, eds. *Global Burden of Disease and Risk Factors.* New York: Oxford University Press; 2006:228–229.

22. Rowley J, Berkley S. Sexually transmitted diseases. In: Murray CJL, Lopez AD, eds. *Health Dimensions of Sex and Reproduction.* Geneva: World Health Organization; 1998:41.

23. Rowley J, Berkley S. Sexually Transmitted Diseases. In: Murray CJL, Lopez AD, eds. *Health Dimensions of Sex and Reproduction.* Geneva: World Health Organization; 1998:42–46.

24. Tinker A. *A New Agenda for Women's Health and Nutrition.* Washington, DC: The World Bank; 1994.

25. Personal communication with Adrienne Germain, March, 2007.

26. Violence Against Women and AIDS. Available at: http://data.unaids.org/GCWA/GCWA_BG_Violence_en.pdf. Accessed February 28, 2006.

27. Heise L, Moore K, Toubiz N. *Sexual Coercion and Reproductive Health.* New York: Population Council; 1995.

28. *World Development Report 1993.* New York: Oxford University Press; 1993.

29. Rape as a Tool of War. *Fact Sheets* Available at: http://www.amnestyusa.org/stopviolence/factsheets/rapeinwartime.html. Accessed June 10, 2006.

30. WHO. *World Health Report 2005.* Geneva: World Health Organization; 2005.

31. Rosenberg ML, Butchart A, Mercy J, Narasimhan V, Waters H, Marshall MS. Interpersonal violence. In: Jamison DT, Breman JG, Measham AR, et al., eds. *Disease Control Priorities in Developing Countries.* 2nd ed. New York: Oxford University Press; 2006:759.

32. Last JM. *A Dictionary of Epidemiology.* 4th ed. New York: Oxford University Press; 2001:110.

33. WHO. *The World Health Report 2005: Make Every Mother and Child Count.* Geneva: World Health Organization; 2005:61–77.

34. WHO. *The World Health Report 2005: Make Every Mother and Child Count.* Geneva: World Health Organization; 2005:4.

35. Graham WJ, Cairns J, Bhattacharya S, Bullough CHW, Quayyum Z, Rogo K. Maternal and perinatal conditions. In: Jamison DT, Breman JG, Measham AR, et al., eds. *Disease Control Priorities in Developing Countries.* 2nd ed. New York: Oxford University Press; 2006:506.

36. Herz BK, Measham AR. *The Safe Motherhood Initiative: Proposals for Action.* Washington, DC: The World Bank; 1987.

37. Tinker A. *A New Agenda for Women's Health and Nutrition.* Washington, DC: The World Bank; 1994:10.

38. AbouZahr C. Antepartum and postpartum hemorrhage. In: Murray CJL, Lopez AD, eds. *Health Dimensions of Sex and Reproduction: The Global Burden of Sexually Transmitted Diseases, HIV, Maternal Conditions, Perinatal Disorders, and Congenital Anomalies.* Cambridge, Ma: Harvard School of Public Health; 1998:169.

39. AbouZahr C. Antepartum and postpartum hemorrhage. In: Murray CJL, Lopez AD, eds. *Health Dimensions of Sex and Reproduction: The Global Burden of Sexually Transmitted Diseases, HIV, Maternal Conditions, Perinatal Disorders, and Congenital Anomalies.* Cambridge, Ma: Harvard School of Public Health; 1998:170.

40. Levine R, Langer A, Birdsall N, Matheny G, Wright M, Bayer A. Contraception. In: Jamison DT, Breman JG, Measham AR, et al., eds. *Disease Control Priorities in Developing Countries.* 2nd ed. New York: Oxford University Press; 2006:1075–1090.

41. The World Bank. *Priorities in Health.* Washington, DC: The World Bank; 2006.

42. WHO. *The World Health Report 2005: Make Every Mother and Child Count.* Geneva: World Health Organization; 2005:41–58.

43. AbouZahr C. Prolonged and obstructed labor. In: Murray CJL, Lopez AD, eds. *Health Dimensions of Sex and Reproduction: The Global Burden of Sexually Transmitted Diseases, HIV, Maternal Conditions, Perinatal Disorders, and Congenital Anomalies.* Cambridge, Ma: Harvard School of Public Health; 1998:243–266.

44. Obstetric Fistula as a Catalyst: Exploring Approaches for Safe Motherhood. Atlanta, GA: Paper presented at: Fistula as a Catalyst Meeting; 2005.

45. Buvinic M, Medici A, Fernandez E, Torres AC. Gender differentials in health. In: Jamison DT, Breman JG, Measham AR, et al., eds. *Disease Control Priorities in Developing Countries.* 2nd ed. New York: Oxford University Press; 2006:197.

46. Buvinic M, Medici A, Fernandez E, Torres AC. Gender differentials in health. In: Jamison DT, Breman JG, Measham AR, et al., eds. *Disease Control Priorities in Developing Countries.* 2nd ed. New York: Oxford University Press; 2006:201.

47. Rosenberg ML, Butchart A, Mercy J, Narasimhan V, Waters H, Marshall MS. Interpersonal violence. In: Jamison DT, Breman JG, Measham AR, et al., eds. *Disease Control Priorities in Developing Countries.* 2nd ed. New York: Oxford University Press; 2006:755–770.

48. The World Bank. *World Development Indicators 2003* Washington, DC: The World Bank; 2003.

49. Wickramasuriya GAW. Maternal mortality and morbidity in Ceylon. *Ceylon Branch British Med Assn.* 1939;36(2):79–106.

50. Population Data Sheet. In: Pacific) EEaSCfAat, ed. Bangkok: United Nations; 1999.

51. ESCAP (Economic and Social Commission for Asia and the Pacific). Population Data Sheet. Bangkok: United Nations; 1999.

52. Manoff R. Getting your message out with social marketing. *Am J Tropical Med Hygiene.* 1997;57(3):260–265.

53. Mitra SN, Al-Sabir A, Cross AR, Jamil K. *Bangladesh Demographic and Health Survey 1996–1997.* Dhaka: National Institute for Population Research and Training; 1997.

54. Khuda B-e, Roy NC, Rahman DM. Family planning and fertility in Bangladesh. *Asia-Pacific Pop J.* 2000;15(1):41-54.

55. Janowitz B, Holtman M, Johnson L, Trottier D. The importance of field workers in Bangladesh's family planning programme. *Asia-Pacific Pop J.* 1999;14(2): 23–36.

56. Routh, Subrata, Barkat-e-Khuda. An economic appraisal of alternative strategies for the delivery of MCH-FP services in urban Dhaka, Bangladesh. *Intern J Health Planning Manage* 2000;15:113–152.

57. The Obstetric Fistula Partnership—Working in Niger, Sudan, Tanzania and Uganda. Available at: http://www.engenderhealth.org/ia/swh/mcfpartnership.html. Accessed June 10, 2006.

58. Bill & Melinda Gates Foundation. Available at: http://www.gates-foundation.org/default.htm. Accessed June 9, 2006.

59. Welcome to Women's Dignity Project. Available at: http://www.womensdignity.org/. Accessed June 9, 2006.

60. WDP in the News: Local Press on WDP. Available at: http://www.womensdignity.org/wdp_localpress.asp#1. Accessed June 9, 2006.

61. Program Highlights: Funds for Fistula Repairs. Available at: http://www.womensdignity.org/highlights_fff.asp. Accessed June 9, 2006.

62. Program Highlights: Participatory Research. Available at: http://www.womensdignity.org/highlights_pr.asp. Accessed June 9, 2006.

63. Mwanamke U. Faces of Dignity: Seven Stories of Girls and Women with Fistula. Available at: http://www.womensdignity.org/Face_of_Dignity.pdf. Accessed June 9, 2006.

64. African Medical and Relief Foundation. Available at: http://www.amref.org/. Accessed June 9, 2006.

65. The Campaign to End Fistula. Available at: http://www.endfistula.org/. Accessed June 9, 2006.

66. UNICEF. *Female Genital Mutilation/Cutting, A Statistical Exploration 2005.* New York: UNICEF; 2005.

67. Rosenberg ML, Butchart A, Mercy J, Narasimhan V, Waters H, Marshall MS. Interpersonal violence. In: Jamison DT, Breman JG, Measham AR, et al., eds. *Disease Control Priorities in Developing Countries.* 2nd ed. New York: Oxford University Press; 2006:761.

68. Rowley J, Berkley S. Sexually transmitted diseases. In: Murray CJL, Lopez AD, eds. *Health Dimensions of Sex and Reproduction.* Geneva: World Health Organization; 1998:95–99.

69. Providing Interventions. In: Jamison DT, Breman JG, Measham AR, et al., eds. *Priorities in Health.* New York: Oxford University Press; 2006:153.

70. Rowley J, Berkley S. Sexually Transmitted Diseases. In: Murray CJL, Lopez AD, eds. *Health Dimensions of Sex and Reproduction.* Geneva: World Health Organization; 1998.

71. Providing Interventions. In: Jamison DT, Breman JG, Measham AR, et al., eds. *Priorities in Health.* New York: Oxford University Press; 2006:154.

72. Tinker A. *A New Agenda for Women's Health and Nutrition.* Washington, DC: The World Bank; 1994:31.

73. Tinker A. *A New Agenda for Women's Health and Nutrition.* Washington, DC: The World Bank; 1994:32–33.

74. Jamison DT. Maternal and perinatal conditions. In: Jamison DT, Breman JG, Measham AR, et al., eds. *Disease Control Priorities in Developing Countries.* 2nd ed. New York: Oxford University Press; 2006:499–529.

75. Tinker A. *A New Agenda for Women's Health and Nutrition.* Washington, DC: The World Bank; 1994:29–30.

76. Graham WJ, Cairns J, Bhattacharya S, Bullough CHW, Quayyum Z, Rogo K. Maternal and perinatal conditions. In: Jamison DT, Breman JG, Measham AR, et al., eds. *Disease Control Priorities in Developing Countries.* 2nd ed. Washington, DC: Oxford University Press and The World Bank; 2006:515–516.

CHAPTER 10

Child Health

By the end of this chapter the reader will be able to:

- Understand the most important causes of child illness and death around the world
- Discuss the importance of neonatal death in overall child deaths
- Understand why some children survive and others die
- Describe the most cost-effective child health interventions
- Describe some examples of successful child health initiatives
- Discuss some of the challenges of further enhancing the health of children

VIGNETTES

Nassiba was born in a remote part of Tajikistan. At 3 years of age, she became very ill with measles. She died before her parents could get her to a health center. Nassiba was never registered when she was born because the registration center was far away from where her family lived. In addition, her parents could not afford to pay the registration fee. When Nassiba died, her death was not recorded either. According to the national records, she never existed.

Esther was born in Capetown, South Africa, several years ago. Esther's mother was HIV positive. Esther's family depended on the public health system for care but at the time that system did not offer drug therapy to stop transmission of HIV from mother to child. Esther's mother breastfed her for most of the first 6 months, but not exclusively. A few months ago, Esther showed signs of HIV disease.

Tirtha was born in the far west of Nepal and was the fourth child in her family. She was 7 months old and was eat-ing some baby foods, as well as breastfeeding. One day Tirtha became feverish and developed persistent diarrhea. Her mother was not sure if she should continue to feed the baby or if that would make the diarrhea worse. She wanted to take Tirtha to the health center but it was 4 hours away by foot so she decided to see how Tirtha was feeling the next day. The next morning Tirtha was dead from dehydration.

Juan was born in the highlands of Bolivia to an indigenous family. The family did what they could to keep the new baby warm but it was very cold in the mountains. Several days after birth, Juan began to breathe heavily. The family called the community health worker for assistance. The health worker treated Juan for pneumonia with an antibiotic that she had just learned to use as part of a new program for "saving newborn lives." She also gave the family advice about taking care of their new baby. The last baby born to the family had died of pneumonia but Juan survived.

THE IMPORTANCE OF CHILD HEALTH

There are a number of reasons why the health of young children deserves its own chapter in a book on global health. First, about 10.8 million children around the world die every year before they reach their fifth birthday. This is equal to an astounding 30,000 children younger than five years who die every day.[1] The second reason to pay special importance to child health is that so many of these deaths are preventable. It has been estimated, for example, that nearly 6 million of the almost 11 million child deaths each year could be avoided through known, simple, and low-cost interventions.[2] Third, children have a special place in the global health agenda because they are so vulnerable. The measures needed to ensure that they are born healthier, breastfed properly, immunized on schedule, and raised in safe and hygienic conditions, for example, can only be taken by others who care for them. Their vulnerability also raises important ethical issues about the responsibility of adults to ensure the health and survival of children.

Child health is also closely linked with poverty. If children had access to safer water and better sanitation, then many of them would not succumb to diarrhea. If their families had more education, especially their mothers, then families would be better equipped to ensure that their children were cared for. If families had more income, then they would have greater access to health, education, and other social services that would also serve children well.

The health of children is also of particular concern because so little progress has been made in some parts of the world in enhancing child health. This has been especially true in parts of Sub-Saharan Africa, where the direct and indirect costs of HIV/AIDS and malaria take a significant toll on the health of children. This is also the case in South Asia, where

poor nutritional status is at the root of so much ill health for children under five years.

For all these reasons, children are featured prominently in the MDGs, as noted in Table 10-1.

This chapter will highlight for you the most important issues concerning the health of children in low- and middle-income countries. It will review the burden of disease for children, with important comments on the first month of life. It will review the risk factors for illness and death that occur in children under five years. The chapter will then examine measures that can be taken to reduce the burden of disease in young children and some successful cases in which that has been done. The chapter will conclude with a review of some of the key challenges to further the health of children in the developing world.

Nutritional factors, often combined with disease, are a major cause of ill health and death in children; however, nutrition was largely covered in Chapter 8. Children also suffer an important burden of morbidity and mortality as a result of conflict. Civil strife and other emergencies will be reviewed in Chapter 14. This chapter will largely cover four causes of illness and death in children: neonatal causes, diarrhea, pneumonia, and malaria. It will also comment briefly on worms, which will also be covered in greater detail in the next chapter.

KEY TERMS

In Chapter 2, you were introduced to some of the key indicators used in measuring and analyzing global health issues. Those terms, which will be used extensively in this chapter, included neonatal mortality rate, the infant mortality rate, and the under-five child mortality rate.

In this chapter, we will continuously speak of four different phases of the lives of young children:

Perinatal—referring to the first week of life
Neonatal—referring to the first month of life
Infant—referring to the first year of life
Under-five—referring to children 0 to 4 years old

In addition, you will read about some of the most important causes of disease, disability, and death in children under five years, as shown in Table 10-2.

THE BURDEN OF CHILDHOOD ILLNESS
Children Under Five Years

As noted earlier, there are almost 11 million deaths each year in low- and middle-income countries of children under five years. As shown in Figure 10-1, about 10 million of those deaths, or about 90% of them, are due to the combination

---

TABLE 10-1 Linkages Between Child Health and the MDGs

Goal 1: Eradicate Extreme Hunger and Poverty
More than 50% of child deaths worldwide are associated with malnutrition.
Goal 2: Achieve Universal Primary Education
Enrollment, attendance, and performance of children in schools is closely linked with their health.
Goal 3: Promote Gender Equality and Empower Women
Empowering women will enhance their health, their education, and their ability to raise more healthy children.
Goal 4: Reduce Child Mortality
This is directly related to child health.
Goal 5: Improve Maternal Health
Maternal health is a major predictor of the birth weight of a child and the child's subsequent health and survival prospects.
Goal 6: Combat HIV/AIDS, Malaria, and Other Diseases
HIV/AIDS and malaria are major killers of young children.
Goal 7: Ensure Environmental Sustainability
An important share of childhood illness and death is related to unsafe water and poor sanitation. Indoor air pollution is also very important to the heath of children.

Source: Author commentary on the UN Millennium Goals. Available at: http://www.un.org/millennium goals. Accessed July 11, 2006.

TABLE 10-2 Selected Terms Relating to Causes of Child Illness and Death

Asphyxia—A condition of severely deficient oxygen supply.

Diahhrea—A condition characterized by frequent and watery bowel movements.

Hookworm—A parasite that lives in the intestines of its host, which may be a mammal such as a dog, cat, or human. Two species of hookworm commonly infect humans, *Ancylostoma duodenale* and *Necator americanus*.

Malaria—A disease of humans caused by blood parasites of the species *Plasmodium falciparum, vivax, ovale,* or *malariae* and transmitted by anopheline mosquitoes.

Pertussis—A highly contagious bacterial disease that is one of the leading causes of vaccine-preventable death.

Pneumonia—An inflammation, usually caused by infection, involving the alveoli of the lungs.

Polio—An infectious disease, caused by poliovirus that can lead to paralysis.

Sepsis—A serious medical condition caused by a severe infection, leading to a systematic inflammatory response.

Tetanus—A bacterial infection usually contracted through a puncture wound with an unclean object. Neonates acquire tetanus when their birth cord is contaminated, often when cut with an unsterile object.

Source: Author created with data from Birley MH. PEEM Guidelines 2—Guidelines for Forecasting the Vector-borne Disease Implications of Water Resources Development. Available at: http://www.who.int/docstore/water_sanitation_health/Documents/PEEM2/english/peem2chap4.htm. Accessed April 14, 2007; Doctors Without Borders. Glossary. Available at: http://www.doctorswithoutborders.org/education/bol/Glossary.htm. Accessed April 14, 2007. Wikipedia. Asphyxia. Available at: http://en.wikipedia.org/wiki/Asphyxia. Accessed April 14, 2007; Wikipedia. Hookworm. Available at: http://en.wikipedia.org/wiki/Hookworm. Accessed April 14, 2007; Wikipedia. Pneumonia. Available at: http://en.wikipedia.org/wiki/Pneumonia. Accessed April 14, 2007; Wikipedia. Sepsis. Available at: http://en.wikipedia.org/wiki/Sepsis. Accessed April 14, 2007.

of neonatal disorders and communicable diseases, including pneumonia, diarrhea, malaria, measles, and HIV/AIDS. Only about one million of them are due to non-communicable causes.[1]

Over 90% of the annual deaths of children younger than five years worldwide happen in 42 low- or middle-income countries. 50% of these deaths occur in only six countries—India, Nigeria, China, Pakistan, Democratic Republic of Congo, and Ethiopia.[1]

According to UNICEF's 2006 *State of the World's Children Report*,[3] on average worldwide, 79 children die before they reach their fifth birthday for every 1000 who are born. When we look at the numbers in a different way, though, we see that, on average, only 6 die per 1000 in developed countries, whereas 87 die per 1000 in developing countries. If we look only at the poorest developing countries, as many as 200 children die before their fifth birthday for every 1000 born.

The largest killer of children under 5 who die every year in low- and middle-income countries is neonatal disorders, which will be explored further later. The next largest killer of children under 5 in these countries is respiratory infections. The third largest cause of death is diarrheal disease. Malaria is the fourth largest cause of death. Another very important cause of death is measles, which is one of a cluster of vaccine-preventable diseases that includes pertussis, polio, diphtheria,

and tetanus. HIV/AIDS in children is growing and is now the sixth largest cause of death in children younger than five years in low- and middle-income countries.

The various causes of childhood deaths are different, however, for children younger than 1 month old, between 1 month and 1 year of age, and different again, between 1 and 5 years. For neonates, the leading causes of death are low birthweight, mostly associated with prematurity, respiratory infections, birth asphyxia, and trauma, followed by tetanus and diarrheal disease. For children between 1 month and 1 year old, the leading cause of death is diarrheal disease, followed by respiratory infection, and then low birthweight. For children between 1 and 5 years, the leading causes of death are measles, respiratory infections, malaria, and pertussis.[4]

The distribution of deaths also varies by region. Although pneumonia and diarrhea are the first and second biggest causes of childhood illness and death globally, in Africa the picture is different. Acute respiratory infections and diarrhea are still prominent causes of illness and death in Africa, but the single biggest cause of childhood death is malaria. In fact, 3000 African children die every day of malaria. As regions become more advanced in their epidemiological transition, the share of child deaths caused by infectious diseases falls. The leading causes of death of children younger than five years are shown for three regions in Figure 10-2.

FIGURE 10-1 Distribution of Deaths of Children Under Five Years, by Cause, 2000

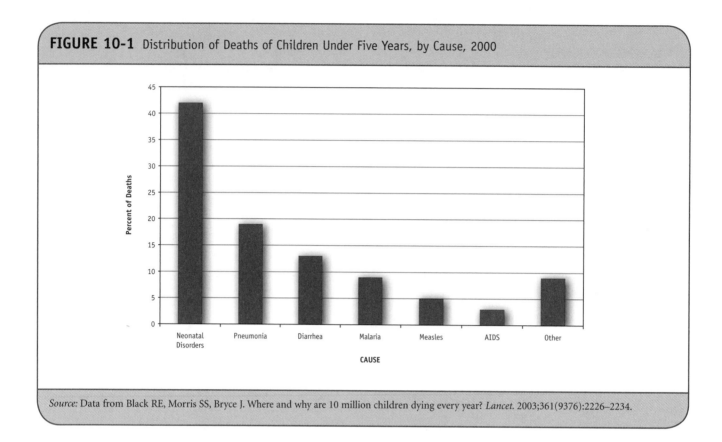

Source: Data from Black RE, Morris SS, Bryce J. Where and why are 10 million children dying every year? *Lancet.* 2003;361(9376):2226–2234.

Figure 10-2 clearly depicts the relative importance of malaria and other infectious diseases in Africa, as well as the shift away from diarrhea and malaria in higher income regions, as you can see in the Latin America and Caribbean Region.

Chapter 2 introduced you to the rates of neonatal, infant, and child mortality. Infant and child mortality are reflected together by region in Figure 10-3.

This figure makes clear what you have seen throughout the book. There are pockets of high rates of infant and child deaths in a number of regions. However, South Asia and Sub-Saharan Africa are the regions of most concern for under-five mortality.

In addition to the significant discrepancies between countries and regions, there can be equally large differences within countries in neonatal, infant, and child mortality. As you read about in the case study of Kerala in Chapter 2, for example, there are only 14 deaths in the first year of life per 1000 children born in the state of Kerala, while 88 per 1000 children die before they reach their first birthday in the state of Orissa.[5] Significant health disparities exist among groups in almost all low- and middle-income countries, and some high-income countries, such as the United States.

Additional Comments on Selected Causes of Morbidity and Mortality

Acute respiratory infections are very common causes of sickness and death in children younger than five years in low- and middle-income countries where children average three to six acute respiratory infections per year. These cases are more severe and cause higher rates of death in developing countries than in developed countries. The most common acute respiratory infections are upper respiratory tract infections, such as the common cold and ear infections. The common lower respiratory infections are pneumonia and bronchiolitis. Pneumonias are caused by both bacteria and viruses. The most common forms of bacterial pneumonia are caused by *Streptococcus pneumoniae* (pneumococcus) and *Haemophilus influenzae,* type b (Hib).[6] This chapter will generally speak only of "pneumonia."

Diarrhea is caused by a number of different infectious agents, including bacteria, viruses, protozoa, and helminths.[7] Diarrhea is transmitted by what is known as the "fecal-oral" route of transmission, from the stool of one individual, eventually to the mouth of another. This is generally the result of unsafe water, poor sanitation, and poor hygiene, as discussed extensively in Chapter 7. Dehydration, loss of nutrition and wasting, or damage to the intestines are all consequences of severe diarrhea.[8] Rapid diarrhea due to dehydration can be fatal quickly. In one study, infants with persistent diarrhea and severe malnutrition were at 17 times greater risk of dying than infants with mild malnutrition.[8] Children younger than five

FIGURE 10-2 Selected Causes of Death Among Children Under Five Years of Age, 2001, for Selected Regions, as a Share of Total Deaths of Under Five Children

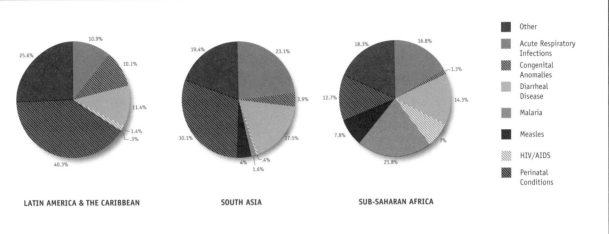

LATIN AMERICA & THE CARIBBEAN   SOUTH ASIA   SUB-SAHARAN AFRICA

Source: Data with permission from The World Bank. Lopez, Alan D, Begg, Stephen, and Bos, Ed. *Demographic and epidemiological characteristics of major regions,* 1990-2001 in Jamison, DT, Breman, JG, and Measham AR, et al, eds. Disease Control Priorities in Developing Countries. 2nd edition. New York: Oxford University Press, 2006.

FIGURE 10-3 Infant and Under-Five Child Mortality Rate, by Region, 2004

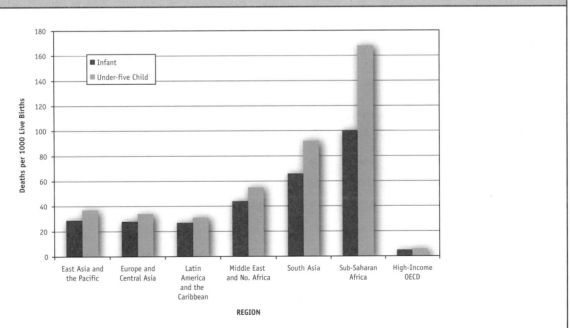

Source: Data with permission from The World Bank. World Development Indicators, Data Query. Available at: http://devdata.worldbank.org. Accessed July 10, 2006.

years in developing countries have around three to four cases of diarrhea per year, with infants 6 to 11 months of age having almost twice as many cases. As noted earlier, this is the age during which they usually stop exclusive breastfeeding and are at most risk of being exposed to unsafe water and foods.[8]

Malaria has an enormous impact on the morbidity and mortality of young children in direct and indirect ways. More than one million children younger than five years are estimated to die yearly from malaria.[9] In addition, the morbidity associated with malaria in young children is staggering. It is estimated that a child in Sub-Saharan Africa is likely to have a case of malaria every 40 days.[10] Moreover, the most severe form of malaria, cerebral malaria, has a case fatality rate of close to 20%, meaning that 20% of the children who get the disease die from it. Beyond the direct consequences of malaria on children are the indirect consequences on them. Malaria is associated with premature birth and intrauterine growth retardation, which are linked with low birthweight and reduced chances of survival.[10]

HIV/AIDS will be discussed at considerable length in Chapter 11, which is on communicable diseases. However, it should be noted here that one route of transmission of HIV is from mother to child. This can either take place during birth or through breastfeeding. The number of HIV infected children in the world has grown, particularly in Sub-Saharan Africa. In Botswana, for example, 37% of pregnant women are estimated to be infected with HIV[11] and child mortality has increased from 58 deaths per 1000 births in 1990 to 116 deaths per 1000 births in 2004, with the increase reflecting the problem of HIV/AIDS.[12]

Measles is an acute respiratory infection that can lead to complications including pneumonia, diarrhea, encephalitis, and blindness. Children who are younger than five years and either vitamin A deficient or HIV infected are more vulnerable to measles complications and are more at risk of death than other children their age. Recent studies in Sub-Saharan Africa suggest that between 0.5%–10% of the children who get measles will die from it. The role of vaccination in preventing measles and other diseases will be discussed later in the chapter. However, it is interesting to note that, in the absence of vaccination, almost 100% of a population will get measles.[13]

Chapter 11 will discuss soil-transmitted helminth infections, and in that chapter you will have an additional opportunity to think about the importance of worms to child health. However, it is important to understand now that it is estimated that two billion people worldwide suffer from helminth infections. About 300 million suffer severe morbidity from these infections, especially iron deficiency anemia, and these worms are also associated with impaired physical and mental development in childhood. The burden of several species of worms is highest in children around 6 or 7 years of age.[14] Few children die directly from these worms. However, the DALYs lost to these worms in children who are 5 to 14 years old are higher than those lost by this age group from almost any other single cause.[15]

Neonatal Mortality

The neonatal period is the first month of life and, as already noted, the largest killers of children younger than five years in the low- and middle-income countries are "neonatal disorders." There has been important progress in reducing the deaths of children younger than five years. However, there has been little progress in reducing the neonatal death rate, except from neonatal tetanus.[16] Of the almost 11 million children under five years who die annually, about 4 million of them actually die in the first month of life. Furthermore, approximately 99% of those 4 million children live in developing countries.[17] Although the rate of neonatal mortality in high-income countries, as discussed in Chapter 2, is about 4 per 1000, it averages about 33 per 1000 in low- and middle-income countries, and goes as high as 70 per 1000.[18] The largest number of neonatal deaths occurs in South Asia, given the relatively poor health circumstances of large numbers of poor families in India, Pakistan, and Bangladesh. China, Nigeria, and Ethiopia are the other countries that have some of the highest numbers of neonatal deaths. However, 80% of the countries with the highest neonatal mortality rates are in Sub-Saharan Africa.[18]

If the world is to further reduce child death rates, then it will have to reduce neonatal death rates. If the world is to do that, then it will have to focus more precisely on when child deaths take place, where they take place, and why they occur. About three million, or 75% of the deaths that take place in the first month of life, actually take place in the first week of life. In addition, about one million, or 25% of the neonatal deaths take place in the first 24 hours of life.[16,18] Clearly, every day that a child lives increases the likelihood that he or she will stay alive. This may help to explain why children in a number of cultures are not named until after their first month of life. It may also help to explain why so many births are not registered with civil authorities, as was the case for Nassiba in the vignette that opened this chapter.

The main causes of neonatal mortality are infections, including pneumonia, diarrhea, and tetanus (36%); preterm birth (28%); and asphyxia (23%). The causes of death in the first few days of life are predominantly preterm birth, asphyxia, and congenital defects. The primary causes of deaths after the first week of life are infections. Despite global efforts to eliminate the problem of neonatal tetanus, it remains a common cause of neonatal death in both South Asia and Sub-Saharan Africa. Just as you would expect, in countries in which the neonatal mortality rate (NNMR) is high, most deaths are caused by infections. As the rate falls, the proportion of deaths due to infection will also fall, and the deaths due to prematurity and congenital defects will become proportionately the most important.[19]

Chapter 2 introduced you to neonatal mortality rates. Table 10-3 shows neonatal mortality rates by WHO Region for 2000. It also shows how those rates vary by highest and lowest income quintile. As we have seen before, the neonatal mortality rate varies between about 50% higher and 100% higher when comparing the poorest income groups to the highest income groups. An enormous number of child lives could be saved if the gap in child deaths between the richest and poorest segments of society were narrowed.

In thinking about neonatal deaths, just as in thinking about the deaths of all infants and children under five years, we must remember the relationship between the health of the mother and the health of the baby. Between 60–80% of neonatal deaths occur in low birthweight babies. This generally reflects the poor health and nutritional status of the mother, including her being undernourished or having malaria, for example.[19]

RISK FACTORS FOR NEONATAL, INFANT, AND CHILD DEATHS

Why do so many children still die and so many others become disabled at such young ages? As mentioned earlier, poverty contributes to poor health and is a major underlying cause of morbidity and mortality among children. Where there is poverty, there is often inadequate nutrition. Where there is poverty, there is less access to safe water and sanitation, health services, and education. All of these are important determinants of child health.

In addition, you already know that there is very strong correlation between family income and the likelihood that a neonate, an infant, or a child will survive. You also know that there is a similar correlation between the health and the educational status of the mother and the prospects that a child will survive birth and the first 5 years of life. Nutritional status, malaria, and HIV are also powerful determinants of the weight the baby will have at birth and of his or her chances for survival.

The Millennium Report 2006, in commenting on progress towards the Millennium Development Goal of reducing child morbidity and mortality, revealed that higher household income and education for mothers doubles child survival rates. In families where the mother had no education or only primary education, child mortality averaged 157 deaths per 1000 live births, whereas in families where the mother had secondary education or higher, mortality rates were close to 50% less, at 82 per 1000 live births.[20]

Related to both income and the educational status of the family is the fact that the survival of a newborn is also closely linked with whether or not the birth is in an appropriate healthcare setting and is attended by a trained healthcare provider.[21] A baby's chances of survival increase greatly when the baby is born in a setting that can deal with obstetric emergencies. The chances of survival also increase if the delivery is attended by a skilled birth attendant who can resuscitate babies who need it and can help to counsel families about

TABLE 10-3 Neonatal Mortality Rates, Total and by Lowest and Highest Income Quintile, for WHO Regions, 2000

Region	NMR per 1000 live births (range across countries)	Median NMR by income quintile by region Poorest Quintile	Richest Quintile
Africa	44 (9-70)	48	34
Americas	12 (4-34)	35	18
Eastern Mediterranean	40 (4-63)	38	28
Europe	11 (2-38)	--	--
South Asia	38 (11-43)	50	28
Western Pacific	19 (1-40)	28	17

Source: Adapted with permission from The World Bank. Lawn JE, Zupan J, Begkoyian G, Knippenberg R. Newborn survival. In: Jamison DT, Breman JG, Measham AR, et al., eds. *Disease Control Priorities in Developing Countries.* 2nd ed. New York: Oxford University Press; 2006:531–549.

keeping babies warm and breastfed. The child's chances of survival also increase if the family has access to appropriate antibiotic treatment for pneumonia if it arises.

The burden of diarrheal disease on child health makes clear that unsafe water and poor sanitation are major risk factors for child health. We have seen how the risk of unsafe hygiene increases greatly as the child begins to eat complementary foods and is no longer exclusively breastfed. We have also seen that better educated families have more awareness about health risks as well as safe behaviors that can improve their children's health and chances of survival.

Chapter 8 reviewed nutrition in detail and made clear the extent to which undernutrition is a risk factor for child morbidity and mortality. However, it is worth reminding ourselves of the profound impact of nutritional status, indirectly, through the mother, and directly, on the health and survival prospects of neonates, infants, and children younger than five years.

- "Infants aged 0–5 months who are not breastfed have seven-fold increased risks of death from diarrhea and pneumonia, respectively, compared to infants who are exclusively breastfed."[22]
- ". . . 35% of all child deaths are due to the effect of underweight status on diarrhea, pneumonia, measles, and malaria and relative risks of maternal body mass index for fetal growth retardation and its risks for selected neonatal causes of death."[22]
- "In children with vitamin A deficiency, the risk of dying from diarrhea, measles, and malaria is increased by 20–24%. Likewise, zinc deficiency increases the risk of mortality from diarrhea, pneumonia, and malaria by 13–21%."[22]

The impact of wars and conflicts on health is covered in Chapter 14. Wars and conflicts take a significant toll on children and are regrettable risk factors for child morbidity and mortality, particularly in Sub-Saharan Africa. UNICEF estimates that in a "typical" 5-year war, under-five mortality increases 13%.[23] In addition, the highest rates of neonatal death occur in conflict ridden countries or countries just emerging from conflict, such as Liberia and Sierra Leone.[24]

THE COSTS AND CONSEQUENCES OF CHILD MORBIDITY AND MORTALITY

One cannot measure "direct losses in productivity" that relate immediately to the morbidity and mortality of young children from the causes discussed in this chapter. There are, however, enormous costs and consequences to these illnesses. Some

of them are short-run and relate to the family. Others are medium-term or longer run and relate to the child directly.

First, the direct and indirect costs of caring for a sick child can be very high. As noted earlier in this chapter, the average child in Africa is infected with malaria every 40 days. In addition, the average child in low- and middle-income countries will get three to six bouts per year of acute respiratory infection, and two to three cases of diarrhea. In this light, it is not surprising that families spend considerable parts of their limited financial resources buying medical care for a sick child.[8] Moreover, caregivers devote special attention to the child who is ill, which prevents them from engaging in their normal income-earning activities.

Second, the medium and long-term consequences of some childhood illnesses can be very high. The consequences of undernutrition and micronutrient deficiency were explored at length in Chapter 8. Problems associated with prematurity, low birth weight, intrauterine growth retardation, and congenital abnormalities can lead to permanent disability and the related costs to families and to society that are associated with it. A study on diarrheal disease in Brazil concluded that intelligence test scores were "25–65% lower in children with an earlier history of persistent diarrhea."[25] The complications of measles can lead to encephalitis and blindness, as indicated earlier. By causing anemia, growth retardation, and the retardation of mental development, helminthic infections reduce enrollment in school, attendance at school, and performance in school and have consequences for later productivity.[26]

Finally, there are a range of social costs and consequences associated with childhood illness and death. Many poor families in low-income countries, knowing the odds are high that their newborn will die, have very high fertility to "compensate" for these deaths. In other words, in the hope of ensuring that the number of children they want will survive, they have more children than they would have otherwise.

CASE STUDIES

Some of the important progress made so far in reducing the burden of disease in children has been associated with the control of diarrheal disease, supplementing children with vitamin A, and the spread of immunization programs. The three cases below look at successful examples in each of these areas that were affordable, effective, and had a substantial impact on reducing morbidity and mortality in young children. You can read about each of these cases in greater detail in *Case Studies in Global Health: Millions Saved*. The case below on diarrheal disease in Egypt complements the case on diarrhea in Bangldesh that was featured in Chapter 5.

Preventing Diarrheal Deaths in Egypt

Background

About 20% of child deaths worldwide are due to complications from diarrheal disease, mostly among children younger than 2 years old. Bacteria, protozoa, and viruses cause diarrhea, which can quickly become deadly as the body expels electrolytes and water and becomes dehydrated. Intravenous infusions can help rehydrate patients in hospitals, and some drugs can help stop the diarrhea. However, these infusions are relatively costly, invasive, and difficult to carry out in many low-income environments.

In the 1960s, oral dehydration therapy (ORT) was developed in Bangladesh and India. As discussed earlier, ORT is a simple solution of water, sugar, and salt that was found to be as effective in stopping dehydration as expensive intravenous therapy. In 1970, it was invaluable in saving lives of many of the millions of refugees camped along the Bangladesh and India borders when cholera struck during a war between Bangladesh and Pakistan. In 1972, the World Health Organization declared ORT the world's standard treatment for diarrhea.

Intervention

In the 1970s in Egypt, infant mortality was as high as 100 per 1000 live births. Diarrheal disease caused at least half of all infant deaths in Egypt in 1977 when ORT was introduced into clinics and pharmacies. Initially there was little take-up of the newly available intervention. However, it was realized that physicians and mothers could play a key role in promoting the program, and they were trained to effectively use ORT. The use of ORT rose dramatically, and in pilot areas where training was conducted, diarrhea-related mortality declined by 45%.

Based on the impact demonstrated in the pilot areas, a nationwide campaign was launched. In 1981, the National Control of Diarrheal Disease Project (NCDDP) was established in partnership with the private sector, professional societies, and international organizations such as WHO and UNICEF. The program had four components. First, there was product design and branding. ORT packets were distributed in a size that Egyptian mothers considered suitable for a child's drink. Second, production and distribution of an uninterrupted supply of ORT by public and private entities was subsidized by UNICEF and NCDDP. The public sector received ORT through a network of distribution centers, including the private homes of community leaders in remote rural areas. Third, private sector distributors were given incentives to sell ORT rather than antidiarrheal drugs. Lastly,

thousands of health workers were trained to teach mothers about ORT and a national media campaign took advantage of the new TV service to expand access to knowledge about ORT. By 1984, the use of ORT to manage cases of child diarrhea had reached 60%.

Impact

Between 1982 and 1987, overall infant mortality dropped by 36% and child mortality dropped by 43%. Diarrhea mortality fell by 82% among infants and by 62% among children during the same period. Challenges remained, however, despite the success: private physicians were slow to convert to ORT and a large number of antidiarrheal drugs continued to be sold.

Costs and Benefits

The average cost per child treated with ORT was estimated at only $6. The cost per death averted was between $100 and $200. The program cost a total of $43 million, of which $17 million came from Egypt and $26 million came from USAID. UNICEF and WHO provided technical support to the program.

Lessons Learned

Research was the key to the success of Egypt's diarrhea control program. Anthropological and market research about cultural practices and consumer preferences shaped the communication program, product design, and branding. Epidemiological and clinical research lead to the appropriate composition of the ORT product. It also contributed to a better understanding of risk factors and kept the medical community engaged in the issue of ORT. Data from ongoing project evaluation and from independent, external evaluations were used continuously to guide decision-making. Different approaches were regularly piloted and the program was flexible and open to change as new, effective strategies were identified to ensure continued success of the program.

Reducing Child Mortality in Nepal Through Vitamin A

Background

As discussed in Chapter 8, vitamin A deficiency is a leading determinant of child mortality in low- and middle-income countries. Vitamin A deficiency compromises the immune systems of nearly 40% of the developing world's children and leads to the deaths of approximately one million young children each year. Additionally, it contributes to 16% of the global burden of disease caused by malaria, 18% of the global burden of diarrheal disease, and a significant proportion of the acute respiratory infections and measles.[27]

Vitamin A deficiency has been an especially important health problem in Nepal, with 2–13% of preschool-aged children experiencing xerophthalmia. Economic and geographic barriers help to explain this high prevalence rate. First, difficult terrain makes it hard to grow or access the types of food that supply vitamin A. Second, 38% of the Nepali population lives in absolute poverty, many of whom are socially excluded lower caste families who frequently lack the means to pay for nutritious foods.

Intervention

Prior to the late 1980s, it was widely held that micronutrient deficiencies were a result of diarrhea and other infant illnesses, rather than a cause of them. Yet, as early as the 1970s, Alfred Sommer noticed in conjunction with studies in Indonesia that vitamin A deficiency appeared to be linked with child death. A later randomized control trial conducted in Nepal by Keith West and Alfred Sommer indicated that periodic vitamin A delivery could reduce mortality in children aged 6 to 60 months by as much as 30%.[28]

In light of these research findings and Nepal's excessive infant mortality rate, the Nepalese Ministry of Health initiated a plan of action on vitamin A in 1992. The Ministry worked closely with other government agencies and NGOs to develop a pilot program to deliver vitamin A capsules throughout Nepal. A technical assistance group was created to assist the health ministry in running the program. His Majesty, the King of Nepal, also demonstrated long-term commitment to this effort by incorporating Nepal's National Vitamin A Program into the Ten Year National Program of Action.

This program aimed to reduce child morbidity and mortality by prophylactic supplementation of high dose vitamin A capsules to children 6 to 60 months of age, twice each year; the treatment of xerophthalmia, severe malnutrition, and prolonged diarrhea; and promotion of behavior change to increase dietary intake of vitamin A and promote exclusive breastfeeding for the first 6 months of a baby's life.

The action plan on vitamin A focused on expanding the intervention in phases as Nepal's administrative capacity for the program was strengthened. The program was expanded to 32 priority districts at a rate of eight districts per year over 4 years. From 1993 to 2001, the program was brought to Nepal's remaining 43 districts. Children and new mothers in districts where the National Vitamin A Program was not yet established received one dose of vitamin A as part of national immunization campaigns. Once the National Vitamin A Program was operating in their district, the children received vitamin A supplementation twice a year.

Nepal's public health system faced severe problems at the time the vitamin A program was developed, from low utilization rates by people who had no confidence in the system to absenteeism by health workers. Consequently, the vitamin A intervention was revised to build upon and improve the existing networks of female community health volunteers (FCHVs) who helped deliver primary health care and family planning services to the villages of Nepal. Before the intervention, there were 24,000 FCHVs throughout 58 districts. However, many were not respected in their communities and had little incentive to remain committed to volunteering. The leader of the program's technical assistance group, Ram Shrestha, changed the way FCHVs were viewed by communities and themselves by focusing on notions of "Respect, Recognition, and Opportunity." Shrestha challenged deeply rooted gender biases by giving women responsibilities valued by their families and communities and the opportunity to make a difference.

A few years later, the number of FCHVs had more than doubled to 49,000 strong, and they were able to reach 3.7 million children twice a year with vitamin A capsules. By directly administering the capsules, the FCHVs served as a critical bridge between the public health sector and the community. Families were urged to bring their children to the distribution site, and many government sectors began to integrate messages about the importance of vitamin A into their programs.

Impact

An evaluation of the program indicated that under-five mortality decreased by almost 48 deaths per 1000 births, on average. Higher literacy rates among women, improved weight and nutritional status of children, and better vaccination rates were also associated with success. About 134,000 deaths were averted between mid-1995 and mid-2000 as a result of Nepal's Vitamin A Program.[29] Although it took nearly 8 years to achieve nationwide distribution, program coverage never dropped below 90% in districts, once they were covered.

Costs and Benefits

Compared to other micronutrient supplement programs, which can cost up to about $5 per child,[30] the vitamin A supplement program in Nepal was a relatively inexpensive approach to ease the burden of a national problem. The cost of the program per child covered was approximately $0.81 to $1.09 for a child receiving one capsule and $0.68 to $1.65 for a child receiving two capsules of vitamin A.[31] Additionally, given the 7500 lives saved annually, the expanded program in 2000 was estimated to cost $345 per death averted or $11 to $12 per DALY gained.[32]

Lessons Learned

The success of Nepal's vitamin A supplementation program demonstrates how a technical innovation, when paired with an equally innovative operational plan, can result in a major population impact. Rather than trying to restructure the health system to accommodate the vitamin A program, Shrestha's adapted the vitamin A program to the preexisting network of FCHVs and then refined it in a way that it could be successful. This approach also reinforced a multi-sectoral effort by involving the government, NGOs, and communities. Other key factors associated with this successful effort were partnership building, regular monitoring of quality, straightforward and effective public messages, and clarity of objectives and operational strategy. These lessons are all the more important given that this successful effort took place in a very poor country with extremely weak governance and poor administrative capacity.

Eliminating Polio in Latin America and the Caribbean

Background

Poliomyelitis is caused by the intestinal poliovirus, which enters through the nose or mouth and multiplies in the lymph nodes. Within days, an otherwise healthy person can become paralyzed for life or possibly not survive the disease. In 1952, Dr. Jonas Salk discovered the inactivated polio vaccine. Mass immunizations between 1955 and 1961 led to a 90% drop in infections in the Western Hemisphere.[54] Ten years later, in 1962, Dr. Albert Sabin developed an oral polio vaccine that cost less, was easier to administer, and reduced the multiplication of the virus in the intestine.

The new oral polio vaccine became part of a package of six childhood vaccines included in an Expanded Program on Immunization (EPI) launched by WHO in 1977. Latin America adopted the Expanded Program on Immunization in 1977, and the coverage of oral polio vaccine reached 80% within just 7 years. Between 1975 and 1981, the incidence of polio was nearly halved and the number of countries reporting polio cases dropped from 19 to 11.[55]

Intervention

Encouraged by the remarkable progress against polio, the Pan American Health Organization (PAHO) launched a program to eradicate polio from Latin America and the Caribbean. Many international organizations joined together in the program and regional and country-level Inter-Agency Coordinating Committees were established to oversee the program. Thousands of health workers, managers, and technicians were trained to implement the strategy for the eradication of polio, which included reaching every child with oral polio vaccination, identification of new polio cases, and aggressive control of any outbreaks. If polio were to be eradicated, then the campaign against it would build on the lessons learned from the smallpox eradication campaign.[56]

Impact

The last case of polio in the Latin America and the Caribbean region was reported in Peru in 1991. Polio reemerged briefly in the year 2000 when 20 vaccine-associated cases were reported in Haiti and the Dominican Republic, but no cases have been reported since the year 2000.

Costs and Benefits

The polio campaign cost $120 million in its first 5 years—$74 million from national sources and $46 million from international donors, and $10 million annually from donor sources thereafter. Taking into account the costs of treating polio and its disabling consequences, the investment paid for itself in only 15 years.[53] The program also generated vast improvements in the region's health infrastructure, and it advanced overall goals for immunization.

Lessons learned

The success of eliminating polio from Latin America and the Caribbean in only 6 years was a result of exemplary political commitment, interagency and regional coordination, and tremendous social and community mobilization. The reemergence of polio in the year 2000 alerted the region to the need for continued vaccination and surveillance. The success in Latin America and the Caribbean prompted a global effort to eradicate polio that was launched in 1998.[57]

The Global Polio Eradication Initiative is an international partnership spearheaded by national governments, the WHO, Rotary International, the U.S. Centers for Disease Control and Prevention, and UNICEF. The importance of building trust with local leaders and working closely with communities that was learned in the polio efforts in the Americas is one of many lessons that is being put to good use in the global polio eradication initiative.

ADDRESSING KEY CHALLENGES IN CHILD HEALTH

As noted earlier, there has been important progress in the last 30 years in reducing morbidity and mortality of children younger than five years. The under-five mortality rate worldwide fell 50% between 1960 and 1990.[33] There was a particularly rapid rate of improvement in the 1970s, including significant declines in child death rates in Sub-Saharan Africa and South Asia, the two regions with the highest rates.

Despite this progress, the challenges to meeting the MDG on child health and to improving the health of children in low- and middle-income countries remain enormous. First, as also discussed earlier, the progress that has been made has largely been in reducing the rate of death of children between 1 and 5 years. By contrast, very little progress has been made in reducing the death rate of neonates.[16,17] In fact, about 40% of the children younger than five years who die are now 1 year old or younger.

In addition, many interventions that are known to be low cost and effective at reducing morbidity and mortality in young children are not being implemented where they are needed most. A large number of births in low-income countries take place without the help of a skilled birth attendant who can assist the mother and, for example, resuscitate the baby if needed. Many families still do not use ORT when their child gets diarrhea. Too often, the pneumonia that kills young children is not diagnosed or treated in a timely way. Coverage with the important life-saving measles vaccination remains low in many countries. In addition, insecticide treated bed nets, which are known to reduce the transmission of malaria, are still not as widely used as they should be.

The experience of the developed countries in reducing neonatal deaths shows that a large proportion of neonatal deaths in the developing countries can be avoided with simple technologies that could be effectively implemented in low-income settings.[21] In fact, almost two thirds of the child deaths that occur every year could be prevented by the effective implementation of measures such as these, that are both low cost and effective.[34]

What can be done to increase the uptake of these approaches, especially in South Asia and Sub-Saharan Africa, the regions with the highest rates of child death? What can be done to decrease as quickly as possible the rate of neonatal deaths, again, largely in these two regions? Can measures be taken that will help children from low-income families with little education die as rarely as children from better-off and better educated families?[35] The section below examines some of what has been learned about cost-effective interventions to prevent child deaths and how these efforts can be scaled up more rapidly. Some of the comments will be organized around the life cycle. Others will be organized by type of intervention. Finally, additional comments will be made about how such interventions might be put into place most rapidly and effectively.

Critical Child Health Interventions

The Mother and Mother-to-Be

As you have read repeatedly, an extremely important factor in determining the health of the newborn and young child is the health and nutritional status of the mother. The chapters on nutrition and on women's health have commented at length on measures that can be taken to ensure that women are getting enough calories and that they are not deficient in key micronutrients. However, it is also very important to pregnancy outcomes that pregnant women not suffer from malaria. Rather, they should be treated appropriately for malaria, as will be discussed in detail in the next chapter.

You have also read about the importance of having a skilled attendant at delivery. Proper monitoring of labor and the fetus can improve pregnancy and birth outcomes. In addition, if the labor is complicated, then access to emergency obstetric care can reduce risks to both mother and child. Preventing infection is also important to the mother and child. Ensuring that the mother is vaccinated against tetanus is also critical to the prospects for child survival.[36]

A substantial number of pregnant women are infected with HIV in parts of central and southern Africa in particular, as will also be discussed further in the next chapter. If an HIV-infected mother does not breastfeed, then there is a 15–30% chance that her child will contract HIV. If the mother breastfeeds her baby for an extended period of time, then the risk of her child becoming infected with HIV increases to 30–45%. The risk of a mother transmitting HIV to her child can be reduced by feeding the child with an alternative to breast milk, although this also carries risks of diarrheal disease in settings where water is unsafe and hygiene is poor.[37]

Measures to prevent HIV infection among women and mothers-to-be are the most cost-effective ways to ensure that HIV is not transmitted from mothers to their children. However, if a mother is HIV infected, then providing drug therapy to prevent transmission can also be cost-effective.[38]

The Newborn

As discussed earlier, most child deaths in the first month of life will be from prematurity, asphyxia, or infections. You also read that prematurity, infection, and asphyxia are the leading causes of death in the first week of life and infections are the leading cause of death in the 3 weeks after that.[19] There are a number of cost-effective measures that can be taken to address these problems. They are largely based on evidence of what works. They focus on: "essential newborn care" for all newborns; "extra care for small babies"; and, "emergency care" and are summarized in Table 10-4.[39] Low-income countries do not need to adopt expensive, high technology solutions to immediately reduce their neonatal death rates.

In terms of essential care of newborns, skilled attendance at delivery is crucial to save both newborn lives, as well as the lives of mothers. It is imperative for the health of the baby, for example, that the delivery attendant cut the umbilical cord in a hygienic manner and practice other infection controls. In addition, the baby needs to be kept warm and not bathed for the first 24 hours. The attendant should also be trained and have the equipment needed to resuscitate the baby if necessary and efforts are underway for that to be done in the simplest possible way in low-income settings. Attendance at delivery is also an appropriate time for a trained practitioner to counsel the family about exclusive breastfeeding and about how to know the danger signs for threats to the baby's health that require immediate attention, such as pneumonia.[40]

Some babies need extra care. If the baby is born prematurely or of low birth weight, then it is especially important that the baby be kept warm, fed properly, and that any complications that arise be managed quickly and appropriately. In developed countries, of course, premature babies would be kept in an incubator. This option, however, rarely exists for the children of poor families in low-income countries. However, a study done in India[41] showed that the neonatal mortality rate among babies born between 35 to 37 weeks, or moderately premature babies, was reduced by 87% by the provision of special "sleeping bags" to keep the baby warm, coupled with the promotion of breastfeeding and early treatment of infections. Another effort at keeping premature and low birth weight babies warm is called "kangaroo mother care." In this approach, continuous skin-to-skin contact is maintained between the mother and baby and exclusive breastfeeding is promoted. This hospital-based program showed a reduction in child morbidity, compared to similar children who did not have kangaroo care.[42]

Despite the above efforts, some babies will become infected and will require emergency care. The question of providing antibiotics to neonates who have infections is a challenging one in many settings. In many places, only physicians are legally allowed to prescribe antibiotics. Yet, physicians may not be accessible, particularly in rural and impoverished settings that will have the highest rates of neonatal mortality. There is some evidence that

---

TABLE 10-4 Essential Interventions for Newborn Care

Essential Newborn Care
- Early and exclusive breastfeeding
- Warmth provision and avoidance of bathing during first 24 hours
- Infection control, including cord care and hygiene
- Postpartum vitamin A provided to mothers
- Eye antimicrobial to prevent opthalmia, inflammation of the eye or conjunctiva
- Information and counseling for home care and emergency preparedness

Extra Care for Small Babies
- Extra attention to warmth, feeding support, and early identification and management of complications
- Kangaroo mother care
- Vitamin K injection

Emergency Care
- Providing supportive care for severe infections; neonatal encephalopathy (brain disease); severe jaundice or bleeding; and, neonatal tetanus

Source: Adapted with permission from The World Bank. Lawn JE, Zupan J, Begkoyian G, Knippenberg R. Newborn Survival. In: Jamison DT, Breman JG, Measham A, et al., eds. *Disease Control Priorities in Developing Countries.* New York: Oxford University Press and World Bank; 2006:537.

---

community health workers can be trained to safely give antibiotics to neonates who have infections that are life threatening.[41,43]

Infants and Young Children

The leading killer of infants and young children in low- and middle-income countries is diarrhea. Such deaths are almost completely unnecessary. As you know, there are many reasons why exclusive breastfeeding until children are 6 months of age is so important, and one of them is to avoid diarrhea in settings that are not hygienic. As children move to complementary foods, there are a number of measures that can be taken to reduce the risk to them of diarrheal disease. The first, of course, is to engage in better personal hygiene and more hygienic food preparation. Second, complementary foods that are fortified can help children meet their requirements for micronutrients.[44] Third, ensuring that children are immunized against measles can help to reduce deaths from diarrhea. It has been estimated, in fact, that measles immunization could eliminate 6–26% of diarrheal deaths of children younger than five years.[45] As discussed in Chapter 7, improving water supply and sanitation can be very important to reducing diarrhea in children. Unfortunately, the infrastructure to do so can be very expensive and health benefits flow mostly when communities adopt safer water and sanitation systems, rather than just having them adopted by individual families.[45]

When young children do get diarrhea that is not of the type that requires antibiotics, there are two measures that are very cost-effective that can be taken to manage the diarrhea. First is the use at home of ORT, as modeled in the cases on Bangladesh and Egypt about which you read earlier. Second is supplementation with zinc, because such supplements have been shown to reduce the duration and severity of diarrhea.[1]

Immunization

In 1974, WHO launched the Expanded Program on Immunization (EPI), which promoted worldwide a package of six basic vaccines for children and "vaccination against childhood communicable diseases through the Expanded Program on Immunization is one of the most cost-effective public health interventions available."[46] The vaccines in standard EPI programs include those against diphtheria, pertussis, tetanus, polio, tuberculosis, and measles. There is a standard schedule for giving these immunizations.

One of the leading goals of the EPI today is to ensure that 80% of the children in 80% of the districts in a country receive the third immunization for diphtheria, pertussis, and tetanus.[47] In light of the immunization schedule, this is a benchmark for good coverage of an immunization program. It is estimated that in 2001, in the absence of the vaccinations that were carried out, deaths from measles would have risen by 60%, deaths from tetanus by about 70%, deaths from pertussis by almost 80%, and deaths from diphtheria would have risen by more than 90%.[48]

Most vaccinations are given in health facilities. However, national authorities also have occasional campaigns to immunize against some diseases, as they have done as part of the global polio eradication program. Some vaccinations are given by outreach workers who travel to people's homes or central locations. In some cases, vaccines are made available through the private sector.

Despite the importance of immunization and the efforts made for EPI in most countries, there are still important gaps in the coverage of the basic vaccines in some countries, especially in Sub-Saharan Africa. In Nigeria, for example, the most populous country in Sub-Saharan Africa, the average immunization coverage is very low at 13% coverage, and in some states only 1% of the children are being immunized.[49] One child in five dies in Nigeria before their fifth birthday and 22% of them died of vaccine-preventable diseases in 2002. In other words, nearly 200,000 child deaths could have been prevented in Nigeria that year with more complete coverage of basic immunization.

In addition, as you have seen in several places in the book, vaccine coverage varies directly with the education of the mother and the income of the family. The children most in need of getting vaccinated will be the children in the poorest families in South Asia and Sub-Saharan Africa. Unfortunately, they will also be the least likely to get vaccinated.

In high-income countries, the number and selection of vaccines for children has increased considerably from just the six basic vaccines, and developing countries are starting to introduce some of the additional vaccines, as well, such as those for hepatitis B and *Haemophilus influenza* type b vaccines. In deciding which newer vaccines to introduce, countries need to assess both the burden of disease in their country as well as what their health budgets can afford and the feasibility of introducing a new vaccine in their existing EPI. To enhance coverage and to introduce in developing countries vaccines against hepatitis B and *Haemophilus influenza* type b, development partners created the Global Alliance for Vaccines and Immunization, or GAVI, in 1999. This organization is discussed in Chapter 15.

Community-Based Approaches to Improving Child Health

As you have seen throughout the book, many of the measures that are needed to reduce the burden of illness and death in neonates, infants, and young children have to do with appropriate knowledge and behavior of individuals and families. You have also read that studies that have been done in a number of places show that community-based approaches to improving health behaviors and providing basic health services with the help of trained members of the community can lead to significant gains in health. In Chapter 5, you read about how a very large share of all primary healthcare services are delivered in Bangladesh by a community-based NGO called BRAC.

The role of the family and community is key to newborn health. Community awareness and the engagement of women's groups have been highly effective in improving the health and survival of newborns. In one project in rural Bolivia, the involvement of local women's groups in raising awareness of maternal, fetal, and neonatal issues lead to increased use of prenatal and postnatal health services, more traditional birth assistants at childbirth, and an overall 62% reduction of perinatal mortality. In another study in rural Nepal, working with local women's groups was key to motivating increased hygiene and health seeking behavior, which contributed to a 30% reduction in neonatal mortality.[4]

In fact, a family and community-based approach to promoting hygiene, including hand washing and umbilical cord care, keeping the newborn warm, and exclusively breastfeeding are all important home measures that could lead to an estimated 10–40% reduction in neonatal mortality. Home based supplementary feeding, using a dropper or a cup, is another important measure to ensure the survival of low birthweight babies, who account for 60–80% of neonatal deaths.[4]

Table 10-5 is a summary of measures that families can take, even in low-income communities, to protect the health of their young children. You can see in the table the extent to which families, if they had better knowledge of good health practices and community support to engage in them, could promote important reductions in child morbidity and mortality. Low-income people in developing countries are not going to have any quick increase in formal education, income, or social and political voice. Thus, it will be very important to take community-based approaches to help families improve their knowledge and practice of good health behaviors.

Integrated Management of Childhood Illness

The need for working closely with communities has emerged again in recent efforts worldwide to encourage a more integrated approach to health services for sick children. In many developing countries, as discussed in the chapter on health systems, a number of health programs have been organized as somewhat separate programs sometimes called "vertical" that are not well linked with other parts of health services. It is quite common, for example, for the vaccination program to operate with limited connections to other parts of the health services. The same has tended to be true of family planning services, as well as services for a variety of other programs.[50]

Given the multiple factors that lead to child illness and, in some cases, death, however, it is widely agreed that no single child intervention is adequate to ensure a child's health. It is also agreed that, given the interrelated factors that effect a child's health and survival, an integrated approach to managing illness is important for newborns, infants, and older children.

Integrated Management of Childhood Illnesses, called IMCI, is an approach that recognizes the importance of looking at the "whole" child and not treating one symptom

TABLE 10-5 12 Key Family Practices

Communities need to be strengthened and families supported to improve child survival, growth, and development. Evidence suggests that families should:

- Breastfeed infants exclusively for at least 6 months (mothers found to be HIV positive require counselling about possible alternatives to breastfeeding).
- Feed children complementary foods starting at about 6 months of age, while continuing to breastfeed up to 2 years or longer.
- Ensure that children receive adequate amounts of micronutrients (vitamin A and iron in particular), either in their diet or through supplementation.
- Dispose of feces, including children's feces, safely, and wash hands after defecation, before preparing meals, and before feeding children.
- Complete a full course of immunizations (BCG, DPT, OPV, and measles) for children before their first birthday.
- Protect children in malaria-endemic areas by ensuring that they sleep under insecticide-treated bednets.
- Promote mental and social development by responding to a child's needs through talking, playing, and providing a stimulating environment.
- Feed and offer more fluids, including breast milk, when children are sick.
- Give sick children appropriate home treatment for infections.
- Recognize when sick children need treatment outside the home and seek care from appropriate providers.
- Follow health worker's advice about treatment, follow-up, and referral.
- Ensure that every pregnant woman has adequate antenatal care, including at least four antenatal visits with an appropriate healthcare provider, and the recommended doses of the tetanus toxoid vaccination. The mother also needs support from her family and community in seeking care at the time of delivery and during the postpartum and lactation period.

Source: Adapted with permission from World Health Organization. Child and Adolescent Health and Development: Prevention and Care of Illness, Neonates and Infants. Available at: http://www.who.int/child-adolescent-health/PREVENTION/12_key.htm. Accessed November 9, 2006.

or providing one intervention without looking at other possible needs. It also recognizes that care is needed at the level of overall health system, local health center, and at the level of family and community. The IMCI approach focuses on training health workers and caretakers at all levels, but pays special attention to home and community-based care, which is increasingly acknowledged as being able to contribute to significant reduction of childhood deaths at minimal cost.

A number of evaluations of IMCI efforts have taken place and reveal that health workers trained in IMCI programs provide higher quality of care than workers trained in other programs. A review of IMCI experience in Tanzania showed that better care could be provided at lower cost than in non-IMCI areas, because better care led to fewer hospitalizations of children. Overall, however, it appears that if IMCI is to meet its promise, then it will have to be carried out in a way that is more closely linked with the communities where it is being done and in a way that ensures that families engage in the practices noted in Table 10-5.[51]

There is widespread agreement about what interventions are needed to improve child health. The key challenge to gaining such improvements, however, is not what to do, but how to do it and how to engage communities in ensuring that needed interventions happen. There are countries, such as Sri Lanka, Cuba, and China, and states within countries, such as Kerala, in which there is widespread knowledge of appropriate health and hygiene behaviors, appropriate nutrition practices, the home management of illness, and when to seek care from health services. In Bangladesh, as you read, there has been widespread adoption of ORT, despite the low educational and income status of a large share of the population. Families and communities are the key to rapid uptake of critical measures to improve child health and a central issue in global health today is to learn from experience about how large scale change in health and child caring behaviors can be promoted as quickly, effectively, and efficiently, as possible.

MAIN MESSAGES

Approximately 10.8 million children around the world die each year before they reach their fifth birthday. Nearly six million die due to causes which are largely preventable, and nearly four million, or 36%, die in their first 4 weeks of life. 90% of the deaths happen in 42 low- or middle-income countries, and 50% of the under-five deaths happen in only six countries—India, Nigeria, China, Pakistan, the Democratic Republic of Congo, and Ethiopia.

As we learned in the vignettes that opened the chapter, the chances of survival for a newborn, an infant, and a young child are vastly different across different settings. The discrepancies within an individual country can be as wide as differences between countries. High-income countries have, on average, 6 deaths per 1000 live births for children younger than five years, while developing countries have on average 87 deaths per 1000 live births in that same age group. In the poorest and most conflict-ridden countries, the under-five child mortality rate can be as high as 200 deaths per 1000 live births.

Communicable diseases are the leading cause of death among children in the developing countries. Pneumonia is the biggest killer of children who are younger than five years. One fifth, or 2 million of the 10.8 million children who die before five years each year, die of pneumonia. The second most important cause of illness and death among children is diarrheal disease. Another significant cause of childhood death is measles, which is responsible for 500,000 deaths annually. In Africa, the single biggest cause of childhood death is malaria, and 3000 children die every day of malaria across Africa.

Poverty is a significant underlying factor of morbidity and mortality among children. Where there is poverty, there is often inadequate nutrition and inadequate access to safe water, sanitation, health services, or education. Drinking or eating food prepared with unsafe water, lack of water for hygiene, and inadequate access to sanitation together contribute nearly 1.5 million child deaths annually.[52]

Although a large part of the population can be reached through the health system in many countries, marginalized groups may not have access to health care for social, economic, or geographic reasons. Some children, like Tirtha in one of the opening vignettes, live too far away for their mothers to be able to take them to a health center. In other cases, families may not be far from a health center but they may not have the information to understand that they need to take their child to one. In addition, they may not have enough money for transportation there or for any fees at the health center. For cultural reasons, a woman may not be allowed to go to a health center alone, and must often wait for her husband's permission or for her husband to accompany her.

Most illness and death among young children is due to multiple illnesses or, more often, malnutrition combined with disease. It is important to ensure that children have the right combination of needed preventive and curative interventions. In the first 6 months of life, exclusive breastfeeding is crucial because there are important antibodies in a mother's breast milk. Appropriate complementary feeding, a full course of immunization, insecticide-treated bed nets for malaria prevention, and ORT for children with diarrhea are the most basic and cost-effective child health interventions available. The basic package of vaccines include vaccines against six major diseases including diphtheria, whooping cough (pertussis), tetanus, polio, tuberculosis, measles, and increasingly, hepatitis B and *Haemophilus influenza* type b vaccines. Safe water and sanitation are also keys to good health, but they are relatively expensive.

There is widespread agreement about the interventions needed to enhance child health. The key challenge facing the global health community is how to help families and communities quickly get the information and the means that they need to engage in safer and more appropriate health behaviors on a large scale, in coordination with what will hopefully be enhanced health services, and improvements in water and sanitation.

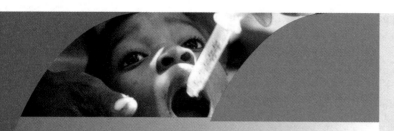

Study Questions

1. What are the most important causes of child death globally?

2. How do causes of death differ for neonates, infants, and children younger than five years?

3. Why are there different levels of child illness and death in different parts of the same country?

4. What is the link between nutrition and child health?

5. How does the health of young children in low-income countries vary with the income of the family?

6. How does the health of young children in low-income countries vary with the mother's level of education?

7. What is the importance to neonatal health of having a skilled birth attendant at delivery?

8. What are some of the most cost-effective interventions for saving the lives of newborns?

9. What are some of the most cost-effective interventions for saving the lives of children younger than five years?

10. What measures can families take, even in the absence of additional income or health services, to keep their children healthy?

REFERENCES

1. Black RE, Morris SS, Bryce J. Where and why are 10 million children dying every year? *Lancet.* 2003;361(9376):2226–2234.

2. Jones G, Steketee RW, Black RE, Bhutta ZA, Morris SS. How many child deaths can we prevent this year? *Lancet.* 2003;362(9377):65–71.

3. UNICEF. *State of the World's Children 2006.* New York: UNICEF; 2006.

4. Lawn JE, Zupan J, Begkoyian G, Knippenberg R. Newborn survival. In: Jamison DT, Breman JG, Measham AR, et al., eds. *Disease Control Priorities in Developing Countries.* 2nd ed. New York: Oxford University Press; 2006:531–549.

5. Babille M. Paper presented at: International Pediatrics Conference, 2005.

6. Simoes EAF, Cherian T, Chow J, Shahid-Salles S, Laxminarayan R, John TJ. Acute respiratory infections in children. In: Jamison DT, Breman JG, Measham AR, et al., eds. *Disease Control Priorities in Developing Countries.* 2nd ed. New York: Oxford University Press; 2006:483–484.

7. Keusch GF, Fontaine O, Bhargava A, et al. Diarrheal diseases. In: Jamison DT, Breman JG, Measham AR, et al., eds. *Disease Control Priorities in Developing Countries.* 2nd ed. New York: Oxford University Press; 2006:371.

8. Keusch GF, Fontaine O, Bhargava A, et al. Diarrheal diseases. In: Jamison DT, Breman JG, Measham AR, et al., eds. *Disease Control Priorities in Developing Countries.* 2nd ed. New York: Oxford University Press; 2006:372.

9. Lopez AD, Mathers CD, Murray CJL. The burden of disease and mortality by condition: data, methods, and results for 2001. In: Lopez AD, Mathers CD, Ezzati M, Jamison DT, Murray CJL, eds. *Global Burden of Disease and Risk Factors.* New York: Oxford University Press; 2006:127–128.

10. Breman JG, Mills A, Snow RW, et al. Conquering malaria. In: Jamison DT, Breman JG, Measham AR, et al., eds. *Disease Control Priorities in Developing Countries.* 2nd ed. New York: Oxford University Press; 2006:418.

11. Centers for Disease Control and Prevention. The Emergency Plan in Botswana. CDC Global AIDS Program. Available at: www.cdc.gov.nchstp/od/gap/countries/Botswana.htm. Accessed July 26, 2006.

12. United Nations. Millennium Development Goals Indicators. Children Under Five Mortality Rate Per 1,000 Live Births. Available at: http://millenniumindicators.un.org/unsd/mdg/SeriesDetail.aspx?srid=561&crid=. Accessed July 26, 2006.

13. Brenzel L, Wolfson LJ, Fox-Rushby J, Miller M, Halsey NA. Vaccine-preventable diseases. In: Jamison DT, Breman JG, Measham AR, et al., eds. *Disease Control Priorities in Developing Countries.* 2nd ed. New York: Oxford University Press; 2006:396–397.

14. Hotez PJ, Bundy DAP, Beegle K, et al. Helminth infections: soil-transmitted helminth infections and schistosomiasis. In: Jamison DT, Breman JG, Measham AR, et al., eds. *Disease Control Priorities in Developing Countries.* 2nd ed. New York: Oxford University Press; 2006:467–482.

15. Lopez AD, Mathers CD, Murray CJL. The burden of disease and mortality by condition: data, methods, and results for 2001. In: Lopez AD, Mathers CD, Ezzati M, Jamison DT, Murray CJL, eds. *Global Burden of Disease and Risk Factors.* New York: Oxford University Press; 2006:180–185.

16. Lawn JE, Cousens S, Zupan J. Four million neonatal deaths: When? Where? Why? *Lancet.* 2005;365(9462):891–900.

17. Lawn JE, Zupan J, Begkoyian G, Knippenberg R. Newborn Survival. In: Jamison DT, Breman JG, Measham AR, et al., eds. *Disease Control Priorities in Developing Countries.* 2nd ed. New York: Oxford University Press; 2006:531.

18. Lawn JE, Zupan J, Begkoyian G, Knippenberg R. Newborn survival. In: Jamison DT, Breman JG, Measham AR, et al., eds. *Disease Control Priorities in Developing Countries.* 2nd ed. New York: Oxford University Press; 2006:532.

19. Lawn JE, Zupan J, Begkoyian G, Knippenberg R. Newborn Survival. In: Jamison DT, Breman JG, Measham AR, et al., eds. *Disease Control Priorities in Developing Countries.* 2nd ed. New York: Oxford University Press; 2006:534.

20. United Nations. *The Millennium Development Goals Report 2006.* New York: United Nations; 2006.

21. Darmstadt GL, Bhutta ZA, Cousens S, Adam T, Walker N, de Bernis L. Evidence-based, cost-effective interventions: how many newborn babies can we save? *Lancet.* 2005;365(9463):977–988.

22. Black RE, Morris SS, Bryce J. Where and why are 10 million children dying every year? *Lancet.* 2003;361(9376):2227.

23. UNICEF. *State of the World's Children 2005.* UNICEF; 2005.

24. Lawn JE, Zupan J, Begkoyian G, Knippenberg R. Newborn survival. In: Jamison DT, Breman JG, Measham AR, et al., eds. *Disease Control Priorities in Developing Countries.* 2nd ed. New York: Oxford University Press; 2006:533.

25. Keusch GF, Fontaine O, Bhargava A, et al. Diarrheal diseases. In: Jamison DT, Breman JG, Measham AR, et al., eds. *Disease Control Priorities in Developing Countries.* 2nd ed. New York: Oxford University Press; 2006:375.

26. Hotez PJ, Bundy DAP, Beegle K, et al. Helminth infections: soil-transmitted helminth infections and schistosomiasis. In: Jamison DT, Breman JG, Measham AR, et al., eds. *Disease Control Priorities in Developing Countries.* 2nd ed. New York: Oxford University Press; 2006:467.

27. WHO (World Health Organization). *The World Health Report 2002: Reducing Risks, Promoting Health Lives.* Geneva: World Health Organization; 2002.

28. West KP, Jr., Pokhrel RP, Katz J, et al. Efficacy of vitamin A in reducing preschool child mortality in Nepal. *Lancet.* 1991;338(8759):67–71.

29. Rutstein SO, Govindasamy P. *The Mortality Effects of Nepal's Vitamin A Distribution Program.* Calverton, MD: ORC Macro; 2002.

30. Caulfield LE, Richard SA, Rivera JA, Musgrove P, Black RE. Stunting, wasting, and micronutrient disorders. In: Jamison DT, Breman JG, Measham AR, et al., eds. *Disease Control Priorities in Developing Countries.* 2nd ed. New York: Oxford University Press; 2006:551–568.

31. Fiedler JL. *The Nepal National Vitamin A Program: A Program Review and Cost Analysis.* Bethesda, MD: Partnerships for Health Reform Project. Abt Associates; 1997.

32. Fiedler JL. The Nepal National Vitamin A Program: prototype to emulate or donor enclave? *Health Policy Plan.* 2000;15(2):145–156.

33. Lawn JE, Cousens S, Zupan J. Four million neonatal deaths: When? Where? Why? *Lancet.* 2005;365(9462):891.

34. Black RE, Morris SS, Bryce J. Where and why are 10 million children dying every year? *Lancet.* 2003;361(9376):2226.

35. Victora CG, Wagstaff A, Schellenberg JA, Gwatkin D, Claeson M, Habicht JP. Applying an equity lens to child health and mortality: more of the same is not enough. *Lancet.* 2003;362(9379):233.

36. Lawn JE, Zupan J, Begkoyian G, Knippenberg R. Newborn survival. In: Jamison DT, Breman JG, Measham AR, et al., eds. *Disease Control Priorities in Developing Countries.* 2nd ed. New York: Oxford University Press; 2006:536–538.

37. UNAIDS. Mother to Child Transmission. Available at http://www.unaids.org/en/Issues/Affected_communities/mothertochild.asp. Accessed July 26, 2006.

38. Bertozzi S, Padian NS, Wegbreit J, et al. HIV/AIDS prevention and treatment. In: Jamison DT, Breman JG, Measham A, et al., eds. *Disease Control Priorities in Developing Countries.* New York: Oxford University Press; 2006:345–346.

39. Lawn JE, Zupan J, Begkoyian G, Knippenberg R. Newborn survival. In: Jamison DT, Breman JG, Measham A, et al., eds. *Disease Control Priorities in Developing Countries.* New York: Oxford University Press; 2006:535–541.

40. Lawn JE, Zupan J, Begkoyian G, Knippenberg R. Newborn survival. In: Jamison DT, Breman JG, Measham AR, et al., eds. *Disease Control Priorities in Developing Countries.* 2nd ed. New York: Oxford University Press; 2006:535–543.

41. Bang AT, Bang RA, Baitule SB, Reddy MH, Deshmukh MD. Effect of home-based neonatal care and management of sepsis on neonatal mortality: field trial in rural India. *Lancet.* 1999;354(9194):1955–1961.

42. Conde-Agudelo A, Diaz-Rossello JL, Belizan JM. Kangaroo mother care to reduce morbidity and mortality in low birthweight infants. *Cochrane Database Syst Rev.* 2000(4):CD002771.

43. Lawn JE, Zupan J, Begkoyian G, Knippenberg R. Newborn survival. In: Jamison DT, Breman JG, Measham AR, et al., eds. *Disease Control Priorities in Developing Countries.* 2nd ed. New York: Oxford University Press; 2006:541.

44. Keusch GF, Fontaine O, Bhargava A, et al. Diarrheal diseases. In: Jamison DT, Breman JG, Measham AR, et al., eds. *Disease Control Priorities in Developing Countries.* 2nd ed. New York: Oxford University Press; 2006:376.

45. Keusch GF, Fontaine O, Bhargava A, et al. Diarrheal diseases. In: Jamison DT, Breman JG, Measham AR, et al., eds. *Disease Control Priorities in Developing Countries.* 2nd ed. New York: Oxford University Press; 2006:377.

46. Brenzel L, Wolfson LJ, Fox-Rushby J, Miller M, Halsey NA. Vaccine-preventable diseases. In: Jamison DT, Breman JG, Measham AR, et al., eds. *Disease Control Priorities in Developing Countries.* 2nd ed. New York: Oxford University Press; 2006:389.

47. Brenzel L, Wolfson LJ, Fox-Rushby J, Miller M, Halsey NA. Vaccine-preventable diseases. In: Jamison DT, Breman JG, Measham AR, et al., eds. *Disease Control Priorities in Developing Countries.* 2nd ed. New York: Oxford University Press; 2006:390.

48. Brenzel L, Wolfson LJ, Fox-Rushby J, Miller M, Halsey NA. Vaccine-preventable diseases. In: Jamison DT, Breman JG, Measham AR, et al., eds. *Disease Control Priorities in Developing Countries.* 2nd ed. New York: Oxford University Press; 2006:398.

49. National Population Commission Federal Republic of Nigeria. *Nigeria Demographic and Health Survey NDHS 2003.* Calverton, MD: ORC Macro; 2003.

50. Victora CG, Adam T, Bryce J, Evans DB. Integrated management of the sick child. In: Jamison DT, Breman JG, Measham AR, et al., eds. *Disease Control Priorities in Developing Countries.* 2nd ed. New York: Oxford University Press; 2006:1177.

51. Victora CG, Adam T, Bryce J, Evans DB. Integrated management of the sick child. In: Jamison DT, Breman JG, Measham AR, et al., eds. *Disease Control Priorities in Developing Countries.* 2nd ed. New York: Oxford University Press; 2006:1177–1192.

52. Black RE, Morris SS, Bryce J. Where and why are 10 million children dying every year? *Lancet.* 2003;361(9376):2228.

53. Musgrove P. Is the eradication of polio in the western hemisphere economically justified? *Bulletin of the Pan American Sanitary Bureau.* 1988;22(1).

54. Henderson DA, de Quadros CA, Andrus J, Olive J-M, Guerra de Macedo C. Polio eradication from the western hemisphere. *Annual Review of Public Health.* 1992;13:239–252.

55. de Cuadros CA. Polio. *Encyclopedia of Microbiology 3*; 3000:762–772.

56. Gawande A. The mop-up: Eradicating polio from the planet. *The New Yorker.* January 12, 2004:34–40.

57. Global Polio Eradication Initiative. Afghanistan, Egypt, India, Niger, Nigeria, and Pakistan, Progress Report. Available at: www.polioeradication.org/content/publication/2003progress.pdf. Accessed August 10, 2004.

Communicable Diseases

VIGNETTES

Henrietta was a 35-year-old Kenyan mother of four who lived in Mombassa. Over the last 4 months, Henrietta was barely able to digest her food, had frequent bouts of diarrhea, and had been losing weight. She worried about having HIV. Henrietta went to a local clinic where she was tested and found to be HIV-positive. She had been infected by her husband, who was a truck driver.

Maria was 33 years old and lived in the mountains of Peru. For some time, she had not been feeling well. She often had a fever, was coughing a lot, and had night sweats. Maria had TB earlier and worried that this might be TB again. Maria was correct. In fact, this time she had drug-resistant TB, which would be difficult and expensive to cure. When Maria was sick the first time, she took most of her drugs. However, because she felt much better after the first 2 months of drugs, she did not take the rest of them.

Wole was 4 years old and lived in southwestern Nigeria. He had flu-like symptoms, a fever, and a headache. His mother suspected he might have malaria but decided she would see if he got better before taking him to the doctor. In another few days, however, Wole was much sicker and weaker. He was also dizzy and, shortly thereafter, lapsed into a coma. His mother then rushed him to the local health center but he died within a few hours. Unfortunately, Wole had the most virulent form of malaria.

Sanjay was 18 months old and lived in Lucknow, India. His mother was a day laborer and his father was a rickshaw driver. They lived in a hut in a large slum with little access to water and no sanitation. Sanjay was below the normal height and weight for his age and looked only 12 months old. Over the past year, Sanjay had four bouts of severe diarrhea.

THE IMPORTANCE OF COMMUNICABLE DISEASES

Communicable diseases are immensely important to the global burden of disease and account for about 40% of the disease burden in low- and middle-income countries.[1] Annually, HIV/AIDS kills about 3 million people, diarrhea kills 1.8 million, tuberculosis kills 1.6 million, and malaria kills 1.2 million.[1] Parasitic infections also account for an enormous burden of disease and disability.

Communicable diseases are the most important burden of disease in Sub-Saharan Africa. They are also especially important in South Asia. These diseases disproportionately affect the poor. Better-off people have the knowledge and income to protect themselves from diseases spread by unsafe water. They do not live in the crowded circumstances that can spread TB, and they also protect themselves as much as possible against malaria. In additon, they immunize their children against vaccine-preventable diseases at rates that are much higher than poor people do.

Communicable diseases are also of enormous economic consequence. These diseases constrain the physical and mental development of infants and young children and reduce their future economic prospects. The impacts on adult productivity of HIV, TB, and malaria are also exceptionally large. In addition, the direct and indirect costs of treatment for the infected person are often a substantial share of their income, causing them to borrow money or sell their already limited assets, and forcing them to sink into poverty. High rates of communicable diseases are also impediments to the investment needed to spur economic growth.

Much of the burden of communicable diseases is unnecessary because many of these diseases can easily be prevented or treated. Vaccines are an extremely cost-effective way to prevent a number of communicable diseases in children. The safe use of water can reduce the burden of diarrhea and certain parasitic diseases. There are inexpensive, safe, and effective treatments for TB, malaria, and some parasitic infections. Unfortunately, these technologies are not sufficiently used in low- and middle-income countries, especially by the poor.

Given their importance and their impact on the poor, the communicable diseases are of immense relevance to the MDGs, as noted in Table 11-1.

This chapter will introduce the reader to some of the major communicable diseases and the burden of morbidity, disability, and mortality associated with them in low- and middle-income countries. It will also outline how selected communicable diseases can be controlled and will elaborate on some success stories in addressing them effectively. The chapter will conclude by reviewing some of the remaining challenges the world faces in the control of these diseases. This chapter will focus on HIV/AIDS, TB, malaria, and a set of parasitic and bacterial infections often referred to as "neglected diseases." It will discuss diarrheal disease in a manner complementary to the discussion in Chapter 10 on child health. Finally, it will offer some brief comments on avian influenza as an example of new and emerging infectious diseases.

This chapter is only introductory. Communicable diseases are a very important topic about which an exceptional amount of material has been written. Those interested in gaining a deeper understanding of these diseases are encouraged to read some of the materials cited in this chapter.

KEY TERMS, DEFINITIONS, AND CONCEPTS

As you begin to explore communicable diseases in greater detail, there are a number of terms and concepts with which one should be familiar. These are defined in Table 11-2. It is also important to recall that a communicable disease is a dis-

ease that is transmitted from an animal to another animal, an animal to a human, a human to another human, or a human to an animal. Transmission can be direct, such as through respiratory means, or indirect through a vector, such as a mosquito as in the case of malaria. Most people use the term "communicable disease" in a manner that is synonymous with "infectious disease." However, others prefer to speak separately about diseases caused by infectious agents, such as TB, and those caused by parasites, such as hookworm. This chapter will consistently use the term "communicable disease" to refer to infectious and parasitic diseases.

As we examine the basic concepts concerning communicable diseases, it is also important to know how such diseases can be spread. This is shown in the following list, which includes examples of diseases spread in each manner:

- Food-borne—Salmonella, *E. coli, Entamoeba histolitica*
- Waterborne—cholera, rotavirus
- Sexual or blood-borne—hepatitis, HIV
- Vector-borne—malaria, onchocerciasis
- Inhalation—tuberculosis, influenza, meningitis
- Non-traumatic contact—anthrax
- Traumatic contact—rabies

In addition, it is critical to understand the ways in which communicable diseases can be controlled. These are noted below, also with examples of relevant diseases:

- Vaccination—smallpox, polio, measles, pediatric tuberculosis, diphtheria, pertussis, tetanus, hepatitis B, yellow fever, meningitis, influenza
- Mass chemotherapy—onchocerciasis, hookworm, lymphatic filariasis
- Vector control—malaria, dengue, yellow fever, onchocerciasis, west nile virus
- Improved water, sanitation, hygiene—diarrheal diseases
- Improved care seeking, disease recognition—maternal health, neonatal health, diarrheal disease, respiratory disease
- Case management (treatment) and improved care giving—diarrheal disease, acute respiratory illness
- Case surveillance, reporting, and containment—avian influenza, meningitis, cholera
- Behavioral change—HIV, sexually transmitted infections

A final concept of exceptional importance when discussing communicable diseases is the concept of "drug resistance." When considering the concerns of this book, this generally refers to the extent to which infectious and parasitic agents develop an ability to resist drug treatment. These agents naturally evolve over time to resist the treatments against them. Penicillin, for example, was previously used as the drug of choice against a variety of bacterial infections. Some of these bacteria over time, however, became resistant to the penicillin and this drug can no longer be used effectively against them. It is critical when considering public health approaches to major burdens of disease to understand that the improper use of drugs hastens the pace at which drug resistance develops. This has contributed to the development of TB strains that are resistant to the drugs normally used to treat TB. Similarly, some strains of malaria are no longer susceptible to treatment with chloroquine. A fundamental goal of interventions in public health is to avoid the development of drug resistance as much as possible. As indicated in the opening vignette about Maria, drug resistant strains of disease are difficult to treat, expensive to treat, and sometimes even impossible to treat.

THE BURDEN OF COMMUNICABLE DISEASES

Communicable diseases account for about 36% of total deaths and about 40% of total DALYs lost annually in low- and middle-income countries.[1] Table 11-3 summarizes the major causes of deaths from communicable diseases for the world and in low- and middle-income countries.

The relative importance of communicable diseases, compared to non-communicable diseases and injuries, varies considerably by region. Figure 11-1 indicates the share of the total deaths by region that is represented by communicable diseases. Figure 11-1 further highlights the fact that South Asia and Sub-Saharan Africa have the highest burden of deaths from communicable diseases, relative to other causes of death. Communicable diseases are the largest cause of death only in Sub-Saharan Africa.

The relative importance to the burden of disease of specific communicable diseases also varies by region. HIV/AIDS

TABLE 11-1 Communicable Diseases and the MDGs

Goal 1: Eradicate Extreme Hunger and Poverty
Communicable diseases are associated with high rates of morbidity and mortality. Communicable diseases can be part of a cycle of disease and malnutrition. In addition, communicable diseases reduce one's ability to work, thereby decreasing productivity and family income. In addition, illness causes people to spend an important share of their income on health care.

Goal 2: Achieve Universal Primary Education
Enrollment, attendance, and performance of children in schools is closely linked with health status. Communicable diseases are the leading cause of illness among the poor in Sub-Saharan Africa and South Asia.

Goal 4: Reduce Child Mortality
The three leading causes of death among children in the developing world are respiratory infections, diarrheal diseases, and malaria.

Goal 5: Improve Maternal Health
Malaria can cause anemia and mortality in pregnant women and is a major cause of poor maternal outcomes.

Goal 6: Combat HIV/AIDS, Malaria, and Other Diseases
Reducing the burden of communicable diseases is at the core of meeting this development goal.

Goal 8: Develop a Global Partnership for Development
The most important communicable diseases are being addressed through public-private partnerships or through product-development partnerships, such as Roll Back Malaria; Stop TB; The Global Fund to Fight Against AIDS, TB, and Malaria; The Global Polio Eradication Program; The Global Alliance for TB Drug Development; The Malaria Vaccine Initiative; and The International Partnership on Microbicides.

Source: Author commentary on the Millennium Development Goals. Available at: http://www.un.org/millenniumgoals/goals. Accessed July 11, 2006.

TABLE 11-2 Communicable Disease Definitions

- **Case**—An individual with a particular disease.
- **Case Fatality Rate**—The proportion of persons with a particular condition (cases) who die from that condition.
- **Control (Disease Control)**—Reducing the incidence and prevalence of a disease to an acceptable level.
- **Eradication (of Disease)**—Termination of all cases of a disease and its transmission and the complete elimination of the disease-causing agent.
- **Palliative Care**—End of life care.
- **Parasite**—An organism that lives in or on another organism and takes its nourishment from that organism.

Source: The Author and Centers for Disease Control and Prevention: Reproductive Health Glossary. Available at: http://www.cdc.gov/reproductivehealth/EpiGlossary/glossary.htm. Accessed April 15, 2007.

TABLE 11-3 Leading Causes of Death from Selected Communicable Diseases, 2001, by Number of Deaths in Thousands

Condition	World	Low- and Middle-Income
Lower Respiratory Conditions	3753	3408
HIV/AIDS	2574	2552
Diarrheal Diseases	1783	1777
Tuberculosis	1606	1590
Malaria	1208	1207
Measles	763	762

Source: Data with permission from The World Bank. Lopez AD, Mathers CD, Ezzati M, Jamison DT, Murray CJL. Measuring the global burden of disease and risk factors 1990–2001. In: Lopez AD, Mathers CD, Ezzati M, Jamison DT, Murray CJL, eds. *Global Burden of Disease and Risk Factors.* New York: Oxford University Press; 2006:8.

FIGURE 11-1 Deaths from Selected Infectious and Parasitic Diseases, as Percent of Total Deaths, by Region 2001 (Includes Infectious and Parasitic Infections and Lower Respiratory Infections)

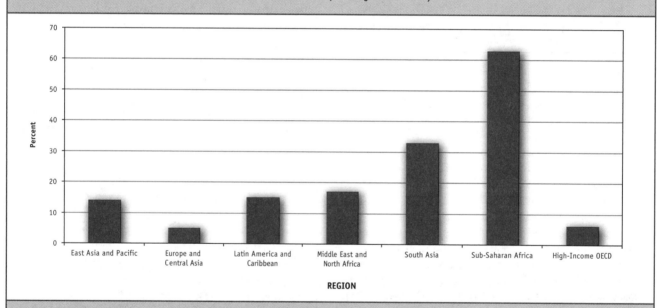

Source: Data with permission from The World Bank. Lopez AD, Mathers CD, Murray CJL. The burden of disease and mortality by condition: data, methods, and results for 2001. In: Lopez AD, Mathers CD, Ezzati M, Jamison DT, Murray CJL, eds. *Global Burden of Disease and Risk Factors.* New York: Oxford University Press; 2006:126–179.

is of exceptional importance in Sub-Saharan Africa, as is malaria. The "neglected" diseases are also much more important in Sub-Saharan Africa than in any other region.

The burden of specific communicable diseases varies by age group. Diarrheal disease, malaria, lower respiratory infections, and measles are most important for young children. HIV/AIDS and TB are most important for people who are 15

to 59 years old, although there is also a substantial TB burden for people older than that. In Table 11-4, one can see the leading causes of deaths from communicable diseases in low- and middle-income countries, by broad age group.

There are relatively small differences in the distribution of deaths from communicable diseases between males and females in low- and middle-income countries. However, it is consistently the case that TB affects males more than females. It is also true that the HIV/AIDS epidemic is being increasingly feminized and that HIV/AIDS is now a more important cause of death for woman than for men. These can be seen in Table 11-5.

The section that follows offers additional comments on the burden of disease from specific communicable diseases.

HIV/AIDS

Human Immunodeficiency Virus (HIV) and Acquired Immune Deficiency Syndrome (AIDS) can justifiably be considered the plague of the 21st century. Rarely has a single pathogen had a greater impact on the human condition than

TABLE 11-4 Leading Causes of Death in Low- and Middle-Income Countries by Broad Age Group, 2001, as Percent of Total Deaths

Aged 0–14		Aged 15–59	
Cause	Percent of Total Deaths	Cause	Percent of Total Deaths
Perinatal conditions	20.7	HIV/AIDS	14.1
Lower respiratory infections	17.0	Ischemic heart disease	8.1
Diarrheal diseases	13.4	Tuberculosis	7.1
Malaria	9.2	Road traffic accidents	5.0
Measles	6.2	Cerebrovascular disease	4.9
HIV/AIDS	3.7	Self-inflicted injuries	4.0
Congenital anomalies	3.7	Violence	3.1
Whooping cough	2.5	Lower respiratory infections	2.3
Tetanus	1.9	Cirrhosis of the liver	2.2
Road traffic accidents	1.5	Chronic obstructive pulmonary disease	2.2

Source: Data with permission from The World Bank. Lopez AD, Mathers CD, Murray CJL. The burden of disease and mortality by condition: data, methods, and results for 2001. In: Lopez AD, Mathers CD, Ezzati M, Jamison DT, Murray CJL, eds. *Global Burden of Disease and Risk Factors.* New York: Oxford University Press; 2006:70–71.

TABLE 11-5 Leading Causes of Death by Sex, Low- and Middle-Income Countries, 2001, as Percent of Total Deaths

Males		Females	
Cause	Percent of Total Deaths	Cause	Percent of Total Deaths
Ischemic heart disease	11.8	Ischemic heart disease	11.8
Cerebrovascular disease	8.5	Cerebrovascular disease	10.7
Lower respiratory infections	6.7	Lower respiratory infections	7.4
Perinatal conditions	5.4	HIV/AIDS	5.2
HIV/AIDS	5.4	Chronic obstructive pulmonary disease	5.1
Chronic obstructive pulmonary disease	4.7	Perinatal conditions	4.9
Tuberculosis	4.1	Diarrheal diseases	3.7
Diarrheal diseases	3.6	Malaria	2.8
Road traffic accidents	3.1	Tuberculosis	2.4
Malaria	2.3	Diabetes Mellitus	1.8

Source: Data with permission from The World Bank. Lopez AD, Mathers CD, Murray CJL. The burden of disease and mortality by condition: data, methods, and results for 2001. In: Lopez AD, Mathers CD, Ezzati M, Jamison DT, Murray CJL, eds. *Global Burden of Disease and Risk Factors.* New York: Oxford University Press; 2006:70.

HIV. No cure exists for it. Although effective drugs are available to keep HIV/AIDS under control, drug regimens require careful adherence and have significant side effects.

Some of the basic facts about HIV/AIDS are presented in Table 11-6. HIV is a virus that can be spread through:

- unprotected sex
- mother-to-child-transmission, during birth or through breastfeeding
- blood, including by transfusion and needle sharing
- transplantation of infected tissue or organs

The main risk factors for HIV are unprotected sex with an HIV-positive person; being born to and breastfed by an HIV-positive woman; exposure to the blood of an infected person through, for example, transfusion, the sharing of needles with an infected person, or a needlestick injury. Being an uncircumcised male also increases risk. Females are also at greater biological and social risk than males of being infected with HIV. Having a sexually transmitted disease also increases the risk of HIV infection.

The efficiency with which the virus is transmitted varies. The virus is spread most efficiently from exposure to infected blood products and through the sharing of infected needles. There is a 90% probability of being infected from a transfusion of blood from an HIV-positive person.[2] The efficiency of

TABLE 11-6 HIV/AIDS—Basic Facts

Number of AIDS cases to date—69 million
Number of AIDS deaths to date—20 million
Number of people living with HIV/AIDS—39.5 million
Number of new HIV infections in 2006—4.3 million
Prevalence among adults—0.1% in East Asia to 5.9% in Sub-Saharan Africa
Prevalence—Two thirds of those living with HIV are in Sub-Saharan Africa
Distribution of infection by sex—21.8 million men; 17.7 million women
Children under 15 with HIV—2.3 million
Number of HIV-positive people on treatment with anti-retroviral therapy—1.6 million

Source: Data from UNAIDS. AIDS Epidemic Update 2006. Available at: http://data.unaids.org/pub/EpiReport/2006/02-Global_Summary_2006_EpiUpdate_eng.pdf. Accessed November 21, 2006. UNAIDS. Global Facts and Figures. Available at: http://data.unaids.org/pub/EpiReport/2006/20061121_EPI_FS_GlobalFacts_en.pdf. Accessed November 21, 2006.

transmission is also relatively high from sharing needles with an HIV-infected person. Sexual transmission depends on the type of sexual act and whether the HIV-positive person is male or female. Male-to-female transmission is higher than female-to-male transmission. The risk of unprotected receptive anal intercourse is about 30 times greater than it is for receptive or insertive vaginal intercourse.[2]

HIV attacks the human immune system. The time from becoming infected until one is diagnosed with AIDS can vary from as little as 1 year to as many as about 15 years. However, without treatment for HIV, about half of those infected will be diagnosed with AIDS in 10 years. Infectiousness is high during the initial period of infection and also increases as the immune system weakens and in the presence of other sexually transmitted infections.[3]

As the immune system of an HIV-positive person deteriorates, that person will suffer from a variety of what are called opportunistic infections, because they take advantage of the person's compromised immunity. As their HIV disease reaches a fairly advanced state, for example, HIV-positive people who are not on antiretroviral therapy may fall ill with TB, herpes infections, a variety of cancers, and an array of significant communicable diseases such as toxoplasmosis and cryptococcal meningitis.[4]

The main routes of transmission of HIV vary by location. In the first phases of the epidemic in high-income countries and in Brail, HIV was largely spread through unprotected sex among men who have sex with men. In Sub-Saharan Africa, the disease has been spread overwhelmingly through unprotected sex between men and women, especially among those engaging in "high-risk behaviors," such as sex workers and their clients and men engaging in sex with multiple female partners. In China, the epidemic was centered originally in a group of people who received transfusions from blood that had been infected with the blood of HIV-positive people. From there, it spread largely through sex between men and women but also through injecting drug use. In Russia and much of the former Soviet Union, the epidemic is being driven by injecting drug users who are HIV-positive and who share needles. The epidemic is spreading from them largely through unprotected sex.

HIV/AIDS epidemics are categorized as either a "concentrated epidemic," in which less than 1% of the population of adults is HIV positive, or a "generalized epidemic," in which more than 5% of the adult population is infected. When HIV first appears in a population, it is generally concentrated in certain groups, such as sex workers, truckers, men who have sex with men, or injecting drug users. If the virus is controlled in these groups, then the spread to the general population can be limited. A generalized epidemic means that HIV/AIDS has spread to the general population, transmission is widespread, and prevalence is high. South Africa and Zimbabwe, for example, have generalized epidemics. India and Vietnam have concentrated epidemics.

It is estimated that about 40 million people worldwide are now infected with the HIV virus, and in the year 2005 about 2.3 million people died of HIV. It is also estimated that about 4.3 million people were newly infected with HIV in 2005.[5] The prevalence of HIV varies considerably by region and by country. The prevalence rate of HIV by country is shown in Figure 11-2.

The highest rates of prevalence of HIV/AIDS are in Central and Southern Africa. Relatively high rates of HIV/AIDS are also found in several other African countries and in parts of the Caribbean. With about 25 million infections, Sub-Saharan Africa has about 62.5% of the total number of infections in the world and about 75% of the AIDS-related deaths.[5] There is also considerable concern that the HIV/AIDS epidemics in China and India could become general-

ized. In addition, there is enormous worry about HIV/AIDS in Russia and other parts of the former Soviet Union. This stems largely from concerns over social disruptions linked with increasing poverty, commercial sex, and injecting drug use, all of which fuel the spread of HIV.

New HIV infections occur predominantly in people aged 15 to 24.[5] They also occur among infants due to maternal-to-child transmission. In the high-income countries, efforts have been made to address maternal-to-child transmission and there are almost no such cases any longer. In the highest prevalence countries, however, infants continue to be infected through maternal-to-child transmission, although efforts have begun to reduce it through drug therapy.

Tuberculosis

Some of the basic facts concerning TB are noted in Table 11-7.

Almost one third of the world, or about two billion people, are infected with tuberculosis. One person is infected with TB every second. This leads to about 30 million new

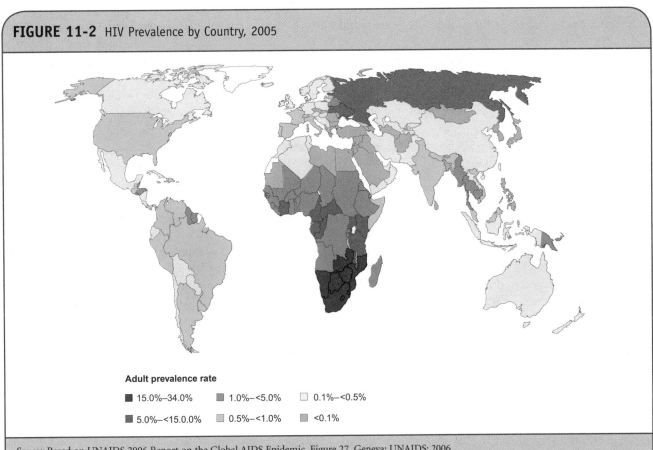

FIGURE 11-2 HIV Prevalence by Country, 2005

Adult prevalence rate

- 15.0%–34.0%
- 5.0%–<15.0.0%
- 1.0%–<5.0%
- 0.5%–<1.0%
- 0.1%–<0.5%
- <0.1%

Source: Based on UNAIDS 2006 Report on the Global AIDS Epidemic, Figure 27. Geneva: UNAIDS; 2006.

TABLE 11-7 TB—Basic Facts

Number of people infected worldwide—2 billion

Number of new TB cases each year—9 million

Growth in incidence—1% per year

Number of TB deaths each year—2 million, equal to 5000 per day

Number of new multi-drug resistant TB cases each year—450,000

Global distribution of prevalence—29% of cases in Sub-Saharan Africa; half of all new cases in Bangladesh, China, India, Indonesia, Pakistan, and the Philippines

Global TB targets—70% detection of smear positive cases and 85% cure of those cases

Recommended approach to treatment—DOTS (Directly Observed Therapy, Short Course)

Source: Data from: WHO. 2006 Tuberculosis Facts. Available at: http://www.who.int/tb/publications/2006/tb_factsheet_2006_1_en.pdf. Accessed November 15, 2006.

infections annually and about 9 million people in the world with active tuberculosis.[6]

Tuberculosis is caused by the bacteria *Mycobacterium tuberculosis*, and it is spread through aerosol droplets. People breathe in the TB bacteria from other infected people. Tuberculosis can affect all organs of the body, but 80% of cases infect the lungs.

Not everyone infected with TB becomes sick with it. Rather, the TB remains latent in the bodies of about 90% of those infected and they do not have active TB disease. People with latent TB do not spread TB to others.

The nature of latent TB is extremely important, especially in an age of HIV, because latent TB can become active when people's immune systems become weak. This could occur because of immune suppressing drugs or because of illness such as some cancers, diabetes, or HIV. Thus, the large pool of people in the world with latent TB infection presents a very significant risk of developing active TB infection if they become infected with HIV.

An untreated person with active pulmonary TB can infect 10 to 15 people annually. If left untreated, about one third of those with active TB will die, one third will self-cure, and one third will remain infectious to others. Pulmonary TB can be spread from person to person, but people with TB in other organs generally do not spread TB. Active TB is characterized by a persistent cough for more than 3 weeks, decreased appetite, general weakness, and profuse night sweats.

In terms of the extent to which people can spread pulmonary TB, there are two forms of TB disease. One is called smear positive and the other is called smear negative. The recommended means for diagnosing TB in low- and middle-income settings is through a microscopic examination of smears of sputum from a person suspected of having TB. Smear positive TB cases are those in which the presence of TB bacteria is confirmed by microscopic examination. They are the most contagious, and in resource-poor settings, they receive priority for treatment.[6]

The TB-HIV interface is a very important public health issue in terms of TB transmission and morbidity and mortality for both TB and HIV. The *lifetime* risk of developing active TB for a person who is *not* infected with HIV is 10%. If a person is HIV-positive, however, the *annual* risk of developing active TB is 10%; thus, after 8 years, the HIV-positive individual has an 80% chance of developing active TB. HIV/AIDS is also associated with a higher proportion of TB that is not pulmonary, compared to TB in people who are not HIV-positive. In addition, TB in HIV-positive people is often very difficult to diagnose.

Tuberculosis kills between two and three million people each year, equal to one person every 10 seconds, and is responsible for 30–40% of the mortality from HIV/AIDS. Most of the infections, cases, and deaths are in adults. Africa has the highest estimated incidence with 356 new cases per 100,000 population, but the most populous countries of Asia, such as Bangladesh, China, India, Indonesia, Pakistan, and the Philippines annually comprise half of the total number of new cases in the world.[6]

TB is the fifth most important cause of death worldwide, with 1.6 million deaths annually. Seventy-five% of the TB infections and deaths occur in the most productive age group—those who are 15 to 54 years old.[6] There are about 8.8 million new cases of TB each year and about half are sputum-smear-positive. TB accounts for 36 million DALYs annually, which is 2.3% of the world's total. Men are more frequently infected than women with TB, possibly because of reporting, but also because of exposure and, perhaps, susceptibility. Nonetheless, TB is also a leading killer of women, with about 550,000 female deaths attributed to TB annually.[7,8]

The number of cases of TB is declining in most high-income countries and new cases there are often among immigrants from low-income countries. However, in much of the developing world the number of cases is increasing, largely fueled by HIV/AIDS. Cases had also been growing in Russia and the former Soviet Union, also driven by HIV/AIDS, the social dislocation noted earlier, and breakdowns in the health system.

The main risk factors for TB are exposure to a person infected with TB, living in crowded circumstances, undernutrition, HIV, inadequate health care, and other conditions that weaken the immune system. TB is overwhelmingly a disease of the poor because it is they who have the most exposure to these risk factors.

There has been an increase in TB infections that are resistant to one or more TB drugs. These forms of TB are called drug-resistant TB, multidrug-resistant TB (MDR TB), and extensively drug-resistant TB (XDR TB). An underlying cause for the development of resistant forms of TB is the failure to complete TB treatment, as was the case for Maria in one of the opening vignettes. However, it is also possible to be infected with drug-resistant TB directly from another person. Drug-resistant strains are found in many countries and are difficult and expensive to treat. Drug resistance is especially important in countries in which TB programs are weak or have fallen into disarray, as in many of the very poor countries, Russia, and in countries with high rates of HIV. In 2006, a number of cases of XDR TB were found in South Africa among HIV patients, and 52 of 53 patients died within 25 days, despite being on HIV treatment. This caused considerable alarm in the public health community.[9] A global effort is now underway to determine the extent of XDR TB.

Malaria

Malaria is caused by parasites in the genus *Plasmodium* and there are four species of malaria parasites that infect humans. They are *Plasmodium falciparum*, *Plasmodium vivax*, *Plasmodium ovale*, and *Plasmodium malariae*. These parasite species exist in different proportions in different regions of the world. *Plasmodium falciparum*, for example, dominates in Africa, *Plasmodium vivax* occurs in temperate zones, and *Plasmodium ovale* is found in South Asia and tropical Africa. The disease is spread by the bite of the female *Anopheles* mosquito. Essentially, the mosquito carries the parasite from an infected person to an uninfected person.

Malaria infects 300 to 500 million people annually, kills 1.2 million people each year, and causes over 40 million DALYs lost annually, which is equal to 2.9% of the global total.[10] Malaria is the ninth leading cause of death in low- and middle-income countries and the fourth leading cause of death in children aged 0 to 14 in those countries. Sub-Saharan African children account for 82% of the malaria deaths worldwide. About 11% of the childhood deaths worldwide are attributed to malaria.[10]

The most important risk factor for malaria is being bitten by mosquitoes that carry malaria. This risk varies with the feeding habits of various species of mosquitoes, the climate, and the time of year. Some people have a degree of immunity to malaria from having grown up in malarial zones and the risks of contracting malaria increase if one does not have such immunity.

Pregnant women are at high risk of giving birth to low birthweight children, and they and their fetuses are at high risk of anemia and death because of malaria. It is estimated that 45 million pregnancies occur annually in malaria endemic areas of Africa and 23 million occur in high malaria transmission areas. 3 to 15% of African mothers suffer severe anemia, accounting for 10,000 malaria-related anemia deaths per year. Globally, malaria causes about 30% of low birth weight in newborns and between 75,000 and 200,000 infant deaths per year.[11]

Diarrheal Disease

As briefly discussed in Chapter 10, diarrhea is caused by certain bacteria, viruses, and/or parasites that are transmitted by contaminated water or food through the fecal-oral route, such as *Shigella sp.*, *Salmonella sp.*, *Cholera vibrio*, rotavirus, and *Escherichia coli*. Diarrheal disease agents can be spread by dirty utensils, dirty hands, or flies. Diarrhea causes severe dehydration and a loss of body water and can kill infants and young children very quickly. Poor recognition of the extent of illness, failed home care, and lack of knowledge about simple therapies increase the severity of diarrhea. Diarrheal diseases can be prevented by access to safe drinking water, improved sanitation, and the carrying out of more hygienic personal behaviors, such as hand washing.

Diarrheal diseases most significantly impact the poor, especially children in developing countries.[12] Poor housing, crowding, lack of safe water and sanitation, cohabitation with domestic animals, lack of refrigeration for food storage, and poor personal and community hygiene all contribute to the transmission of diarrheal disease agents. In addition, poor nutrition contributes to poor immunity and increases the frequency and severity of diarrhea.

Diarrheal disease mortality has decreased significantly since the 1980s from an estimated 4.6 million deaths to the 1.8 million estimated today, which is about 17% of all childhood deaths. The decline is due to improved nutrition of infants, better disease recognition, improved care seeking, and appropriate use of oral rehydration therapy, as discussed in the case studies in Chapters 5 and 10. Nonetheless, the burden of diarrheal disease remains very substantial. Diarrhea is a major cause of death and sickness for children younger than five years. Children suffer about 3.2 episodes of diarrhea annually but rates vary worldwide.[13] It is estimated that there are 113 million episodes of bloody diarrhea in children under 5 each year caused by *Shigella*.[12]

Neglected Diseases

Another set of diseases, which are increasingly referred to as neglected diseases, are associated with significant morbidity and economic loss. About 4.2 billion people are at risk of these diseases in 142 countries. These diseases account for 24% of total DALYs lost annually from communicable diseases, and 20% of the communicable disease deaths.[14] Those most affected are children. Ascaris, trichuris, and hookworm infect 1.2 billion, 800 million, and 740 million people worldwide, respectively.[14] As with other tropical infectious diseases, Africa bears the brunt of morbidity and mortality.

Neglected diseases include helminthic worm, protozoan, and bacterial infections, a few of which are discussed here.

Helminth Infections:

Soil-transmitted Helminth infections:

Ascariasis-Trichuriasis-Hookworm
Lymphatic Filariasis (Elephantiasis)
Onchocerciasis (River Blindness)
Schistosomiasis
Dracunculiasis (Guinea Worm)

Protozoan Infections:

Leishmaniasis (Kala-azar)
African Trypanosomiasis (Sleeping Sickness)
Chagas' Disease

Bacterial Infections:

Leprosy
Trachoma
Buruli Ulcer

The life cycles of the soil transmitted helminth infections are similar. The worms live in the gastrointestinal tract of humans. They produce eggs, which are passed out with the human feces. Those who ingest them are at risk of becoming infected. Hookworms can produce anemia in their human hosts. In addition, children with the heaviest burden of worms are at risk of impaired mental and physical development.[15] The burden of worms varies, with 20% of those infected harboring 80% of the worms.[15]

The most important risk factors for soil-transmitted helminths are:

- being an agricultural worker
- poverty, poor sanitation, lack of clean water
- living near wet, warm areas[15]

Lymphatic filariasis is caused by a nematode worm that is carried from an infected to an uninfected person with the bite of a mosquito. The nematode *Wucheria bancrofti*, which is the cause of this illness, is present in many of the humid and tropical parts of the world. Female worms produce microfilariae that enter the bloodstream and can cause a variety of manifestations. Among the most disabling of these problems are swelling of the genitalia and of the limbs, which are both debilitating and stigmatizing.[16]

Schistosomiasis is another neglected disease of importance. It is caused by the liver fluke, a trematode. People with schistosomiasis release fluke eggs in their urine or their feces. The flukes enter into fresh water snails, from which they emerge into the water. The flukes penetrate the skin of a human when they are wading, bathing, or working in water that has been infected. One form of the fluke causes manifestations in the intestinal track and liver. Another form causes problems in the urinary track. Over time, these can lead to severe disease of the urinary track or liver, among other things.[17]

The burden of some of the most important neglected diseases in Africa is shown in Table 11-8. Additional comments on onchocerciasis appear in the case study in Chapter 15.

THE COSTS AND CONSEQUENCES OF COMMUNICABLE DISEASES

The economic and social costs of the enormous burden of communicable diseases are very high. First, these diseases constrain the health and development of infants and children, often by having an impact on their schooling and on their productivity as adult workers. Second, stigma and discrimination against people with HIV, those with TB, and those with a variety of other debilitating communicable diseases, such as leprosy and lymphatic filariasis, are strong and pervasive. Third, adults who suffer from the diseases discussed in this chapter suffer substantial losses in productivity and incomes. Fourth, families spend considerable sums of money trying to treat these illnesses. Fifth, high rates of infectious diseases in any country reduce investments in that country's development. Some of the economic and social consequences that relate more specifically to AIDS, TB, malaria, and the neglected diseases are discussed briefly here.

HIV/AIDS

HIV/AIDS has enormous social and economic consequences, especially in high prevalence countries in Sub-Saharan African countries, which go beyond the usual impact of diseases on morbidity and mortality. Rather, HIV/AIDS affects family

TABLE 11-8 Burden of Selected Helminthic and Protozoan Infections in Africa, by Percent of Global Burden of Condition

Condition	Cases in Africa	% of Global Burden of Condition
Hookworm	198 million	27–34%
Ascariasis	173 million	14–22%
Schistosomiasis	166 million	89%
Trichuriasis	162 million	20–26%
Trachoma	33 million	40%
Lymphatic Filariasis	46 million	38%
Onchocerciasis	18 million	99%
Afr. Trypanosomiasis	0.5 million	100%
Dracunculiasis	< 0.1 million	100%

Source: Reprinted with permission from The World Bank. Hotez PJ, Bundy DAP, Beegle K, et al. Helminth infections: soil-transmitted helminth infections and schistosomiasis. In: Jamison DT, Breman JG, Measham AR, et al., eds. *Disease Control Priorities in Developing Countries*. 2nd ed. New York: Oxford University Press; 2006:467–482.

cohesion, business, trade, labor, the armed forces, agricultural production, education systems, governance, public services, and even national security.

In the absence of treatment, the person infected with HIV will eventually become sicker, progress to full blown AIDS, and suffer from a variety of opportunistic infections, as noted previously. As this happens, the person becomes less able to work, loses part or all of his or her income, and becomes dependent on others for care. The caretaker may also lose his or her income.

This cycle has caused enormous economic losses to individuals and their families, especially in Sub-Saharan Africa. A study done in Tanzania, for example, indicated that men with AIDS lost an average of 297 days of work over an 18-month period and women lost an average of 429 days of work over that same period, which implies that these women were essentially unable to attend to any of their normal tasks.[18] A study in Thailand showed that families that suffered from AIDS lost an average of 48% of their income as a result of their illness.[18]

Another important consequence of HIV/AIDS is the creation of an exceptional number of orphans. When speaking of HIV/AIDS, an orphan is defined as an individual 15 years old or younger who has lost one or both parents to the disease. It is estimated that there are 15 million HIV/AIDS orphans and that this number could rise to 25 million by 2010.[5] Despite efforts by many families to care for their relatives, many orphans do not have anyone with whom to live and may resort to living on the street, where they fall into commercial sex and crime.

HIV/AIDS is a highly stigmatized condition, as are a number of other communicable diseases. HIV/AIDS, how-ever, has a special stigma because people in many societies believe that people acquire HIV/AIDS because they engage in behaviors that society does not sanction, such as men who have sex with men, commercial sex work, or injecting drug use. Understanding the notion of stigma and discrimination against people with HIV is central to understanding the HIV/AIDS epidemic.

In fact, stigmatization of HIV in many societies has led to unwillingness to allow people with HIV to attend schools or be employed, get health care, live in certain places, or even live with their families. Stigma has also been a major constraint to people's getting tested or treated for HIV. It has also complicated prevention efforts in some settings by driving underground some of the very people it is important to reach, such as sex workers and injecting drug users.

For the poorest developing countries, the direct cost of AIDS treatment is very expensive compared to per capita income and per capita health expenditure, even at the reduced prices for those drugs that have been agreed upon globally. In fact, the cost of providing drugs and related laboratory and clinical services costs is generally at least $300 per patient, per year. Yet, many of the low-income countries that are providing AIDS drugs to people living with HIV/AIDS normally spend only about $5 per person per year on health. It will be difficult for low-income countries with high HIV prevalence to support the treatment of a large share of people living with HIV/AIDS without considerable and sustained external assistance.

The increasing attention paid to HIV has been positive in many ways. However another cost of HIV/AIDS is the extent to which attention to it diverts human and financial resources away from other health priorities, such as child health or the neglected diseases. Striking an effective and equitable balance between HIV/AIDS and other public health priorities is a challenge for many countries.

Many studies of the impact of HIV/AIDS have been used to help convince governments that failure to address HIV early could result in lower economic growth of their country. Overall, the studies suggest that HIV/AIDS will have a large impact on the economic growth of high-prevalence countries in Africa, largely because it tends to strike people in their most productive years.[19] The higher the prevalence and the more families that use their savings to help pay for the costs of illness, the more likely HIV is to have a negative impact on the growth of per capita income.[20]

TB

The cost of TB to families, communities, and countries is very high, given the large number of people who are sick with TB, the relatively long course of the illness, and the losses people face when they do have TB. A study of TB in India suggested that those sick with TB lost about 3 months of wages, spent an amount equal to about one quarter of national income per capita on care and treatment, and took on debts to pay for this care that were equal to about 10% of per capita income.[21] A similar study on Bangladesh indicated that those sick with TB lost 4 months of wages.[22] A Thai study showed that TB patients spent more than 15% of their annual wages on TB, that 12% of them took out bank loans to help make up for the costs of their illness, and that 16% sold part of their property to finance the costs of dealing with their illness.[23]

There are also significant social costs associated with TB. Because of the stigma associated with TB, females who get infected are often shunned by their families. In one Indian study, 15% of the women with TB faced familial rejection.[24] In another Indian study, 8% faced rejection.[21]

A study of the macroeconomic impact of TB suggested that the economic growth of a country is inversely correlated with the rate of TB. Every increase of 10% in the incidence of TB was associated with lower annual economic growth of 0.2–0.4%.[25] A study of the economic costs of TB in the Philippines indicated that the annual economic loss due to morbidity and premature mortality from TB was equal to almost $150 million. In addition, the cost to the Philippines of treating all of the expected cases of TB would be between $8 million and $29 million.[26]

Malaria

The cost of malaria at the family level is significantly less than the costs of HIV/AIDS and TB but is still substantial because individuals often have malaria up to five times per year. In one study in Ghana, for example, there were 11 cases of malaria per household, per year, on average.[18] These same studies showed that individuals lost one to five work days per episode of malaria, that the indirect cost of dealing with their illness was greater than the direct costs of treatment, and that each episode of malaria probably cost an adult about 2% of his annual income.[18] In many African countries, malaria typically accounts for 20–40% of outpatient visits at health facilities and 10–15% of hospital admissions.[27]

Over $3.5 billion is lost annually due to malaria in Africa alone.[27] Roll Back Malaria suggests that the economic costs of malaria in countries with a high malaria burden is about 1.3% per year loss of GDP. One study suggested that a 10% reduction in malaria was associated with a 0.3% higher increase in economic growth. Clearly, malaria in Sub-Saharan Africa is a deterrent to trade, business development, tourism, and foreign investment.[28,29]

Neglected Diseases

As noted earlier, neglected diseases cause over 500,000 deaths and 57 million DALYs annually. They also cause a great deal of long-term disability, disfigurement, and suffering.[30] Studies of the economic costs of these diseases have been limited. However, an extensive study done in Kenya indicated that de-worming improved school attendance better than any other investment, which should ultimately lead to higher earnings for the students than they would otherwise have.[31] A study of hookworm in the southern part of the United States in the early part of the 20th century showed that hookworm infection was associated with a 23% reduction in school attendance.[32] It has already been noted that parasitic infections are associated with reduced weight gain, lower height, anemia, and lower productivity and capacity for wage earning.

ADDRESSING THE BURDEN OF DISEASE
HIV/AIDS

Despite considerable and increasing efforts, there is not yet either a preventive or therapeutic vaccine for HIV/AIDS. In the absence of such a vaccine, halting the spread of HIV will have to focus on the prevention of new infections. Yet, despite 25 years of efforts to prevent HIV, there is little rigorous evidence about the most cost-effective approaches to prevention. Nonetheless, some evidence is emerging, as discussed below.

The few successful prevention efforts that have occurred, such as in Thailand and Uganda, have consistently been associated with a number of factors related to strong political leadership and commitment and open communications including:

- Sustained political leadership at the highest levels
- Involvement of a broad range of civil society efforts to address HIV/AIDS, including opinion leaders and religious leaders
- Broad-based programs to change social norms in the population
- Open communication about HIV/AIDS and related sexual matters
- Programs to reduce stigma and discrimination[33]

In addition, we also know that to be successful, prevention efforts need to include:

- Good epidemic surveillance
- Information, education, and communication
- Voluntary counseling and testing
- Condom promotion
- Screening and treatment for sexually transmitted infections
- Prevention of mother-to-child-transmission through avoiding pregnancy, antiretroviral treatment, and breast milk substitutes
- Interventions that target populations that transmit the virus from high-risk to low-risk populations
- Prevention of blood-borne transmission through blood safety, harm reduction for injecting drug users, and universal precautions in healthcare settings.[34]

Some additional comments on prevention efforts follow.

First, the approach to prevention will need to vary with the nature of the epidemic. In low-level and concentrated epidemics, the focus can be on changing the behaviors of those who engage in high-risk behaviors. The approach to prevention in a more generalized epidemic, however, will need to be much broader.[34]

Second, there is an emerging consensus globally that an integrated "ABC" approach to HIV/AIDS prevention is needed but that the weights given to different parts of the approach must vary depending on the nature of the epidemic and the cultural background of each country. "ABC" stands for abstinence, being faithful, and correct and consistent condom use. Major elements of this approach include the promotion of safe sexual behavior, correct and consistent use of condoms for those practicing high-risk behaviors, delay of sexual debut for youth, abstinence until marriage, partner reduction, and fidelity. There is a concern globally, however, to ensure that such an approach, and the weights given to different parts of it, is evidence-based, especially relating to the promotion of abstinence.

There has been a considerable degree of discussion in recent years of appropriate approaches to testing and counseling. From the inception of the HIV/AIDS epidemic, concern for stigmatization of HIV-positive people has caused governments to undertake testing and counseling with complete confidentiality of the person being tested and only on a voluntary "opt in" basis. Recently, however, there has been an increasing concern that it is important to raise the share of people who are tested, particularly in high prevalence settings, because most people do not know their status and most infections are spread at the early stages of infection. Therefore, a number of countries, led by Botswana, now offer an HIV test whenever people have contact with the health system, with the possibility of "opting out" of testing. The advocates of this approach hope that it will lead to more people knowing their HIV status as early as possible, thereby enabling them to avoid infecting others.

There has also been increasing attention to trying to stem maternal-to-child transmission of HIV. The most cost-effective measure to reduce maternal-to-child transmission of HIV is to avoid unwanted pregnancies of HIV positive women through contraception. Providing antiretroviral therapy to pregnant women infected with HIV is also cost-effective because this may prevent about one third of the women from having a baby who is HIV-positive. Little information is available on the cost-effectiveness of breast milk substitutes. However, if a women is going to breastfeed her baby, the baby is less likely to be HIV-positive if the mother exclusively breastfeeds, weans early, and then provides food to the baby because mixing breast milk and food raises the risk that the baby will become HIV-positive.[35]

The promotion, distribution, and social marketing of condoms encourages correct and consistent use of condoms and lowers the rates of sexually transmitted infections (STIs) and HIV. However, there are limited data on the cost-effectiveness of these approaches. At least in the early stages of an HIV epidemic, it appears that screening for and treatment of STIs can be a cost-effective way of preventing HIV.[36]

There is good evidence that needle exchanges are effective in high-income countries, but there are little data on such programs in low- and middle-income countries. There is widespread agreement that blood safety is cost-effective and must be a high priority in all settings. There is evidence that circumcised males are 40–60% less likely to be infected with HIV than uncircumcised males;[37] however, there are little data about how one can manage a cost-effective program for adult circumcision, especially in the face of cultural obstacles in many settings.[38] Thus, a number of efforts are now underway to design programs for adult circumcision as a component of HIV/AIDS prevention activities.

There is also considerable support for linking treatment and prevention programs. The question of what is the most cost-effective approach to treatment, however, is complicated by the limited available evidence. It appears that community-based approaches to palliative care of people who are HIV-affected are likely to be highly cost-effective, and certainly more cost-effective than care provided by healthcare professionals in the homes of the affected. Community-based food supplementation programs can also be cost-effective.[39] In addition, there is good evidence that putting people who are affected with HIV on the antibiotic cotrimoxazole can be a cost-effective way to reduce the risk and delay the onset of opportunistic infections.[40]

Widespread use of antiretroviral therapy has only begun in the developing world, outside of a small number of countries such as Thailand and Brazil, in the last several years. It is too early, therefore, to have definitive evidence about the most cost-effective regimens for treatment of HIV infection. Calculating cost-effectiveness of these drugs will not be simple because there are many different regimens, each drug has different side effects, and patients have to change regimens when they develop side effects or resistance. Nonetheless, evidence needs to be gathered continuously on the cost-effectiveness of various regimens.

As a rule of thumb, low-income countries should aim to place about 15% of those infected on drug therapy, because they will be the ones most in need clinically and because these countries are unlikely to be able to place all of their patients with HIV on treatment as soon as they are diagnosed. Once the patient is under treatment, it is exceptionally important that they take all of their drugs exactly as prescribed in order to avoid developing resistance. If the drugs are discontinued because of interrupted supply, poor compliance by the patient, or poor performance of the health system, then resistance may develop and the patient may require more expensive second-line drugs. Drug resistant strains of HIV also pose risks to others, who can become infected with them directly from others and then face difficulties finding effective drug regimens for their strain of HIV.

Overall, effective HIV/AIDS therapy depends on individuals accessing counseling and testing, a definitive HIV test, a clinical diagnosis of the patient, a laboratory assessment of the individual's immune status with a CD4 cell count, patient adherence to their drug regimen, sound nutrition of the patient, and sound and continuous monitoring and evaluation of the patient. About 1.6 million people in the developing world are now receiving antiretroviral therapy.[5] The world has set a goal of universal access to treatment for HIV by 2010.

TB

There is a vaccine for TB called BCG that is a standard part of the Expanded Program of Immunization for Children. The vaccine reduces severe TB in children but because children are not important transmitters of TB, the vaccine has little impact on the overall incidence or prevalence of TB.[41] Rather, the control of TB depends on effective treatment of active tuberculosis. In many respects, implementing a poor TB program is worse than not having a TB program at all because a poor TB program can give rise to drug-resistant TB.

The treatment strategy for TB is called DOTS: Directly Observed Therapy, Short-Course. DOTS consists of a 6-month regimen that normally includes four drugs—isoniazid, rifampin, pyrazinamide, and ethambutol—for the first 2 months—and then isoniazid and rifampin for the following 4 months. DOTS is just what it says—a relatively short course of therapy directly observed by a local care provider or community member, compared to the longer course that had previously been given without such observation.

The DOTS strategy has five essential components:

- Sustained political commitment to a national TB program;
- Access to quality-assured sputum smears and microscopy;
- Standardized regimens of short-course chemotherapy under direct observation;
- Regular uninterrupted supply of quality-assured anti-TB drugs; and,
- Monitoring and evaluation for program supervision.[6]

Once an active case of TB is identified, appropriate drugs are required in adequate supply for 6 months. Patient compliance with the TB regimen is required for effective therapy and direct observation is meant to ensure appropriate treatment for the entire course. Healthcare workers, NGO staff, community volunteers and leaders, such as teachers, religious leaders, and other community members, provide observation. They are sometimes the holders of the medicine, as well as the persons who observe TB patients taking their medicines.

The TB drugs needed to cure a single case of active TB can be purchased in low- and middle-income countries for as little as $15. Treating active TB with DOTS is very cost-effective and ranges from $5 to $50 per DALY gained in most regions.[41] BCG is cost-effective in reducing severe cases of childhood TB in high prevalence settings. Treating multi-drug-resistant TB is also relatively cost-effective.

HIV and TB

There is a direct relationship between HIV in adults who are 15 to 49 years old and TB. In many countries with high HIV prevalence, 60% or more of those with active TB are HIV-positive, as noted earlier. TB control programs can help to identify HIV-positive patients and AIDS programs should always determine if an HIV-positive person has TB. Unfortunately, the treatment of a person who is co-infected with HIV and TB is complicated. Efforts are underway to see if DOTS or a "DOTS-like" approach to antiretroviral therapy can be helpful to ensuring high patient adherence with their HIV drug regimen, even if HIV drugs need to be taken for a lifetime.

Malaria

Despite many years of effort, there is still no vaccine against malaria. However, there is widespread agreement on the key interventions required to "roll back" malaria. These include:

- Prompt treatment of those infected
- Intermittent preventative therapy for pregnant women
- Insecticide-treated bed nets for people living in malarial zones
- Indoor residual spraying of the homes of people in malarial zones

The Abuja Declaration of 2000 has three objectives for reducing malaria mortality and morbidity in Africa, with the understanding that their achievement by 2005 will be challenging. The Declaration states that 60% of children should receive prompt and effective treatment, 60% of pregnant women should receive intermittent preventive therapy, and 60% of children and pregnant women should sleep under an insecticide-treated bed net.[42] Each intervention holds great promise but a great deal remains to be done before these goals can be realized.

Appropriate treatment of malaria is essential to reduce malaria morbidity and mortality. If people with malaria are treated promptly, then mosquitoes that bite them will not carry malaria to another person. Drugs such as cholorquine, fansidar, and mefloquine are being used but face growing levels of drug resistance.

Artemisinin, a new drug for malaria, is now being used in combination with other anti-malarial drugs in areas where malaria is resistant to other drugs. Efforts are also underway to get artemisinin into use as soon as possible in all malarial areas, so that the advent of resistance can be delayed. Treatment with artemisinin plus other anti-malarial drugs is referred to as ACT, which stands for artemisinin-based combination therapy. Effective therapy depends on accurate laboratory diagnosis and appropriate case management. In addition, pregnant women are being treated with intermittent preventive therapy from between 18 and 24 weeks of their pregnancy through delivery to reduce complications and deaths from malaria among this group of people.

The use of bed nets and eliminating mosquito breeding sites represent additional means of malaria control. Bed nets, impregnated with a biologically safe insecticide, are being widely distributed and sold by governments, donors, and the private sector. Spraying the inside of homes, or indoor residual spraying, is also to be carried out. Reducing the number of mosquitoes that carry malaria at the community level relies on effective communication and commitment by local leaders, the identification of breeding sites, and the availability of appropriate larvicides and/or tools to drain potential breeding sites. However, reducing the number of mosquitoes, called source reduction, is particularly difficult in Africa because the vector, *Anopheles gambiae*, is ubiquitous and breeds in all types of standing water.

Diarrhea

There are five major disease prevention strategies for diarrhea. Perhaps most effective is the promotion of exclusive breastfeeding for 6 months. This is advantageous to the child and mother because the child receives both maternal antibodies and a nutritious and uncontaminated meal. Mothers benefit from an increased birth interval and a healthier child. The second prevention intervention is improved complementary feeding, introduced with breastfeeding after 6 months. Third, is rotavirus immunization, which will be increasingly cost-effective as the vaccines are more affordable in low- and middle-income countries. Diarrhea from rotavirus kills about 600,000 children under five years each year.[43] The next strategy is increased measles immunizations. Data indicate a clear link between measles immunization and reduced incidence and deaths from diarrhea. If measles coverage is increased, especially in Africa, then the burden of diarrheal disease will decline. The fifth prevention strategy is improving access to safe water supply and sanitation. Clean water and appropriate sanitation will reduce diarrheal disease incidence. Furthermore, hand washing can reduce diarrhea incidence by 3%.[44]

Three case management interventions can significantly reduce the severity and mortality of diarrheal disease. The use of oral rehydration therapy (ORT) is the most cost-effective case management intervention, especially if homemade solutions are administered. Although the use of ORT has expanded globally, only about 49% of the diarrhea cases worldwide are managed with ORT or home fluids.[12] Second, it is estimated that zinc supplementation during an acute diarrhea episode for 10 to 14 days during and after diarrhea could prevent 300,000 deaths per year.[45] Third, antibiotics can be given for bloody diarrhea, primarily caused by *Shigella* infection. However, delivering this intervention where it is most needed may depend on careful training of non-physician healthcare personnel because most low-income and many middle-income countries do not have enough physicians living in places where they are most needed.

Neglected Diseases

Many poor people in low- and middle-income countries suffer from more than one of the neglected diseases. A "rapid-impact" package can simultaneously treat seven of the major neglected diseases including ascariasis, hookworm, trichuriasis, lymphatic filariasis, onchocerciasis, schistosomiasis, and trachoma. For less than $1 per person per year, plus donations of five key drugs, scaling-up a rapid-impact package is feasible. Integrating the control of neglected diseases and malaria control in Africa is also feasible. This package, aimed at a large and underserved population, could reduce disease burden significantly and could enhance productivity in many African nations.

Many policy makers have ignored neglected tropical diseases in favor of HIV/AIDS, TB, and malaria. However, the geographic overlap of many neglected diseases with HIV/AIDS, TB, and malaria makes an integrated control effort possible. Drugs for neglected diseases could be deployed through existing health systems and communities and linked to other disease control efforts. In this case, the burden of neglected diseases could be reduced for over 500 million people at an estimated cost of $0.40 per person treated, including the donated drugs, which would be extremely cost-effective.

CASE STUDIES

The control of communicable diseases remains challenging. However, important progress has been made against some of these diseases. Given the exceptional importance of communicable diseases in low-income countries, this chapter includes five case studies. One of them examines the efforts of Thailand to address sexually transmitted diseases and HIV/AIDS. Another discusses China's attempt to control TB through DOTS. The third reviews the exceptional global effort to eradicate polio. The last two cases concern neglected diseases, one on Chagas disease in Latin America and another on trachoma in Morocco. Those interested in more detail

on the cases can consult *Case Studies in Essential Health: Millions Saved.*[46]

HIV/AIDS in Thailand

Preventing HIV/AIDS and Sexually Transmitted Infections in Thailand

Background

In Thailand, approximately 1 in every 60 persons is infected with HIV/AIDS and 75,000 children have been orphaned by AIDS.[47,48] Between 1989 and 1990, HIV among sex workers tripled, from 3.1% to 9.3% and a year later reached 15%. Over the same period, the proportion of male conscripts already infected with HIV when tested on entry to the army at age 21 rose six-fold, from 0.5% in 1989 to 3% in 1991.[48]

The Intervention

In 1989, Dr. Wiwat Rojanapithayakorn, director of a regional office in Communicable Disease Control in Thailand's Ratchaburi province, sought to curb AIDS by making sex in brothels safe, going well beyond the government's approach of raising awareness through mass advertising and education campaigns. Knowing that he could only be effective with political support, he sought the cooperation of the provincial governor. The steep rise in AIDS persuaded the governor to acquiesce, even though prostitution is illegal in Thailand and the government's intervention could imply that it tolerated or even condoned it.

A program was launched with one straightforward rule for all brothels in Ratchaburi: no condom, no sex. Until then, brothels had been reluctant to insist that their clients use condoms for fear of losing them to other establishments where condoms were not required. However, with condoms mandatory in all brothels, the competitive disincentive to individual workers and brothels was removed. Health officials, with the help of the police, held meetings with brothel owners and sex workers to provide them with information and free condoms. Men seeking treatment for sexually transmitted infections (STIs) were asked to name the brothel they had last visited and health officials would then visit the establishment to provide more information. This pilot program had dramatic results, bringing down STIs in Ratchaburi within just a few months.[49] In 1991, the National AIDS Committee, chaired by Prime Minister Anand Panyarachun, adopted this "100% condom program" at the national level.

The Impact

Condom use in brothels nationwide increased from 14% in early 1989 to more than 90% by June 1992.[50] An estimated

200,000 new infections were averted between 1993 and 2000. New STI cases fell from 200,000 in 1989 to 15,000 in 2001, while the rate of new HIV infections fell fivefold between 1991 and 1993–1995.[51] Such dramatic results have raised questions about their accuracy, as well as about their real causes, but independent studies have found the program to be genuinely effective.

The program did little to encourage the use of condoms in casual but noncommercial sex. Interventions among injecting drug users also did not expand to the national level, and the prevalence of HIV among this group is now as high as 50%.[52]

Costs and Benefits

Total government expenditure on the AIDS program has remained steady at approximately $375 million from 1998 to 2001, representing 1.9% of the health budget. Of this, 65% was spent on treatment and care.

Lessons Learned

The success of the program is due, in part, to the sheer scale and level of organization of the sex industry in Thailand, assisting officials in tracing and co-opting brothel owners. Thailand also had a good network of STI services within a well-functioning health system, providing treatment and advice, as well as crucial data for decision makers both at the baseline and when the program took effect. Cooperation between health authorities, governors, and the police was critical to success. Strong leadership from the prime minister, backed by significant financial resources, also made swift action possible. Maintaining Thailand's remarkable results in slowing the AIDS epidemic needs continued vigilance. Due to the high cost of treating STIs, the HIV prevention budget declined by two thirds between 1997 and 2004.[53] Although the Thai experience provides no blueprint for other countries with very different starting conditions, it does demonstrate that targeted strategies and political courage can effect change in deeply entrenched behaviors.

TB in China

Background

Although China established a National Tuberculosis Program in 1981, inadequate financial support hindered its success. In 1991, with $58 million from the World Bank, China embarked on the largest informal experiment in TB control in history: a 10-year Infectious and Endemic Disease Control project in 13 of its 31 mainland provinces.[54] The project adopted the DOTS strategy. Individuals demonstrating TB symptoms were referred to county dispensaries, where they received free diagnosis and treatment. Village

doctors were given financial incentives for enrolling patients and completing their treatment. Efforts were also made to strengthen the institutions involved with the establishment of a National Tuberculosis Project Office and a Tuberculosis Control Center. Quarterly reports were submitted by each county to the province, the central government, and the National Tuberculosis Project Office, which strengthened monitoring and quality control.

Impact

China achieved a 95% cure rate for new cases within 2 years of adopting DOTS, and a remarkable cure rate of 90% for those who had previously undergone unsuccessful treatment.[55] The number of people with TB declined by over 37% between 1990 and 2000, and 30,000 TB deaths have been prevented each year. More than 1.5 million patients have been treated, leading to the elimination of 836,000 cases of pulmonary TB.[56]

Costs and Benefits

The program cost $130 million. The World Bank and the WHO estimated that successful treatment was achieved at a cost of less than $100 per person. One healthy life was saved for an estimated $15 to $20, with an economic rate of return of $60 for each dollar invested.[57]

Lessons Learned

The success of China's program can be attributed to strong political commitment, leadership, adequate funding, and a sound technical approach delivered through a relatively strong health system. It was found that DOTS could be scaled up rapidly without sacrificing quality. Free diagnosis and treatment served as an effective incentive for patients and incentives for doctors to diagnose and complete treatment also worked well. However, the overall rate of case detection proved disappointing, mainly due to the inadequate referral of suspected TB cases from hospitals to TB dispensaries; hospitals charging for services had no incentive to refer patients to dispensaries where services were provided for free.[58] In addition, patients at hospitals often abandoned treatment prematurely. Despite the program's success, TB remains a deadly threat in China and efforts continue to maintain cure rates as well as to expand DOTS coverage to the remaining population.

Controlling Chagas Disease in the Southern Cone of South America

Background

Chagas disease, or American trypanosomiasis, was Latin America's most serious parasitic infection in the early 1990s.

Endemic in all seven countries of the southern cone, it caused an estimated 16 million to 18 million infections and 50,000 deaths each year. In Brazil alone, it was estimated that over a 2-year period the economic costs of the disease were almost $240 million and that $750 million would have been needed to treat its main health effects.[65]

The Intervention

The disease is named after Carlos Chagas, the Brazilian doctor who first described it in 1909 and subsequently discovered its cause: the parasite *Trypanosoma cruzi*. The parasites are found in the feces of "kissing bugs" that live within house walls in poor, rural areas and emerge at night to suck human blood. The parasites enter the bloodstream when insect bites are rubbed or scratched, or when food is contaminated. They can also enter via infected blood, or be transmitted from mother to fetus.

The first phase of the disease, the acute phase, is marked by fever, malaise, and swelling, and can sometimes be fatal, especially in young children. But most cases enter the second, chronic phase when the parasite damages vital body organs, resulting in heart failure, stomach pain, constipation, and swallowing difficulties that can lead to malnutrition.[66] A third of the cases are fatal.

In the absence of a vaccine or cure, control efforts needed to focus on eliminating the vector and screening the blood supply. Early attempts at control entailed methods such as dousing house walls with kerosene or scalding water, or enclosing and filling houses with cyanide gas.[67] The introduction of synthetic insecticides offered a more plausible solution, and spraying campaigns began in several countries in the 1950s and 1960s. Brazil launched a national eradication campaign in 1983, involving nationwide spraying and volunteer schemes. Brazil's early success demonstrated the technical feasibility of vector control. However, it also highlighted the need for regional efforts against border-crossing insects, and the need for sustained political commitment.[67]

In 1991 a new control program called INCOSUR (Southern Cone Initiative to Control/Eliminate Chagas) was launched to bolster national resolve and prevent cross-border reinfestations. Led by the Pan American Health Organization (PAHO), the initiative was jointly adopted by Argentina, Bolivia, Brazil, Chile, Paraguay, Uruguay, and later, Peru. The countries financed and managed their own programs but met annually to share operational aims, methods, and achievements. Intercountry technical cooperation agreements fostered the sharing of information among regional scientists and governments, with additional scientific support from a network of researchers in 22 countries. Between 1992 and 2001, more than 2.5 million homes were sprayed. Canisters that release insecticidal fumes when lit were also provided. Houses were improved to eliminate hiding places for insects, adobe walls were replaced with plaster, and metal roofs were constructed. The screening of blood donors for the parasite is now virtually universal in 10 South American countries.[68]

Impact

Incidence in the seven INCOSUR countries fell by an average of 94% by 2000. Overall, the number of new cases on the continent fell from 700,000 in 1983 to fewer than 200,000 in 2000.[69] The number of deaths each year from the disease was halved from 45,000 to 22,000. By 2001, disease transmission was halted in Uruguay, Chile, and large parts of Brazil and Paraguay. Surveys indicate an improved sense of well-being, domestic pride, and security. Central America and the Amazon region remain the next major challenges.

Costs and Benefits

Financial resources for INCOSUR, provided by each of the seven countries, have totaled more than $400 million since 1991. The intervention is considered among the most cost-effective interventions in public health, at just $37 per DALY saved in Brazil.[69]

Lessons Learned

Chris Schofield, a researcher at the London School of Hygiene and Tropical Medicine, attributes INCOSUR's success to three factors: it was big and designed to reach a definitive end point; it had a simple, well-proven technical approach; and, it gained political continuity from a close coordination between researchers and governments. Alfredo Solari, Uruguay's former minister of health, mentions four elements: peer pressure from neighboring countries in an exercise dealing with border-crossing insects; commitment by all participating countries, backed by international organizations like PAHO and WHO; an international technical secretariat at PAHO that verified surveillance, shared information about progress, processed certification requests and organized annual meetings; and, a favorable economic and institutional environment that allowed resources for expensive national health programs. Sustaining the achievements of INCOSUR will require vigilance, since premature curtailment of active surveillance against the disease could lead to disease resurgence.

Controlling Trachoma in Morocco
Background

Trachoma is the second leading cause of blindness, after cataract, and the number one cause of preventable blindness in the world. Although it has been eliminated in North America and Europe, trachoma still afflicts more than 150 million people in 46 countries, especially in hot, dry regions where access to clean water, sanitation, and health care is limited.[70] In Morocco, trachoma was once widespread, but in the 1970s and 1980s, treatment with antibiotics lowered its incidence in urban areas. A 1992 survey found that 5.4% of Moroccans still suffered from trachoma, mainly in five rural provinces in the southeast, where 25,000 people showed a serious decline in vision, 625,000 needed treatment for inflammatory trachoma, and 40,000 urgently required surgery.

The Intervention

Caused by the bacterium *Chlamydia trachomatis*, trachoma is highly contagious, spreading mainly among children through direct contact with eye and nose secretions, infected clothing, and fluid-seeking flies. Transmission of the disease is rapid in overcrowded conditions of poor hygiene and poverty. In endemic areas, prevalence rates in children aged 2 to 5 years can reach 90%.[71] Women are infected at a rate two to three times that for men because of their close contact with children. Repeated trachoma infections can lead to a painful in-turning of the eyelash which can cause blindness.

In 1991, Morocco formed the National Blindness Control Program (NBCP) with several international and other agencies to eliminate trachoma by 2005. Between 1997 and 1999, this program implemented a pilot strategy to treat trachoma, developed by the Edna McConnell Clark Foundation, called SAFE (surgery, antibiotics, face washing, and environmental change). SAFE differed from earlier approaches by emphasizing behavioral and environmental change, in addition to medication. Under this four-part strategy, a quick and inexpensive surgery to prevent blindness was provided for large numbers of patients in small towns and villages. Antibiotics were used to treat infection and prevent scarring. Face washing, especially among children, was promoted through an education campaign. Living conditions and community hygiene were improved by constructing latrines, drilling wells, storing dung away from flies, and providing health education.[72]

In the mid-1990s, Pfizer discovered Zithromax®, a one-dose cure to replace the six-week course of tetracycline that had been used for treatment, ensuring a higher compliance rate. Pfizer pharmaceutical company donated the drug for Morocco, as well as for other poor countries, through the International Trachoma Initiative (ITI), a private-public partnership that it forged along with the Clark Foundation.

Impact

Between 1999 and 2003, the SAFE strategy led to a 75% decline in trachoma in Morocco. Overall, the prevalence of active disease in children under 10 was reduced by 90% since 1997.[71]

Costs and Benefits

The Moroccan government provided most of the financing for the program. ITI supplemented this with several grants, while UNICEF contributed $225,000. Pfizer's donation of tens of millions of dollars worth of Zithromax® to Morocco and other countries represents one of the largest donations of a patented drug in history.

Lessons Learned

Government commitment to the program was critical to its success, in addition to the array of effective interventions. Four key factors were also listed by ITI: the program was based on solid scientific evidence; it was locally organized and therefore responded well to local circumstances; it fit within a broader agenda of health promotion, disease control, and health equity; and, treatment was closely linked with prevention and the development of a strong public health infrastructure. ITI and its many partners have helped ensure that Morocco's success with SAFE, like the disease that it has nearly eliminated, is contagious.

AVIAN INFLUENZA

Prevention and control of communicable diseases face a number of significant challenges. One of these challenges relates to the spread of existing communicable diseases to places that had previously not seen them. This has been the case, for example, in the last decade with the spread of the West Nile virus and dengue fever to and within some countries.

Another issue relates to the spread of resistant forms of disease. Comments were made earlier about strains of TB that have emerged in Southern Africa that appear to be resistant to most first- and second-line TB drugs and that have had unusually high case fatality rates. Will equally difficult strains of HIV emerge? There are a number of hospital-based infections that are very difficult to treat. Will they become more difficult to treat as they become increasingly resistant to the available antibiotics? Will the development of new antibiotics stay ahead of the development of new resistant forms of bacteria?

Finally, there is the possibility that new diseases will emerge that previously had been unknown, such as Legionnaire's disease, the Ebola virus, and Sudden Acute

Respiratory Syndrome (SARS). New and emerging diseases are the subject of much discussion and study. Some comments will be offered here on only one disease, avian influenza, before returning to a discussion of the challenges faced in addressing HIV/AIDS, TB, malaria, diarrhea, and the neglected diseases.

One challenge of extreme importance is the risk of a major influenza pandemic and the influenza of greatest concern is avian flu. Most of those involved in global work on communicable diseases believe it is not a question of "if" there will be a major global outbreak of avian flu, but only a question of "when" it will occur and how severe it will be.

Avian influenza is caused by the H5N1 strain of the influenza virus. It is transmitted bird-to-bird mainly through fecal contact and from bird-to-human by aerosol transmission. H5N1 is a virus of birds and infects humans irregularly. However, when humans do become infected, severe disease develops. Coughing and fever are the symptoms of the disease in humans, and these symptoms can develop rapidly after initial infection. The development of an avian influenza pandemic among humans would require the emergence of a variant of the H5N1 virus that would be able to replicate in humans, cause serious disease in humans, and be efficiently transmitted from one human to another.

Human influenza pandemics have occurred in the past and will continue to occur in the future. There were three major influenza pandemics is the 20th century, the great Spanish flu of 1918–1919 that killed 40 to 50 million people, the Asian Flu of 1957, and the Hong Kong flu of 1968 that together killed an estimated 4.5 million people. In 1918, two epidemic "waves" occurred. The first wave was contagious, but not very deadly. The second wave spread rapidly as well, and took only 2 months to circle the globe, but had a 10 fold greater mortality. In 3 weeks, two million people died in Africa and an estimated 30% of the world's population fell ill, with most mortality occurring in the 15 to 35 year age group.

Although the 1918 pandemic was extraordinary, influenza continues to cause substantial mortality and morbidity annually. In the United States, in a typical influenza year, about 30 million people are infected and 50,000 are hospitalized with 20,000 to 40,000 deaths occurring, mostly in the elderly.[73] Worldwide, between 250,000 and 500,000 die annually from non-pandemic influenza. It is expected that deaths from a new influenza virus would dwarf those numbers. If 30% of the world were infected, with a case fatality rate of 5%, then about two billion people would be infected and potentially ill, with deaths approaching 100 million.[74]

In addition, this scenario would completely overwhelm health systems in most, if not all, countries. It would also cause incalculable economic loss due to absenteeism, medical expenses, business closings, and the disease control strategies that would keep people, workers, and students at home until transmission and risk of infection subsided. In the United States, the severe epidemic scenario implies 90 million will fall ill, 45 million will require outpatient care, 10 million will need hospitalization, and two million will die.[74]

The key to controlling the risk from a new virus is to prepare carefully for it, and that preparedness depends on four elements: accurate perception of risk, problem identification, rapid response to mitigate impacts, and sustained access to services for recovery. In addition, preparedness requires sound and executable plans, communication, surveillance and case detection, comprehensive situation analyses, and containment. Time is a limiting factor in preparedness and response because a pandemic virus could spread rapidly and overwhelm health systems within 40 days after its appearance. Global preparedness planning is now underway, under the auspices of the United Nations.

Developing a vaccine to address a virus that might cause a pandemic of avian influenza is also a challenging problem and there is a fear that a new avian influenza virus will spread before a vaccine for it could be developed, produced, and distributed. It usually takes 5 to 6 months for a new influenza vaccine to be developed, tested, produced, and distributed and a vaccine can not be produced until a new influenza virus emerges and is identified. In hopes of being more ready for avian influenza, vaccines based on existing strains of H5N1 are being developed collaboratively by governments and industries.

While vaccines are clearly part of the solution to an avian influenza pandemic, laboratory studies suggest some prescription antiviral medicines for human influenza should help to treat avian influenza.[75] With this in mind, governments are stockpiling medicines in order to deliver a comprehensive response to a pandemic if it should occur.

FUTURE CHALLENGES TO THE CONTROL OF COMMUNICABLE DISEASES

A number of challenges constrain efforts to address the burden of the most important communicable diseases. Some of these relate to the need for countries to cooperate to combat communicable diseases. Some concern the ability of weak health systems in low- and middle-income countries to tackle communicable disease problems effectively. Others relate to the issues raised by specific diseases.

First, it is imperative to enhance political commitment to the prevention and control of these diseases. You read earlier that sustained political support at the highest levels is essential if progress is to be made against HIV/AIDS, and this is also true for the other leading causes of communicable disease. Countries will only be successful in acting against these diseases if they make them a real priority both politically and financially.

Second, the underlying causes of communicable diseases in low- and middle-income countries relate to poverty, people's lack of empowerment, people's lack of knowledge of appropriate health behaviors, and a lack of access to basic infrastructure such as safe water, sanitation, and health services. These issues will take many years to address in most low-income countries. Thus, in the short- and medium-run, success against some communicable diseases will depend on community-based efforts.

It is likely that health systems in many low- and middle-income countries will continue to be weak for many years, as well. This suggests that efforts to address communicable diseases will also have to be based on partnership with a variety of actors. This includes communities, religious groups and other non-governmental organizations, the private sector, and government. The great successes in the control of infectious diseases to date have all been built on the foundation of public-private partnerships. The polio eradication effort includes, for example, a remarkable amount of public-private collaboration, as does, for example, the campaign against onchocerciasis. It is especially important that these actors work together in the future across an array of diseases and health systems issues and not just on individual diseases.

Strengthening the surveillance of disease at the local, national, and global levels is also fundamental to effective disease control. A competent body of public health professionals need to be responsible for managing surveillance networks. Appropriate laboratory infrastructures must be an essential part of any improved surveillance efforts. Continuous sharing of surveillance information within and across countries is necessary to prepare for special problems, to know when they arise, and to respond to them effectively.

The lack of adequately trained and appropriately deployed human resources for health will also remain an issue, especially in lower-income countries. There will not be enough personnel, the incentives for their performance will be lacking, and the personnel that do exist will largely be available only in the larger cities. Thus, it will be important to have the lowest level of worker possible handle various health services so that scarce higher-level workers can focus on those things they alone can do. In addition, many services can be devolved to community-based workers. This will be an important point, for example, in countries with high HIV/AIDS prevalence but few trained doctors and nurses, as they spread AIDS treatment beyond the largest cities.

Another important issue will be the balance that needs to be struck between prevention and treatment. This will be especially challenging in the field of HIV/AIDS. There is considerable commitment in the world today to ensuring that all people needing treatment with antiretroviral therapy get it as soon as possible. There are many reasons why this is important. However, it is unlikely to stop transmission because people are most infective early in the disease and usually infect others before they know they have it. Prevention must remain at the core of efforts to address HIV/AIDS.

The challenge of financing enhanced efforts in the control of communicable diseases will also be formidable. Without major changes in their spending patterns and rapid economic growth, many low- and middle-income countries will not be able to pay for the stepped up efforts they need to combat the major communicable diseases. Rather, they will have to depend for some time on financial assistance from the developed countries and private sector partners.

Scientific and technical challenges also remain. There is no effective vaccine for any of the diseases that have been the focus of this chapter, except for rotavirus for some forms of diarrhea. Drug resistance is a constant issue in HIV, a threat in the control of diarrhea and some parasitic infections, and a major issue in the control of TB and malaria. It will be imperative that new drugs are developed that can prevent or overcome such resistance. In HIV, it will be important to continue to have new drugs that are easier to take, easier to transport and store, have fewer side effects, and are less likely to allow resistance to emerge than the present drugs.

Another challenge will be the need to develop models in low- and middle-income countries to provide chronic care of people with HIV. Most health service efforts in low-income countries focus on acute care. The treatment of HIV with antiretroviral therapy creates the possibility that people who are HIV-positive can have full and productive lives for many years. However, it also means that countries with very weak health systems that are mostly accustomed to treating acute illnesses will have to develop effective and efficient models for treating some people for many years of their life.

Another important issue is how low-income and resource-poor countries will be able to financially sustain the progress that they do make in AIDS treatment and several other areas related to the prevention and control of communicable diseases. Successful efforts to prevent and control these diseases will reduce prevalence and, ultimately, reduce the demands on the health system. As the prevalence of hookworm declines, for example, countries will be able to spend less money for hookworm treatment programs. However, the demands on health systems for treatment for HIV/AIDS will continue to be great for many years to come. Low- and middle-income countries with high HIV/AIDS prevalence will have to plan carefully how AIDS treatment can be financed in the future. This is especially important because once people start taking antiretroviral therapy, it is imperative that they continue to take it.

Monitoring and evaluation is an essential tool of public health programming. If the world is to make progress against the most important communicable diseases and continue to learn what is most cost-effective in addressing these diseases, then it is important to enhance the quality of monitoring and evaluation of health investments. All activities require a monitoring and evaluation component to track project progress, estimate cost-effectiveness of the effort, and assess the impact of the activities that are being financed.

MAIN MESSAGES

Communicable diseases account for about 44% of total deaths and 40% of DALYs in low- and middle-income countries. Among the communicable diseases, HIV/AIDS and malaria take an enormous toll on Sub-Saharan Africa. The neglected diseases are also a relatively more important burden of disease in Sub-Saharan Africa than in any other region. The toll from communicable diseases is similar for men and women, but the AIDS epidemic is taking an increasing toll on women, and TB generally affects men more than women.

HIV is an especially important burden. About 40 million people are now infected with HIV; in 2005 about 2.3 million people died from the disease, and another 4.3 million were infected with it that same year. Besides concerns for the African region, there are major concerns that the epidemic will grow in India, China, and the former Soviet Union.

The AIDS epidemic is helping to fuel TB. About one third of the world is infected with TB and there are about nine million people in the world with active TB disease. Both HIV/AIDS and TB mostly affect people in their productive years.

Malaria kills more than one million people a year, mostly young children in Africa. It also causes a huge burden of morbidity because cases of malaria are so common and people may get more than one case a year. Malaria also poses very substantial risks to pregnant women. Diarrhea is an especially important burden of disease for children, as well, and is also responsible for about 1.8 million child deaths a year. A number of parasitic and infectious diseases are often called the neglected diseases and they pose an exceptional burden of disease, again largely in Sub-Saharan Africa and South Asia.

The worm *Ascaris*, for example, infects more than one billion people worldwide. Trichuris and hookworm infect 800 million and 740 million, respectively.

The economic and social consequences of the communicable diseases are very considerable. Diarrhea and worms can cause children to fail to develop properly, delay their entry into and performance in school, and lessen their productivity as adults. HIV/AIDS, TB, and malaria also greatly affect adult productivity. The direct and indirect costs of these diseases to individuals and families are very high and often cause people to borrow money, sell their limited assets, and fall below the poverty line. There is good evidence that high levels of malaria are an important impediment to economic growth in low-income countries in Africa.

Addressing HIV/AIDS will require redoubled efforts on prevention and continued efforts to learn what can prevent transmission in the most cost-effective ways. There is an increasing understanding that strong political leadership, focusing on the groups most at risk, and addressing the needs of "bridge populations" are parts of successful prevention efforts. Other key parts of prevention are maintaining a clean blood supply, testing and counseling, and condom promotion, in connection with efforts to delay sexual debut and reduce the number of sexual partners. It is also important to stem the transmission of HIV from mother to child. There are an increasing number of people on treatment for HIV worldwide, and efforts are underway to ensure that all people who need treatment get it, although meeting this goal will be very challenging in low-income countries.

Although TB incidence and the presentation of TB are being dramatically affected by HIV, the mainstay of efforts to address TB has been DOTS, which stands for Directly Observed Therapy, Short-Course. This is a very cost-effective way of treating TB. Malaria can be addressed through prompt diagnosis and treatment, intermittent treatment of pregnant women, the use of insecticide-treated bed nets, and indoor residual spraying. Proper treatment to avoid the development of resistance is central to efforts in TB, HIV/AIDS, and malaria.

The burden of diarrhea can be reduced through immunization against rotavirus and measles and supplementation with zinc. Oral rehydration therapy is a cost-effective way of managing diarrhea in infants and children. The best approach to diarrhea, of course, would be to try to avoid it through improved hygiene. Better access to safe water and sanitation will help to reduce the burden of some of the parasitic and bacterial infections that make up the neglected diseases. In the short-run, however, there is a package of drug therapy that can be integrated with other disease control efforts to reduce the burden of the neglected diseases in a cost-effective way.

The challenge of addressing the burden of communicable diseases effectively is enormous. They are mostly diseases of poverty that also reflect a lack of access to safe water and sanitation, poor knowledge of appropriate health behaviors, and a lack of health services that are geared to meet the highest priority needs. In addition, several of these diseases are highly stigmatized, efforts to control them must be carried out in countries with weak health systems, and considerably more financing is needed for these efforts than has been available. Nonetheless, there has been major progress in the last 40 years in addressing smallpox, onchocerciasis, and a number of vaccine-preventable diseases in children. The lessons from those experiences suggest that it is possible through concerted efforts and partnerships and greatly enhanced disease surveillance efforts to continue making such progress.

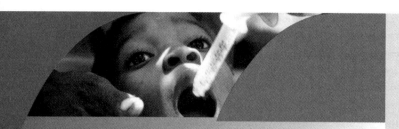

Study Questions

1. What are the most important infectious diseases in terms of deaths in low- and middle-income countries? In terms of DALYs?

2. In what regions will the deaths from HIV/AIDS be most important? In what regions will malaria be most important?

3. What is driving the HIV epidemic in Russia? In Sub-Saharan Africa?

4. In Sub-Saharan Africa, what would be the most cost-effective measures to try to prevent further transmission of the HIV virus? What approach would you take to prevention in South Asia, and why would it differ from what you would do in Sub-Saharan Africa?

5. What groups are especially at risk for malaria? What steps would you take to try to reduce the burden of malaria?

6. What is DOTS? What are the key focuses of this approach? Why has it been more effective than previous approaches to TB control?

7. If relatively few people die as a direct result of parasitic diseases, why are they so important?

8. What are the concerns about drug resistance for malaria and TB? How can resistance be kept to a minimum?

9. Why is it important to develop a vaccine for HIV?

10. What risks would the world face in a pandemic of avian influenza, and how can the world prepare for it?

REFERENCES

1. Lopez AD, Mathers CD, Ezzati M, Jamison DT, Murray CJL. Measuring the global burden of disease and risk factors, 1990-2001. In: Lopez AD, Mathers CD, Ezzati M, Jamison DT, Murray CJL, eds. *Global Burden of Disease and Risk Factors.* New York: Oxford University Press; 2006:8.

2. Bertozzi S, Padian NS, Wegbreit J, et al. HIV/AIDS Prevention and Treatment. In: Jamison DT, Breman JG, Measham AR, et al., eds. *Disease Control Priorities in Developing Countries.* 2nd ed. New York: Oxford University Press; 2006:331–370.

3. Chin J, ed. *Control of Communicable Diseases Manual.* 17th ed. Washington, DC: American Public Health Association; 2000.

4. Bertozzi S, Padian NS, Wegbreit J, et al. HIV/AIDS Prevention and treatment. In: Jamison DT, Breman JG, Measham AR, et al., eds. *Disease Control Priorities in Developing Countries.* 2nd ed. New York: Oxford University Press; 2006:353.

5. UNAIDS. 2006 Report on the Global AIDS Epidemic Available at: http://www.unaids.org/en/HIV_data/2006GlobalReport/default.asp. Accessed November 15, 2006.

6. World Health Organization. Fact Sheet No. 104: Tuberculosis. Available at: http://www.who.int/mediacentre/factsheets/fs104/en/. Accessed November 20, 2006.

7. Stop TB. Fact Sheet—Socioeconomic Impact of TB—Impact of TB on Women and Families. www.stoptb.org/stop_tb_initiative/amsterdam_conference_documents/pfs-imp. Accessed November 15, 2006.

8. Stop TB. TB—A Leading Killer of Women. Available at: http://www.searo.who.int/LinkFiles/Tuberculosis_right5.pdf. Accessed November 15, 2006.

9. Centers for Disease Control and Prevention. Extensively Drug-Resistant Tuberculosis (XDR TB)—Update. Available at: http://www.cdc.gov/nchstp/tb/xdrtbupdate.htm. Accessed November 19, 2006.

10. Lopez AD, Mathers CD, Murray CJL. The burden of disease and mortality by condition: data, methods, and results for 2001. In: Lopez AD, Mathers CD, Ezzati M, Jamison DT, Murray CJL, eds. *Global Burden of Disease and Risk Factors.* New York: Oxford University Press; 2006:70.

11. Breman JG, Mills A, Snow RW, Mulligan J-A. Conquering malaria. In: Jamison DT, Breman JG, Measham AM, Alleyne G, eds. *Disease Control Priorities in Developing Countries.* 2nd ed. New York: Oxford University Press; 2006:413–432.

12. Keusch GT, Fontaine O, Bhargava A, Boschi-Pinto C. Diarrheal Diseases. In: Jamison DT, Breman JG, Measham AM, Alleyne G, eds. *Disease Control Priorities in Developing Countries.* 2nd ed. New York: Oxford University Press; 2006:371–388.

13. Parashar UD. Global illness and deaths caused by rotavirus disease in children. *Emer Infect Dis.* 2003;9(5):565–572.

14. Hotez P, Molyneux DH, Fenwick A, Ottesen E., Sachs SE, Sachs JD. Incorporating a rapid-impact package for neglected tropical diseases with programs for HIV/AIDS, tuberculosis and malaria. *PLos Medicine.* 2006;3(5):576–584.

15. Hotez PJ, Bundy DAP, Beegle K, et al. Helminth infections: soil-transmitted helminth infections and schistosomiasis. In: Jamison DT, Breman JG, Measham AR, et al., eds. *Disease Control Priorities in Developing Countries.* 2nd ed. New York: Oxford University Press; 2006:467–482.

16. Chin J, ed. *Control of Communicable Diseases (Manual).* 17th ed. Washington, DC: American Public Health Association; 2000.

17. Chin J, ed. *Control Of Communicable Diseases (Manual).* 17th ed. Washington, DC: American Public Health Association; 2000.

18. Russell S. The economic burden of illness for households in developing countries: a review of studies focusing on malaria, tuberculosis, and human immunodeficiency virus/acquired immunodeficiency syndrome. *Am J Trop Med Hyg.* 2004;71(2 Suppl):147–155.

19. Brown LR. The potential impact of AIDS on population and economic growth rates. Available at: http://ideas.repec.org/p/fpr/2020br/43.html. Accessed November 22, 2006.

20. Ainsworth M, Over M. AIDS and African Development. *The World Bank Research Observer.* 1994:9(2)203–240.

21. Chand N, Singh T, Khalsa JS, Verma V, Rathore JS. A study of socio-economic impact of tuberculosis on patients and their family. *CHEST.* 2004:126(4)832S.

22. Croft RA, Croft RP. Expenditure and loss of income incurred by tuberculosis patients before reaching effective treatment in Bangladesh. *Int J Tuberc Lung Dis.* 1998;2(3):252–254.

23. Kamolratanakul P, Sawert H, Kongsin S, et al. Economic impact of tuberculosis at the household level. *Int J Tuberc Lung Dis.* 1999;3(7):596–602.

24. Rajeswari R, Balasubramanian R, Muniyandi M, Geetharamani S, Thresa X, Venkatesan P. Socio-economic impact of tuberculosis on patients and family in India. *Int J Tuberc Lung Dis.* 1999;3(10):869–877.

25. Grimard F, Harling G. The Impact of Tuberculosis on Economic Growth. Available at: http://neumann.hec.ca/neudc2004/fp/grimard_franque_aout_27.pdf. *World Bank Res Observer.* Accessed November 22, 2006.

26. Peabody JW, Shimkhada R, Tan C, Jr., Luck J. The burden of disease, economic costs and clinical consequences of tuberculosis in the Philippines. *Health Policy Plan.* 2005;20(6):347–353.

27. Lynch M. Malaria Presentation. 2005.

28. Roll Back Malaria Partnership. Economic Costs of Malaria. Washington: USAID; Available at: http://www.rbm.who.int/cmc_upload/0/000/015/363/RBMInfosheet_10.htm. Accessed November 22, 2006.

29. Gallup JL, Sachs JD. The economic burden of malaria. *Am J Trop Med Hyg.* 2001;64(1-2 Suppl):85–96.

30. Sachs JD, Hotez PJ. Fighting tropical diseases. *Science.* 2006;311(5,767):1521.

31. Miguel EA, Kremer M. Worms: identifying impacts on education and health in the presence of treatment externalities. *Econometrica.* 2003;71(1):159–217.

32. Bleakley H. Disease and development: evidence from hookworm eradication in the American South. *Eur Econ Assoc.* 2003;1(2–3):376–386.

33. Bertozzi S, Padian NS, Wegbreit J, et al. HIV/AIDS Prevention and treatment. In: Jamison DT, Breman JG, Measham AR, et al., eds. *Disease Control Priorities in Developing Countries.* 2nd ed. New York: Oxford University Press; 2006:332.

34. Bertozzi S, Padian NS, Wegbreit J, et al. HIV/AIDS Prevention and treatment. In: Jamison DT, Breman JG, Measham AR, et al., eds. *Disease Control Priorities in Developing Countries.* 2nd ed. New York: Oxford University Press; 2006:331–170.

35. Bertozzi S, Padian NS, Wegbreit J, et al. HIV/AIDS Prevention and treatment. In: Jamison DT, Breman JG, Measham AR, et al., eds. *Disease Control Priorities in Developing Countries.* 2nd ed. New York: Oxford University Press; 2006:345–346.

36. Bertozzi S, Padian NS, Wegbreit J, et al. HIV/AIDS Prevention and treatment. In: Jamison DT, Breman JG, Measham AR, et al., eds. *Disease Control Priorities in Developing Countries.* 2nd ed. New York: Oxford University Press; 2006:345.

37. Centers for Disease Control and Prevention. Male Circumcision and Risk for HIV Transmission: Implications for the United States. Available at: http://www.cdc.gov/hiv/resources/factsheets/circumcision.htm. Accessed March 6, 2007.

38. Bertozzi S, Padian NS, Wegbreit J, et al. HIV/AIDS Prevention and treatment. In: Jamison DT, Breman JG, Measham AR, et al., eds. *Disease Control Priorities in Developing Countries.* 2nd ed. New York: Oxford University Press; 2006:344–346.

39. Bertozzi S, Padian NS, Wegbreit J, et al. HIV/AIDS Prevention and treatment. In: Jamison DT, Breman JG, Measham AR, et al., eds. *Disease Control Priorities in Developing Countries.* 2nd ed. New York: Oxford University Press; 2006:351–353.

40. Bertozzi S, Padian NS, Wegbreit J, et al. HIV/AIDS Prevention and treatment. In: Jamison DT, Breman JG, Measham AR, et al., eds. *Disease Control Priorities in Developing Countries.* 2nd ed. New York: Oxford University Press; 2006:355.

41. Dye C, Floyd K. Tuberculosis. In: Jamison DT, Breman JG, Measham AR, et al., eds. *Disease Control Priorities in Developing Countries.* 2nd ed. New York: Oxford University Press; 2006:289–312.

42. The Abuja Declaration and the Plan of Action. Available at: http://www.rbm.who.int/docs/abuja_declaration_final.htm. Accessed November 15, 2006.

43. Centers for Disease Control and Prevention. Rotavirus. Available at: http://www.cdc.gov/ncidod/dvrd/revb/gastro/rotavirus.htm. Accessed October 15, 2006.

44. Huttly SR, Morris SS, Pisani V. Prevention of diarrhoea in young children in developing countries. *Bulletin of the World Health Organization.* 1997;(75):163–174.

45. Black RE. Zinc deficiency, infectious disease, and mortality in the developing world. *J Nutr.* 2003;133 (5 Suppl 1):1485S–1489S.

46. Levine R. *Millions Saved.* Washington, DC: Center for Global Development; 2004.

47. UNAIDS. *AIDS Epidemic Update (December).* Geneva: UNAIDS; 2002.

48. U.S. Centers for Disease Control and Prevention. Global AIDS Program, Country Profiles: Thailand. www.cdc.gov/nchsp/od/gap/countries/thailand.htm. Accessed February 6, 2004.

49. UNAIDS. *Evaluation of the 100% Condom Programme in Thailand.* Geneva: UNAIDS, in collaboration with the Ministry of Public Health, Thailand; 2000. Document 00.18E.

50. Rojanapithayakorn W, Hanenberg R. The 100% Condom Programme in Thailand. *AIDS.* 1996;10(1):1–7.

51. Celentano D, Nelson K, Lyles C, et al. Decreasing incidence of HIV and sexually transmited diseases among young Thai men: evidence for success of the HIV/AIDS control and prevention program. *AIDS.* 1998;12(5):F29-F36.

52. Chitwarkorn A. HIV/AIDS and sexually transmitted infections in thailand: lessons learned and future challenges. In: Narain JP, ed. *AIDS in Asia: The Challenge Continues.* New Delhi: Sage Publications; 2004.

53. UNAIDS. *Report on the Global AIDS Epidemic.* Geneva: UNAIDS; 2004.

54. China Tuberculosis Control Collaboration. Results of directly observed short-course chemotherapy in 112,842 Chinese patients with smear-positive tuberculosis. *Lancet.* 1996;347:358–362.

55. World Health Organization Regional Office for the Western Pacific. *DOTS for All: Country Reports.* Geneva: World Health Organization; 2002.

56. Zhao F, Zhao Y, Liu X. Tuberculosis control in China. *Tuberculosis.* 2003;85:15–20.

57. The World Bank. *Implementation Completion Report for the China Infectious Diseases Control Project.* Washington, DC: The World Bank; 2002.

58. Chen X, Zhao F, Duanmu H, Wan L, Wang X, Chin DP. The DOTS strategy in China: results and lessons after 10 years. *Bulletin of the World Health Organization.* 2002;80(6):430–436.

59. Musgrove P. Is the eradication of polio in the western hemisphere economically justified? *Bulletin of the Pan American Sanitary Bureau.* 1988;22(1):1–16

60. Henderson DA, de Quadros CA, Andrus J, Olive J-M, Guerra de Macedo C. Polio eradication from the western hemisphere. *Ann Rev Public Health.* 1992;13:239–252.

61. de Cuadros CA. Polio. *Encyclopedia of Microbiology 3.* 2000:762–772.

62. Gawande A. The Mop-Up: Eradicating Polio from the Planet. *The New Yorker.* January 12, 2004:34–40.

63. Jamison DT, Torres AM, Chen LC, Melnick JL. Poliomyelitis. In: Jamison DT, Mosley H, Measham A, Bobadilla JL, eds. *Disease Control Priorities in Developing Countries.* Oxford: Oxford Univesity Press; 1993.

64. Global Polio Eradication Initiative. Afghanistan, Egypt, India, Niger, Nigeria, and Pakistan, Progress Report. www.polioeradication.org/content/publication/2003-progress.pdf. Accessed August 10, 2004.

65. World Health Organization. *Control of Chagas Disease. Report of a WHO Expert Committee. WHO Technical Report Series: 811.* Geneva: World Health Organization; 1991.

66. U.S. Centers for Disease Control and Prevention. Fact Sheet: Chagas Disease. Available at: http://www.cdc.gov/ncidod/dpd/parasites/chagasdisease/factsht_chagas_disease.htm. Accessed July 29, 2003.

67. Dias JCP, Silveira AC, Schofield CJ. The impact of Chagas disease control in Latin America—a review. *Memorias do Instituto Oswaldo Cruz.* 2002;97:603–612.

68. Schmunis GA, Zicker F, Cruz J, Cuchi P. Safety of blood supply for infectious diseases in Latin American countries, 1994–1997. *Am J Trop Med Hygiene.* 2001;65:924–930.

69. Moncayo A. Chagas disease: current epidemiological trends after interruption of vectorial and transfusional transmission in the southern cone countries. *Memorias do Instituto Oswaldo Cruz.* 2003;98(5):577–591.

70. Kumaresan J, Mecaskey J. The global elimination of blinding trachoma: progress and promise. *Am J Trop Med Hygiene.* 2003;69(Supplement 5):S24-S28.

71. Mecaskey J, Knirsch C, Kumaresan J, Cook J. The possibility of eliminating blinding trachoma. *Lancet.* 2003;3:728–734.

72. West S. Blinding trachoma: prevention with the SAFE strategy. *Am J Trop Med Hygiene.* 2003;69(Supplement 5):S18-S23.

73. Centers for Disease Control and Prevention. Key Facts about Influenza and the Influenza Vaccine. Available at: http://www.cdc.gov/flu/keyfacts.htm. Accessed November 15, 2006

74. United States Government. Pandemic Planning Assmptions. Available at: http://www.pandemicflu.gov/plan/pandplan.html. Accessed November 15, 2006.

75. United States Government. Pandemic Flu—General Information. Available at: http://www.pandemicflu.gov/general/. Accessed November 15, 2006.

CHAPTER 12

Non-communicable Diseases

By the end of this chapter the reader will be able to:

- Describe the most important non-communicable diseases
- Discuss the importance of these diseases to global health
- Discuss the burden of non-communicable diseases worldwide
- Outline the costs and consequences of non-communicable diseases, tobacco use, and excessive drinking of alcohol
- Review measures that can be taken to address the burden of non-communicable diseases in cost-effective ways
- Describe some successful cases of dealing with non-communicable diseases

VIGNETTES

Roberto was 45 years old and lived in Bogota, Colombia. He had been overweight for most of his adult life. He enjoyed eating and had a government desk job. Because he lived in the heart of the city, he got little exercise. He had read about increasing rates of diabetes but thought this was largely a disease of people in rich countries. Last year, Roberto started feeling thirsty all the time, had dry mouth, and felt weak after any exertion. He went to his doctor and was diagnosed as having adult onset diabetes.

Shanti was 35 years old and lived in Sri Lanka. She had grown up in a village, had worked hard on her family's small farm, and had been healthy for all of her adult life. She had two children and had not had any problems during either pregnancy. During a recent visit to the local health center, however, the doctor discovered that Shanti had high blood pressure. The doctor talked with Shanti about changing her diet and also prescribed medication for her. The medicine she needed is not expensive, but, unfortunately, Shanti has to take this medicine for the remainder of her life.

Alexei was 47 years old and lived in Moscow, Russia. Alexei had been smoking one pack of cigarettes a day since he was 16 years old. He heard on television and on the radio about the bad effects that cigarettes have on health. Urged by his children to stop smoking, he tried unsuccessfully on several occasions to quit. Over the last few months, Alexei developed a continuous cough and was often short of breath. Alexei had lung cancer.

Lai Ying lived in Guandong Province, China, and was a factory worker. Until recently she had been a happy and healthy young woman. More recently, however, Lai Ying had felt very unhappy. She did not feel like getting out of bed in the morning, did not want to go to work, and had no energy when she was at work. She thought from time to time of death and considered suicide. Lai Ying's family noticed that she was not eating properly and that she was "not herself." However, they thought she was having a difficult time at work or with a boyfriend and that she would soon be fine. After some months of this behavior, Lai Ying committed suicide by taking an overdose of sleeping pills.

THE IMPORTANCE OF NON-COMMUNICABLE DISEASES

Non-communicable diseases are of considerable and growing importance worldwide. In fact, the burden of non-communicable diseases is now greater than the burden of communicable diseases in low- and middle-income countries, as well as in high-income countries. This is a relatively recent fact which contradicts the notion that low-income countries are so overwhelmed with the burden of communicable disease that they do not face a significant burden of non-communicable disease. Among the most important of the non-communicable health conditions that low- and middle-income countries face are cardiovascular disease, diabetes, cancers, and mental disorders.[1]

The risk factors for non-communicable diseases relate in significant ways to lifestyle, much of which is within people's control. We will discuss, for example, the importance of diet, physical activity, tobacco use, and alcohol abuse to the onset of certain non-communicable diseases. By engaging in appropriate health behaviors, it is possible for people to considerably reduce the risk of getting heart disease, some cancers, or diabetes.

Some non-communicable diseases can be prevented at relatively low cost, but these diseases are often very expensive to treat. It is possible, for example, to significantly reduce the chances of getting lung cancer by making a modest investment in smoking cessation therapy and by quitting smoking. By contrast, the cost of treating lung cancer through drugs and surgery is considerably more.

This chapter will focus on non-communicable diseases. It will pay particular attention to cardiovascular disease, can-

---

TABLE 12-1 Key Terms and Definitions

Blood Glucose—Blood sugar, the main source of energy for the body.
Cancer—One of a large variety of diseases characterized by uncontrolled growth of cells.
Cardiovascular Disease—A disease of the heart or blood vessels.
Cholesterol—A fat-like substance that is made by the body and is found naturally in animal-based fods such as meat, fish, poultry, and eggs.
Diabetes—An illness caused by poor control by the body of blood sugar.
Hypertension—High blood pressure, with a reading of 140/90 or greater.
Ischemic Heart Disease—A disturbance of the heart function due to inadequate supply of oxygen to the heart muscle.
Stroke—Sudden loss of function of the brain due to clotting or hemorrhaging.

Source: The Author. Modified from: Global Cardiovascular Infobase Glossary. Available at: http://www.cvdinfobase.ca/cvdbook/En/Glossary.htm. Accessed 14, 2007; National Institutes of Health. Obesity, Physical Activity, and Weight-control Glossary. Available at: http://win.niddk.nih.gov/publications/glossary/AthruL.htm. Accessed April 14, 2007.

---

cer, diabetes, and mental disorders because of their important and growing contribution to the global burden of disease, including in low- and middle-income countries. Because of the importance of tobacco and alcohol as risk factors for non-communicable diseases, the chapter will also contain specific sections on these topics.

The chapter will first introduce you to definitions of selected health conditions. It will then examine the burden of non-communicable diseases and the risk factors for those diseases. Following that, it will comment on some of the most important costs and consequences of these diseases. It will then review what steps can be taken to address the burden of non-communicable diseases effectively and efficiently, and will discuss several examples of successful efforts to prevent and deal with non-communicable diseases. The chapter will conclude with comments on some of the future challenges that must be addressed if the burden of non-communicable diseases is to be reduced.

KEY DEFINITIONS

Communicable diseases are illnesses caused by an infectious agent that spread from a person or an animal to another person or animal. Non-communicable diseases are, in many respects, the opposite of communicable diseases. First, they can not be spread from person to person by an infectious agent, even if they might be associated with one. Second, they tend to last a long time. Third, they can be very disabling, can seriously impair the ability of people to engage in day to day activities, and they often lead to death if they are not treated appropriately.

The terms "chronic disease" and "degenerative disease" are often used interchangeably with non-communicable disease. In this book, however, we shall consistently use the term "non-communicable disease." The most recent studies of the burden of disease include the following under non-communicable diseases: malignant neoplasms (cancers); diabetes; endocrine disorders; neuropsychiatric disorders, such as mental disorders, epilepsy, and Alzheimer's disease; and sense organ disorders, such as hearing loss, glaucoma, or cataracts.

You are already familiar with most of the terms used in this chapter. However, a few key terms with which you may be less familiar are defined in Table 12-1.

THE BURDEN OF NON-COMMUNICABLE DISEASES

Cardiovascular Disease

Cardiovascular disease (CVD) caused 16.4 million deaths in 2001 and is now the leading cause of death in the world.[1]

CVD is the cause of about 30% of all deaths worldwide, and it is predicted that by 2020, more than half of all deaths worldwide will be associated with CVD.[1] As noted earlier, it is now the leading cause of death in low- and middle-income countries, as well as in richer countries. CVD is associated with about 30% of all deaths in high-income countries and about 28% of deaths in low- and middle-income countries.[1]

CVD is the largest cause of death in all regions, except in Sub-Saharan Africa. CVD is the cause of about 58% of all deaths in Europe and Central Asia and about 30% of all deaths in East Asia and the Pacific, but only about 10% of the total deaths in Sub-Saharan Africa.[1] CVD rates are higher in Eastern Europe than in Western Europe, although the rates of CVD are falling in some Eastern European countries. The highest rates of CVD are in the former Soviet Union, where they are contributing to declines in life expectancy.[1] The rate of prevalence of CVD tends to be higher in urban than in rural areas.

About 80% of the burden of CVD worldwide is due to three conditions: ischemic heart disease (IHD), stroke, and congestive heart failure.[1] In most regions, ischemic heart disease is the most important contributor to death due to all cardiovascular diseases. In the Middle East and North Africa, for example, three people die from IHD for every one who dies from stroke. Stroke, however, is the dominant contributor to deaths in both Sub-Saharan Africa and in China.[2] In India, CVD appears in people at younger ages more than in high-income countries. Whereas in high-income countries only about 22% of CVD deaths are in people under 70 years of age, in India, about 50% of the CVD deaths occur in people under 70.[3]

To help get a better understanding of the importance of CVD to the burden of disease, Table 12-2 shows the burden of deaths and DALYs worldwide and by regions that are associated with CVD, compared to some of the other leading causes of death and DALYs lost, including diabetes, cancer, TB, HIV, and malaria.

Diabetes

There are several types of diabetes. The two most common are called type I and type II diabetes. Type I diabetes is "a life-long condition in which the pancreas stops making insulin. Without insulin, the body is not able to use glucose (blood sugar) for energy. To treat the disease, a person must inject

TABLE 12-2 Death and DALYs from Leading Causes, by Region, 2001 as Percentage of Total Deaths and DALYs

Region	CVD	Diabetes	Cancer	TB	HIV	Malaria
East Asia & Pacific						
Deaths	31%	2%	16%	4%	1%	<1%
DALYs	15%	1%	9%	3%	<1%	<1%
Europe & Central Asia						
Deaths	58%	1%	15%	1%	<1%	0%
DALYs	33%	1%	10%	1%	1%	<1%
Latin America & the Caribbean						
Deaths	28%	5%	15%	1%	3%	<1%
DALYs	11%	3%	7%	1%	2%	<1%
Middle East & No. Africa						
Deaths	35%	2%	9%	1%	<1%	1%
DALYs	14%	1%	4%	1%	<1%	1%
South Asia						
Deaths	25%	1%	7%	4%	2%	<1%
DALYs	13%	1%	3%	3%	2%	1%
Sub-Saharan Africa						
Deaths	10%	1%	4%	3%	19%	10%
DALYs	4%	<1%	2%	2%	16%	10%

Source: Data with permission from The World Bank. Lopez AD, Mathers CD, Murray CJL. The burden of disease and mortality by condition: data, methods, and results for 2001. In: Lopez AD, Mathers CD, Ezzati M, Jamison DT, Murray CJL, eds. *Global Burden of Disease and Risk Factors.* New York: Oxford University Press; 2006:126–233.

insulin, follow a diet plan, exercise daily, and test blood sugar several times a day."[4] Type I diabetes usually begins before the age of 30. This type of diabetes was previously known as 'insulin-dependent diabetes mellitus' or 'juvenile diabetes.'[4] 'Type II diabetes was previously known as 'noninsulin-dependent diabetes mellitus' or 'adult-onset diabetes.' Type II diabetes is the most common form of diabetes mellitus, present in about 90–95% of all diabetics. People with type II diabetes produce insulin; however, they either do not make enough insulin or their bodies do not use the insulin they do make."[4] As will be examined further later, type I diabetes is genetic; type II is related to "lifestyle" issues, particularly obesity.

It is estimated that about 5.1% of adults aged 20 to 79 worldwide had diabetes in 2003.[5] The prevalence rate of diabetes among this group was generally higher in high-income countries than in low- and middle-income countries. It ranged from a low of 2.4% in Sub-Saharan Africa to a high of 7.6% in Europe and Central Asia.[5] Almost 200 million people worldwide suffered from diabetes in 2003.[5]

Diabetes has a number of important and costly complications. Among the most common are eye problems that can cause blindness, kidney problems, circulatory problems that can result in amputation of the lower extremities, stroke, and coronary heart disease. About two thirds of the people with diabetes have some disability, compared to less than one third of the people without diabetes.[6] For this reason, the DALYs lost from diabetes are far greater than would be suggested just by the prevalence of the disease. In fact, it is estimated that almost 20 million DALYs were lost to diabetes worldwide in 2001, which is similar, for example, to the DALYs lost for

measles; a little less than is lost due to maternal conditions; and about 50% less than are lost due to nutritional deficiencies. The prevalence of diabetes worldwide is increasing at a rapid rate, mostly associated with the rapid increase in the amount of obesity in the world.[7] Some students of global health now refer to diabetes as being an "epidemic." Table 12-3 shows the number of people with diabetes in 2000 and the number of people projected to have diabetes in 2030.

Type I diabetes appears to have an important genetic component. Studies have been done on other factors that might be linked with type I diabetes, but they are not conclusive. The risk factors for type II diabetes may also include a genetic component. However, they do include low birth weight and having been bottle-fed. The best studies of the risk factors associated with diabetes include obesity and weight gain, as well as physical inactivity.[8] In high-income countries, less-educated and lower-income individuals have higher rates of diabetes than better-educated and wealthier people.[9]

Cancer

There are many different types of cancers. Among the most important in terms of the burden of disease worldwide are cancers of the lung, colon, breast, prostate, liver, stomach, and cervix. There are many risk factors for cancer and they vary by type of cancer. Some cancers are associated with tobacco use, such as lung and esophageal cancers. Other cancers are associated with infectious agents. Liver cancer, for example, is associated with the hepatitis B virus, cervical cancer is associated with the human papillomavirus, and stomach cancer is

TABLE 12-3 Number of People with Diabetes, 2000, and Projected Number with Diabetes in 2030

Region	2000 Number of People with Diabetes	2030 Number of People with Diabetes	Percentage of Change in Number of People with Diabetes	Percentage of Change in Total Population
Established Market Economies	44,268	68,156	54	9
Former Socialist Economies	11,665	13,969	20	−14
India	31,705	79,441	151	40
China	20,757	42,321	104	16
Sub-Saharan Africa	7,146	18,645	161	97
Latin America & the Caribbean	13,307	32,959	148	40
Middle Eastern Crescent	20,051	52,794	163	67
World	171,228	366,212	114	37

Source: © 2004 American Diabetes Association for *Diabetes Care.* Vol. 27. 2004;1047–1053. Reprinted with permission..

associated with the bacteria *Helicobacter pylori*. Liver cancer is associated with schistosomiasis, a parasitic worm that is also called *bilharzia*, which infects more than 200 million people worldwide.[10] There are also numerous environmental and occupational carcinogens, such as asbestos, which was the cause of lung cancer in many roofing workers in the United States, for example.

In 2001, it was estimated that about seven million people worldwide died of cancer, with about five million of those in low- and middle-income countries.[11] At the same time, there were about 10 million new cases of cancer worldwide. The number of deaths caused by different types of cancers varies by region, as shown in Table 12-4, which indicates the first, second, and third leading causes of cancer deaths in each region.

It is clear from the table that lung and breast cancers are two of the five most common types of cancers in both developed and developing countries.

Generally, the higher the income of a country, the more likely it is that the leading forms of cancer deaths will be associated with tobacco use, environmental factors, diet, and lifestyle, whereas there will be a higher preponderance of cancers linked with infectious agents in low-income countries. In high-income countries, for example, lung cancer is the predominant cause of cancer deaths and colon and breast cancer are the next most common causes of cancer deaths. East Asia

and the Pacific is the only region in which stomach cancers, often linked with infection with *Helicobacter pylori*, are the most common cause of cancer deaths. As you can also see, the leading cause of cancer deaths in Sub-Saharan Africa is liver cancer, linked in many cases to infection with the hepatitis B virus. In South Asia, the leading cause of cancer deaths are oral cancers, often associated with the use of betel, a nut that is chewed by many people in the region.[12]

Mental Disorders

As noted earlier, one of the major categories of non-communicable diseases is neuropsychiatric disorders. This includes a number of neurological disorders, such as epilepsy. It also includes alcohol and drug abuse. Mental disorders are also included in this category. Together, neuropsychiatric disorders are very important to the burden of disease, causing about 10% of all DALYs lost in low- and middle-income countries in 2001.[13] Covering a wide range of neuropsychiatric disorders, however, is beyond the scope of this book. This part of the book, therefore, will only cover selected mental disorders.

Mental disorders have generally been given less attention in global health than they deserve when considering their contribution to the overall burden of disease. One reason for this is the extent to which health providers and global health actors have historically underestimated the burden

TABLE 12-4 Leading Causes of Cancer Deaths by Region, Number of Deaths in Thousands, 2001

Region	Cancer Type	Deaths	Cancer Type	Deaths	Cancer Type	Deaths
East Asia & Pacific	Stomach	442	Trachea, Bronchus & Lungs	387	Liver	373
Europe & Central Asia	Trachea, Bronchus & Lungs	165	Other Malignant Neoplasms	82	Stomach	101
Latin America & the Caribbean	Other Malignant Neoplasms	82	Stomach	57	Trachea, Bronchus & Lungs	55
Middle East & No. Africa	Other Malignant Neoplasms	26	Trachea, Bronchus & Lungs	20	Stomach	18
South Asia	Mouth & Oropharynx	140	Trachea, Bronchus & Lungs	129	Other Malignant Neoplasms	99
Sub-Saharan Africa	Other Malignant Neoplasms	55	Liver	46	Prostate	40
High Income Countries	Trachea, Bronchus & Lungs	456	Other Malignant Neoplasms	257	Colon & Rectal	257

Source: Data with permission from The World Bank. Lopez AD, Mathers CD, Murray CJL. The Burden of Disease and Mortality by Condition: Data, Methods, and Results for 2001. In: Lopez AD, Mathers CD, Ezzati M, Jamison DT, Murray CJL, eds. *Global Burden of Disease and Risk Factors.* New York: Oxford University Press; 2006:126-233.

of mental disorders. Recent work on the global burden of disease, however, indicates that four of the most common mental disorders contribute about 5% of the total DALYs lost in low- and middle-income countries, about equal to the burden of HIV/AIDS, diseases of vision and hearing, or ischemic heart disease.[14] Depression alone is estimated to be associated with 3.4% of the DALYs lost, which would make it the fourth most important burden[15] of any health condition globally.[16] One reason for this large burden is the large number of people who suffer mental disorders. Another, however, is that mental disorders start at relatively young ages, they go on for a long time, they are often not "cured," and they, therefore, produce large amounts of disability. There is also some mortality, largely from suicide, that is associated with mental disorders.

Four mental disorders contribute the largest share to the burden of mental disorders. These are unipolar depressive disorders, which will be referred to here as depression, schizophrenia, panic disorder, and bipolar affective disorder. These conditions are defined briefly in Table 12-5.

There is only limited data on the burden of mental disorders from low- and middle-income countries. Nonetheless, when assessing the burden of these four disorders per million people, it is clear that South Asia has the highest rate of depression among all regions. The rate of depression is fairly consistent across better-off regions, somewhat lower in East Asia and the Pacific, and only about half as high in Sub-Saharan Africa as in Europe and Central Asia.[15] The rates of

schizophrenia range from about 1600 DALYs per one million people in Europe and Central Asia to about 2100 DALYs per one million people in East Asia and the Pacific.[15] Bipolar disorder ranges from 1400 DALYs per million people in Europe and Central Asia to 1830 DALYs per million people in the Middle East and North Africa.[15] The range for panic disorders is very narrow, with all regions clustering in the range of 700 to 800 DALYs per million people.[15]

There appear to be both genetic and non-genetic risk factors for mental disorders. It is clear that women suffer from depression more than men, as noted earlier. Early childhood abuse, violence, and poverty may be important environmental risk factors for depression. However, there is still very little definitive evidence on the risk factors for schizophrenia, depression, bipolar disorder, or panic disorders.

Tobacco Use

Tobacco is such an important risk factor for cardiovascular disease and diabetes that it bears specific mention of its own. It is estimated that about five million deaths annually are associated with the use of tobacco, of which about half are in low-income countries.[17] It is also estimated that 1 in 5 males over 30 and 1 in 20 females over 30 who die worldwide, die of tobacco-related deaths.[18] Ultimately, one half to two thirds of those who smoke will die of causes related to tobacco.[17] In addition, half of all tobacco-related deaths occur among people aged 35 to 69.[17] The most common tobacco-related deaths are from CVD; diseases of the respiratory system, such as emphysema; and from cancers.

Most tobacco is used through smoking either cigarettes or *bidis*, which are hand-rolled cigarettes used largely in South Asia. It is estimated that about 1.1 billion people smoke worldwide.[19] The rate of prevalence of smoking for all adults varies from 18% in Sub-Saharan Africa to 35% in Europe and Central Asia. In all regions of the world, men smoke more than women do. This is most pronounced in low-income countries, in which a relatively small share of women smoke. Prevalence for men varies from 29% in Sub-Saharan Africa to 63% in East Asia and the Pacific. The rates for women vary from 5% in East Asia and the Pacific and the Middle East and North Africa to 24% in Latin America and the Caribbean.[17]

The extent to which people take up smoking varies not only by sex, but also by socioeconomic status and level of educational attainment. The higher the socioeconomic status and the higher the level of education, the less likely a person is to smoke. Most people who smoke start when they are teens. In addition, it is important to note that tobacco is physically addictive and once one starts to smoke, it is difficult to stop.[20]

TABLE 12-5 Key Mental Health Terms and Definitions

Bipolar Disorder—A serious mood disorder characterized by swings of mania and depression

Depression—A mental state characterized by feelings of sadness, loneliness, despair, low self-esteem, and self-reproach

Panic Disorders—An anxiety disorder characterized by attacks of acute intense anxiety

Schizophrenia—A mental illness, the main symptoms of which are hallucinations, delusions, and changes in outlook and personality

Source: Modified from Ohio Psychological Association Psychological Glossary. Available at: http://www.ohpsych.org/Public/glossary.htm. Accessed April 14, 2007; The Royal College of Psychiatrists. Diagnoses or conditions. Available at: http://www.rcpsych.ac.uk/mentalhealthinformation/definitions/diagnosesorconditions.aspx. Accessed April 14, 2007.

In some countries, the use of tobacco has been declining, such as Canada, Poland, Thailand, the United Kingdom, and the United States. However, usage is increasing among men in developing countries and among women in all regions. Unless steps are taken to stop the spread of tobacco use, we are likely to see continued growth in CVD and cancers related to smoking, many of which are avoidable.

Abuse of Alcohol

Although we may be familiar with the idea that "a glass of red wine a day is protective against heart disease," on balance alcohol is a major public health problem. About 4% of the global burden of disease, in fact, is attributable to alcohol, which is about the same amount as that related to tobacco and hypertension and somewhat more than is attributed to depression.[21]

High risk drinking is defined as drinking 20 grams or more per day of pure alcohol for a woman and 40 grams a day for a man.[22] This is equal to about one quarter of a bottle of wine for a woman and one half a bottle of wine for a man. High-risk drinking may also be defined to include the total amount that is consumed, the frequency with which it is consumed, and the extent to which one engages in binge drinking.

High-risk drinking has a negative effect on people's health in a number of ways. Among other things, it increases the risks for hypertension, liver damage, pancreatic damage, hormonal problems, and heart disease.[21] In addition, alcohol intoxication is associated with accidents, injuries, accidental death, and a variety of social problems, including the first sexual encounters of teens, unprotected sex, and intimate partner violence. It is also possible to become dependent on alcohol, with a number of negative psychological and physical consequences. Moreover, fetal alcohol syndrome is associated with low birth weight babies who are at risk of developmental disabilities.

The prevalence of high risk drinking varies by region. Men in Europe and Central Asia have the highest rates of high risk drinking: 21.4% between ages 45 to 59. People in the Middle East and North Africa have the lowest rates, which are reported to be very low. South Asia also has a very low prevalence of high risk drinking.[23] The prevalence rate of high risk drinking also varies by age, with fewer people engaging in high risk drinking after age 60 than at younger ages. In each region, high-risk drinking is higher among men than in women, except in South Asia.[23]

There is very little evidence about the determinants of high risk drinking, especially in low-income settings. Studies done in high-income countries suggest that lower socioeconomic status and lower educational attainment are risk factors for drinking to the level of intoxication.[24]

THE COSTS AND CONSEQUENCES OF NON-COMMUNICABLE DISEASES, TOBACCO USE, AND ALCOHOL ABUSE

The economic costs of non-communicable diseases are substantial and are growing, given the increasing burden of cardiovascular disease and diabetes. These costs include the direct costs of treating non-communicable diseases, which by their nature require many years of treatment. They also include indirect costs that result from lost productivity. These are also very substantial, given that non-communicable diseases often start at relatively younger ages, often cause substantial disability, and then persist for many years.

In addition, many actors in the global health arena previously carried out their work as if rich countries faced the burden and costs of non-communicable diseases and poor countries faced only the burden and costs of communicable diseases. However, in light of the increasing amount of non-communicable disease and injury and accidents in developing countries, it is clear that most low-income countries do not have the luxury of facing *either* communicable *or* non-communicable disease. Rather, even low-income countries now *simultaneously* face the burden and costs of communicable diseases, non-communicable diseases, and injuries. Some additional comments follow on the costs and consequences of non-communicable diseases.

Cardiovascular Disease

Only a small number of studies have been done on the direct and indirect costs of CVD in low- and middle-income countries. A study conducted in South Africa suggested that the direct costs of treating cardiovascular disease were about 25% of all healthcare expenditures, which was equal to between 2–3% of GDP in that country.[25] The indirect costs of cardiovascular disease on the economy are likely to be substantial, given the relatively low age at which such diseases affect people in many countries. South Africa is a middle-income country, with a section of the economy that is very advanced. We should, therefore, expect that the costs of cardiovascular disease in most low-income countries will be a lower share of GDP than it is in South Africa. However, we should also expect that the costs of addressing cardiovascular disease in low- and middle-income countries will increase as the burden of such diseases continues to grow in those countries.

Diabetes

It is estimated that the direct costs of treating diabetes vary between 2.5% and 15.0% of health expenditures in different countries, depending on the prevalence of disease and the extent and costs of treatment available.[5] Given the level of development of different regions, it is likely that the Latin America and the Caribbean region has the highest expenditure on diabetes per capita and Sub-Saharan Africa the lowest such expenditures.[5] The indirect costs of diabetes in low- and middle-income countries are probably substantial because many people in those countries are living with diabetes without proper treatment and therefore suffer from disability and loss of productivity. The direct and indirect costs of diabetes will continue to grow for some time in all regions as the number of people with diabetes increases, as noted earlier.

Mental Disorders

There are relatively few reliable data on the direct and indirect costs of mental disorders. In addition, the studies that have been done largely refer to developed countries. Nonetheless, they are indicative of the large and usually unappreciated costs of mental illness in all countries. A study done in the United States estimated that the direct and indirect costs of mental illness were equal to about 2.5% of GNP, and a similar study done in Europe estimated that the costs of mental illness there was between 3–4% of GNP.[26] Studies done in Canada, the United Kingdom, and the United States showed that about half of the total costs of mental illness were direct costs and about half were indirect costs. These indirect costs are so substantial for mental illness that one study done in the United States estimated that almost 60% of the productivity losses that come from illness, accidents, or injuries are linked with mental illness.[26] Studies done in the United States and the United Kingdom showed, in addition, that workers suffering from depression lost 40 to 45 days of work in a year as a result of their illness.[26]

Tobacco Use

Calculating the costs of smoking to an economy can be very complicated.[27] The simplest way to do so is to calculate gross costs, which includes all the costs that are associated with smoking-related diseases. Studies on the costs of smoking have largely focused on the costs of smoking in the developed world. These studies suggested that the gross costs of smoking to various economies in high-income countries range from 0.1–1.1% of GDP and that the costs to low- and middle-income countries might be just as high.[27] The prevalence rates of smoking are increasing among women everywhere and among men in low-income countries. We should expect, therefore, that the economic costs of smoking in those countries will increase for some time to come. In fact, it is estimated that 70 million people died of smoking-related causes between 1950 and 2000 but that, if present trends in tobacco use continue, an additional 150 million people will die of smoking-related causes between 2000 and 2025. Of course, the economic costs of this will be enormous. In addition, it is important to note that the economic burden of smoking in the future is likely to have a disproportionate impact on relatively poorer people, in relatively poorer countries, because they smoke at higher rates than do better-off people.[28]

Alcohol Abuse

For the economic costs of alcohol abuse, as for many other issues, there are relatively few data for low- and middle-income countries. Excessive alcohol use, as discussed earlier, is linked with health problems of the drinker. In addition, it is linked with violence and injuries caused by the drinker, such as when driving while intoxicated. When calculating the economic costs of excessive alcohol drinking, therefore, one has to take account of the costs of health care of the user and on others whose injuries or health condition were caused by the user. The indirect costs of excessive alcohol drinking will include the productivity losses not only of the drinker, but also of people hurt by the drinker because of excessive drinking. The limited studies that have been done on the costs of alcohol abuse can only be considered indicative because they did not follow any standard methodology. However, they all reveal substantial costs of alcohol abuse, as a share of GDP:

> Canada—1.1%
> France—1.4%
> Italy—5.6%
> New Zealand—4.0%
> South Africa—2.0%[29]

ADDRESSING THE BURDEN OF NON-COMMUNICABLE DISEASES

There are also relatively few data available about cost-effective investments to address the burden of non-communicable diseases, including tobacco and alcohol-related illness, in the developing world. However, there is an increasing amount of information about efforts to address these issues in developed countries. Although the circumstances in these high-income countries may be quite different from those in low- and middle-income countries, the efforts undertaken to date may provide some useful lessons for low- and middle-income countries as they seek to prevent the burden of non-communicable diseases from growing. In considering how to address non-communicable diseases, it is important to note that some interventions can be made at the level of the population, whereas others are based on personal contact with an individual. Since smoking tobacco and excessive alcohol drinking are such important risk factors for cancer, cardio-vascular disease, and diabetes, the following section starts with a discussion about measures that can be taken to reduce smoking and excessive alcohol consumption.[30]

Tobacco Use

Experiences in the developed world suggest a number of steps can be taken to reduce the use of tobacco. Almost all countries tax cigarettes; however, low- and middle-income countries tend to tax cigarettes at lower rates than do higher income countries. Public demand for cigarettes is sensitive to price, and the poorer the country, the more price increases will affect demand. Studies conducted in low- and middle-income countries indicate that a 10% increase in cigarette taxes can lead to an 8% reduction in the demand for cigarettes. Under these circumstances, taxing cigarettes would be an effective policy for reducing cigarette consumption.[31]

For countries where there is weak government enforcement of laws, it will be more difficult to enforce restrictions on smoking; however, an increasing number of countries are undertaking these measures. Studies suggest that countries that can enforce legal restrictions can reduce the number of cigarettes smoked between 5–25% and can reduce smoking uptake by about 25%.[31] The effectiveness of these actions is likely to be enhanced in settings in which there are also strong social norms against smoking.

There is also evidence from high-income countries that consumption of cigarettes can be reduced by about 6% through a total ban on cigarette advertising, which is another step that low- and middle-income countries might consider.[31] Countries should also provide the public with information about the negative effects of smoking tobacco. There is evidence from high-income countries that such efforts led to short run reduction in cigarette consumption of between 4–9% and long-run declines of 15–30%.[31]

High-income settings that have had the biggest impact on reducing tobacco consumption have undertaken comprehensive tobacco control programs that generally included efforts to prevent young people from starting smoking, encourage all smokers to quit smoking, reduce exposure to passive smoking, and eliminate disparities in smoking among different population groups by helping those most at risk to reduce tobacco consumption.[32] It remains critically important to stop people from taking up smoking. However, in order to reduce tobacco-related deaths in the near future, it is essential to reduce consumption among those already smoking. Preventing young people from taking up smoking will only have an impact on tobacco-related deaths in the more distant future.

Abuse of Alcohol

Despite the high burden of disease and economic costs that are related to excessive drinking of alcoholic beverages, very few countries have embarked on coherent efforts to reduce alcohol consumption. Those that have done so generally focused their attention on policy and legislative actions, such as taxation, laws on drunk driving, and restricting alcohol sales to selected places, times, and age limits. Controlled advertising and tightened law enforcement, such as through more widespread breath testing of drivers, have also been imposed. Another successful part of their program was to encourage counseling by healthcare providers through "brief interventions with individual high risk drivers."[33]

Just as is the case for cigarette taxation, increased taxation on alcohol will likely lead to a decrease in the purchase and consumption of alcohol. Whereas in the case of tobacco, increased taxation can lead to the smuggling of untaxed cigarettes, in the case of alcohol, increased taxation can lead to a rise in the consumption of illicit alcohol. This is an issue that countries must take into account in considering raising taxes on alcohol.

In selected high-income countries, studies suggest that reducing the number of hours when alcohol can be sold can lead to a 1.5–3% decrease in high risk drinking and to a 1.5–4% decrease in alcohol-related traffic deaths.[34] Government authorities have to assess the extent to which such measures could be implemented effectively, especially in low- and middle-income countries with weak governance, as well as the extent to which such measures might also drive people to seek illicit alcohol.

Bans on alcohol advertising can be put into effect, as discussed for tobacco; however, it appears that such bans have had relatively little effect on the consumption of alcohol.[35] In health care settings in a number of countries, efforts have been made to engage high-risk drinkers in brief but specific education and counseling about the risks of excessive drinking. Even when taking relapses into account, it appears that such counseling is effective in reducing excessive consumption by 14–18%, compared to no treatment at all.[35] Although this approach might be effective in middle-income countries, it is unlikely to be effective in many low-income countries, given the scarcity of effective health services, the lack of health providers, and the already excessive demands on their weak health systems.

High Blood Pressure, High Cholesterol, and Obesity

The majority of risk associated with cardiovascular disease relates to a combination of high blood pressure, high cholesterol, high body mass index, low intake of fruits and vegetables, physical inactivity, and tobacco and alcohol use. The single most important risk factor for type II diabetes is obesity. The following section comments on measures that can be taken to improve diet and to reduce obesity.

To reduce the burden of CVD and diabetes, healthy eating and maintaining a healthy weight is key. Generally, this requires eating more fruits and vegetables and decreasing the intake of salt and foods that are high in saturated fat and trans fats. It also entails limiting the intake of sugar and replacing refined grains with whole grains. People who are overweight generally need to consume fewer calories each day and need to become more active physically.[53]

The lack of regular physical activity, in fact, is associated, among other things, with CVD, stroke, type II diabetes, and colon and breast cancer. Urbanization, motorization, and television watching all reduce physical activity. Countries can use public policies to try to limit the role of automobiles, promote walking and biking, and design communities in ways that encourage healthy lifestyles. In Singapore and London, for example, taxes are levied on cars that enter the center of the city to reduce the use of vehicles and their attendant traffic and pollution. Many cities promote the use of bicycles and have bicycle lanes, as one can see in a number of European cities such as Amsterdam. Some communities in the United States, for example, have no sidewalks, little public transport, and services that are very spread out, all of which provide an incentive for people to use automobiles to get from place to place, rather than to walk or bicycle.[53]

One way to promote healthier diets is through population-based "health education." Large-scale education efforts of this type, often through the mass media, have had mixed results because it is difficult on a large scale to successfully promote the reduction of obesity.[36] Generally, mass programs are more effective when they are combined with direct communication with individuals.

Few efforts to undertake population-based education measures have been studied. However, a study on a project to reduce salt intake among men in one part of China found a reduction in both hypertension and obesity after 5 years. In another effort, the government of Mauritius encouraged the population to switch from cooking with palm oil, which is high in saturated fat, to soybean oil, which has less saturated fat. Over a 5-year period, the intake of saturated fat decreased and the total cholesterol levels of the population fell.[37] Regulations and legislation on labeling food products and the reduction of unhealthy ingredients in commercial food products can also contribute to reducing obesity.

Studies suggest that if large scale health education efforts are to succeed in changing what people eat, then it is important that such programs:

- have a realistic time frame that takes account of the time it takes to change deeply ingrained behaviors;
- be carried out by a respected organization and headed by a competent manager, with clear responsibility;
- encourage different organizations and agencies to work together to maximize the reach of the program and ensure that messages get disseminated in appropriate ways; and
- involve the food industry and enhance food labeling.[38]

Some countries, such as Brazil and Mexico, simultaneously face substantial burdens of underweight and overweight children and women. It may be politically and socially difficult for countries that face such a double burden to get the support they need to address problems of overweight, as many people believe that obesity is a problem that only affects wealthier people. There are few examples to date of best practices for addressing the two problems simultaneously.

Even as countries undertake the steps noted, they will still need to treat those who already have CVD, or who have some of the key risk factors for CVD, including hypertension. Most low- and some middle-income countries do not have the level of health system or the financial resources needed to carry out sophisticated medical procedures. In such settings, however, an important reduction in risks and in the burden of disease can be realized through preventive interventions such as getting people to take an aspirin a day and to get people with high cholesterol and hypertension to take inexpensive medicines to lower blood pressure and cholesterol.

Further Addressing Diabetes

There is no evidence that type I diabetes can be prevented; however, avoiding being overweight is the single most important way to avoid type II diabetes. Although large scale efforts to reduce obesity have generally not been very successful, a pilot project that used intensive personal counseling to promote weight loss through healthier eating and more physical activity was successfully carried out in China, Finland, Sweden, and the United States. The average weight loss after almost 3 years of participation in this study was about 10 pounds more than in the control group. In addition, the study group had a 58% lower rate of type II diabetes than the control group.[9]

Treatment for people with diabetes is needed in all countries. Treating people with type I diabetes with insulin is a cost-effective investment, although difficult to afford or manage in the poorest countries, especially for people living outside of the main cities. For all diabetics, it is cost-effective to control hypertension because the combination of the two diseases can produce major vascular complications. Diabetics are also subject to foot problems from circulation difficulties associated with their diabetes, and appropriate foot care is another cost-effective investment. The cost of not doing this can be ulcers and eventual amputation of the foot.[9] Those countries with greater resources and a health system that can deliver additional interventions can also consider other cost-effective measures for treating diabetes, including vaccination against influenza and pneumococcal infections, diagnosis and treatment of retinal problems associated with diabetes, and treating hypertension with ACE inhibitors to prevent kidney problems from getting worse.[9]

Cancer

Tobacco control is overwhelmingly the first priority for preventing cancer, as noted earlier. Countries can also try to reduce the burden of cancer by addressing infectious agents that are associated with cancers, such as hepatitis B, which is vaccine-preventable; *H. pylori*, which is treatable with antibiotics; and schistosomiasis, which is also treatable with drugs.[39] An increasing number of countries are adding the hepatitis B vaccine to their national immunization programs. This is especially important in countries where a relatively large share of the population carries hepatitis B. Many countries have schistosomiasis control programs, and some of the most successful efforts against schistosomiasis have been undertaken in Egypt and China. *H. pylori* is important in settings like Japan, China, or Colombia where there is a significant amount of stomach cancer linked with this bacteria. In these settings, it might be cost-effective to carry out a screening and treatment program for *H. pylori*.

Mental Disorders

Unfortunately, there are few public health measures that can prevent mental disorders. For the mental disorders that have been discussed, treatment through medication, combined with psychosocial support, is the best way to try to address these illnesses. Providing such treatment and psychosocial support, however, will be difficult in many low- and middle-income countries, given their weak health systems, a historic lack of attention to mental disorders, and a lack of staff at every level to address mental health in effective and efficient ways.

Given the important burden of disease associated with mental disorders, the World Health Organization recommends that countries take a number of steps to address mental health issues. These include:

- Having a mental health policy
- Ensuring there is a unit of government responsible for mental health
- Budgeting for mental health programs—including program development, training, drug procurement, and program monitoring
- Training primary healthcare workers in mental health
- Integrating mental health into the primary healthcare program[39]

In addition, a number of public health measures can be taken to address some of the factors that are associated with mental disorders. Reducing abuse of women and children can reduce the burden of mental illness among the abused. Curtailing bullying of students in schools can also be important. Improving parenting skills is helpful to the healthy development of children. Appropriate care and counseling for children and adults affected by war, conflict, and other complex emergencies can also reduce the risks of mental illness.

To the extent possible, treatments should be made available for the different mental disorders discussed in this chapter. Of the different treatments available, the most cost-effective include those for:

Schizophrenia—combining an older antipsychotic drug with psychosocial treatment

Bipolar disorder—providing an older mood stabilizing drug, plus psychosocial treatment

Depression—providing a newer antidepressant drug

Panic disorder—providing a newer antidepressant drug[40]

It is estimated that including the above in primary healthcare packages could cost between about $3 in Sub-Saharan Africa and $9 per capita in Latin America.[40] This represents a significant share of the current level of public health expenditure in the poorest countries of Sub-Saharan Africa and would be difficult to finance from their own resources. Other developing countries with more resources may be better able to provide needed treatments with their own funds.

Unfortunately, there is often an inadequate understanding of the importance of mental health, a lack of funds, a shortage of people who understand mental health issues, and stigma around mental disorders. As a result, there has been little progress in most low-income countries in addressing mental disorders.[41]

CASE STUDIES

Most efforts to try to reduce the burden of non-communicable diseases, alcohol abuse, and tobacco use have taken place in high-income countries. However, middle- and low-income countries are beginning to gather evidence about what works most effectively in preventing non-communicable diseases. The following section examines efforts to reduce tobacco use in Poland. It will be followed by a review of the cataract blindness control program in India. The last case study is about a program to integrate mental health into primary health care in Uganda.

The Challenge of Curbing Tobacco Use in Poland

Background

More than three quarters of the world's 1.2 billion smokers live in low- and middle-income countries, where smoking is on the rise.[42] In the late 1970s, Poland had the highest rate of smoking in the world, with the average Pole smoking 3500 cigarettes a year and nearly three quarters of Polish men smoking daily. The impact on the nation's health was staggering. In 1990, the probability of a 15-year-old boy in Poland reaching his 60th birthday was lower than in most countries, including China and India.[43] Lung cancer rates were among the highest in the world. But because tobacco production, run by the state, provided a significant source of revenue, the government did not fully disclose to the population the negative consequences of smoking. The fall of communism further exacerbated smoking because tobacco, the first industry to be privatized, was taken over by powerful multinational corporations who flooded the market with international brands, spent vast sums on advertising, and kept prices so low that cigarettes cost less than a loaf of bread.

The Intervention

As the tobacco epidemic escalated, Poland's scientific community laid the foundation of the anti-tobacco movement. Research in the 1980s by the Marie Sklodowska-Curie Memorial Cancer Centre and Institute of Oncology contributed to the first Polish report on smoking, highlighting the link between tobacco and the country's alarming rise in cancer. A series of international workshops and scientific conferences in Poland further strengthened these findings. Civil society was experiencing a renewal at the time, with the formation of anti-tobacco groups such as the Polish Anti-Tobacco Society that began to interact with international bodies, such as WHO and the International Union Against Cancer. In addition, the Health Promotion Foundation was established to lead public efforts on health issues and anti-tobacco education efforts.

With the fall of the Berlin Wall, the media became free to cover health topics and played an important role in dissemi-

nating information, raising awareness about the dangers of smoking, and shaping public opinion. When tobacco control legislation was introduced in 1991, a heated public debate ensued between health advocates and the powerful tobacco lobby, increasingly viewed by the public as a contest between David and Goliath. In 1995, groundbreaking legislation was finally passed, requiring sweeping measures such as large health warnings on cigarette packs and bans on smoking in enclosed workspaces and health centers, on electronic media advertising, and on tobacco sales to minors. A 30% increase in taxes levied on cigarettes was subsequently passed in 1999 and 2000, and advertising was completely banned. In parallel, the Health Promotion Foundation also launched extensive health education and consumer awareness efforts. These included an annual "Great Polish Smoke-Out" competition to encourage smokers to quit, with incentives like winning a week-long stay in Rome and a chance to meet the Polish-born Pope John Paul II. In a decade of smoke-outs, nearly 2.5 million smokers have quit smoking. Since the first smoke-out in 1991, more than 2.5 million poles have permanently snuffed out their cigarettes because of the campaign.

The Impact

Cigarette consumption dropped 10% between 1990 and 1998, and the number of smokers declined from 14 million in the 1980s to under 10 million by the end of the 1990s. The reduction in smoking led to 10,000 fewer deaths each year, a 30% decline in lung cancer among men aged 20 to 44, a nearly 7% decline in CVD, and a reduction in infant mortality and low birth weight.[44] Life expectancy in the 1990s increased by 4 years.

Lessons Learned

Poland's experience shows that once smoking is seen for what it is—the leading cause of preventable deaths among adults worldwide—then governments do act. Working in concert with civil society and using state-of-the-art communication strategies, the Polish government succeeded in countering the powerful economic influence of the tobacco industry and inducing major shifts in smoking, an addictive behavior that was also then an ingrained social norm. Poland's sweeping legislative measures came to serve as a model for other countries. The experience of South Africa provides an interesting parallel: once the African National Congress came to power in 1994, the antismoking movement gained a powerful ally in Nelson Mandela and his first health minister, ultimately leading to the passage of strict tobacco control legislation and dramatic price control measures that increased the real value of cigarette taxes by 215%. As a result, cigarette consumption fell by more than 30%, from 1.9 billion packs in 1991 to 1.3 billion packs in 2002. As a South African researcher noted, "You need the right combination of science, evidence, and politics to succeed. If you have one without the other, you don't see action."[45] For a more detailed discussion of these Polish efforts see *Case Studies in Global Health: Millions Saved.*

Cataract Blindness Control in India

This chapter has focused on a limited number of the leading causes of deaths and DALYs lost due to non-communicable diseases. This chapter, however, does not cover vision disorders, despite the large number of DALYs lost to them in low- and middle-income countries. As you would expect, there are few people who die of diseases related to vision disorders. However, the burden of disability of these diseases, especially in low- and middle-income countries in which they are not generally treated in a timely manner, is great. In fact, about 45 million people worldwide are blind and another 135 million people are visually impaired.[46] The total number of DALYs lost from cataracts alone in low- and middle-income countries is almost the same as those lost to nutritional deficiencies, is slightly more than those lost to maternal conditions, and is about 15% fewer than the amount lost to TB. It is also just under the number of DALYs lost to road traffic injuries.[47]

Background

About one quarter of the total number of people in the world who are blind live in India and the case study that follows deals with controlling cataract blindness there.[48] The blindness control program in India has been one of the most extensive such programs in low-income countries for many years. In addition, over the last decade, this program has emerged, in many respects, as a public health "success story." Those wishing to examine this case in greater detail can read further about it in *Case Studies in Global Health: Millions Saved.*

History

Cataracts are the leading cause of blindness in India. About 80% of all of the people in India who are blind are blind due to cataracts. In addition, there are another 10 million people in India who are visually impaired due to untreated cataracts.

In the simplest terms, a cataract is a clouding of the lens of the eye. It blurs the image on the retina, producing a visual effect that is like looking through a window that is frosted or fogged with steam. Cataracts form when protein clumps in the lens of the eye. This is associated with age, excessive exposure to sunlight, diabetes, undernutrition, and other risk factors. Cataracts can affect one or both eyes.

Cataracts are treatable through surgery. One form of surgery requires a large incision in the eye and the removal of the lens and lens capsule. This form of surgery (ICCE) is relatively easy to perform and relatively inexpensive; however, it requires that the patient wear thick eyeglasses after surgery, and it has a high rate of complications. Nonetheless, it has been the form of surgery traditionally done in low-income settings. The other form of surgery is more technically sophisticated (ECCE); however, it has a lower rate of complications when done by trained surgeons. In addition, recent research in India showed that those having ECCE surgery were 2.8 times more likely to have a good outcome than those having ICCE surgery.[49]

Intervention

India's response to the problem of blindness has been impressive in breadth and duration. India's first intervention in 1963 aimed specifically at controlling trachoma, a highly contagious eye infection. By the end of the decade, the government expanded its approach to include all visual impairment. In 1975, the Central Council of Health declared that "one of the basic human rights is the right to see. In 1976, India formed the National Program for the Control of Blindness (NPCB) to expand access to surgical treatment of vision disorders and to increase ophthalmologic services.

India's first international collaboration in eye care was with DANIDA, the Danish International Development Assistance Agency. Until 1989, DANIDA assisted India in funding the improvement and expansion of its cataract blindness control program through the provision of equipment, mobile units, training, and enhancements of monitoring and evaluation. The program focused then on mass ECCE surgeries in camps that were mostly set up in areas with limited health infrastructure. This demonstrated the ability of the government to lead mass screening and treatment camps, even in rural areas. It also generated enormous demand for cataract surgeries, even among the poor and rural. However, the limited amount of time a camp was stationed in a particular location, as well as the nature of field work, meant that post-surgical follow-up was difficult to implement. Consequently, although the efforts succeeded in reaching many people, only about 75% of those who got surgery returned to an acceptable level of vision.[50]

In 1994, building on its experience with DANIDA, the Government of India began to collaborate with the World Bank to finance a 7-year Cataract Blindness Control Project.

The project focused on seven Indian states that had the highest prevalence of blindness and, in simple terms, it meant to assist India in moving its cataract blindness control program from a focus on quantity to a focus on quality and outcomes. The aims of the program were to improve surgical outcomes by shifting from ICCE to ECCE, strengthen India's capacity to provide high quality surgery done by competently trained staff, and increase the coverage of the program to areas which had previously been underserved. Much greater attention was paid than before to monitoring the outcomes of surgery.

The program also focused on trying to achieve its aims through enhancing collaboration between the public and the private sectors. Some surgeries were done in public facilities. The government financed other surgeries that were conducted by the private and NGO sectors. In addition, NGOs such as Sight Savers International, Lions Clubs International, and Christoffel Blinden Mission also financially supported eye hospitals, training institutes, and the development of school vision-screening programs and outreach. The Aravind Eye Hospital in Madurai, India, was a world famous leader in eye care and became increasingly involved in training and other assistance to the NPCB.

Impact

Over 15 million cataract operations were performed in connection with the Cataract Blindness Control Project. In addition, ECCE surgeries increased as a share of the total surgeries from between 15–65% across different states in 1998–1999 to between 44–91% in 2001–2002.[50] Moreover, by 2001, 92% of surgeries occurred in fixed facilities where better outcomes can be expected. Most importantly, surgical outcomes have improved, with the introduction of improved procedures, well-equipped surgical procedures, and trained personnel. The ability to see at an acceptable level after surgery grew from 75% in 1994 to 82% from 1999 to 2002. The number and quality of surgeries was associated with a decrease in the prevalence of cataract blindness by 26%.

Cost Effectiveness

The World Bank-assisted intervention cost $136 million, with close to 90% coming from the Bank and the remainder from the government of India. When done correctly and in areas of high prevalence, cataract surgery is among the most highly cost-effective interventions.[51] ECCE surgery is estimated to cost about $60 per DALY averted in the South and East Asia regions. Through the combination of serving those most in need and their educational and awareness raising campaigns, NGOs operating under the project used their financial resources very effectively.

Lessons Learned

The efforts in India demonstrate the benefits of collaboration among different public and private sectors and international institutions. The government of India and its political commitment to the problem in the 1960s was a requirement for success, as it offered a "big push" to combating cataract blindness. In addition, even though the government's early efforts were not always at the level of quality desired, they provided a baseline for further studies of how the program could be improved and expanded in a higher quality manner. Finally, the involvement of the NGOs helped to bring innovative approaches to the project and continually encouraged the government to improve and maintain quality services.

Integrating Mental Health into Primary Care in Uganda

Mental disorders are neglected in most developing countries. They are difficult to diagnose and treat, they carry considerable stigma, and low-income countries often lack the skilled personnel and financial resources needed to address mental health issues. Uganda is one of the few low-income countries that has made an effort to tackle the important burden of mental disorders and the case study that follows describes this effort and some of the outcomes associated with Uganda's move to integrate mental health concerns into its primary healthcare program.

Background

In 1986, Uganda came out of a 5-year civil conflict that had been preceded by 8 years of government led by General Idi Amin, which were characterized by misrule and violence. Although the civil conflict was for the most part over in the southern parts of the country, the conflict continued in the north, with abduction of children and terrorizing of the communities carried out by the Lord's Resistance Army. At about the same time, Uganda was increasingly being impacted by the emerging HIV/AIDS epidemic.

According to the 1995 Uganda Burden of Disease study, over 75% of life years lost from premature deaths was the result of preventable communicable disorders.[47] However, it was also recognized that there was a simultaneous surge in the occurrence of non-communicable disorders, such as hypertension, diabetes, cancer, and mental disorders. It was also becoming clearer that HIV/AIDS and the prolonged armed conflict created an increased need for attention to be paid to mental health.

In order to address the increasing burden of mental disorders, the Ministry of Health decided to promote the integration of mental health into primary health care. This involved developing standards and guidelines for the management of eight priority mental disorders for the community, district, and national referral levels of care. This was part of Uganda's efforts to address health care in an effective and efficient manner through the establishment of a minimum healthcare package.

The Intervention

The process of integrating mental health into primary health care was to be implemented through training all healthcare workers to recognize and manage common mental disorders, as well as establishing and strengthening a referral and supportive supervision system. The initiative was outlined in the Uganda Health Sector Strategic Plan 1999 to 2004.[52]

Central level activities included the creation of a Mental Health Coordinating Committee whose main responsibilities were the development of standards and guidelines for the management of common mental disorders, developing materials for the training of health workers, and developing and participating in the referral and supervision system. Central level activities also included participation in the creation of a Core Team on Psychosocial Disorders, a group of representatives of two government sectors; the Ministry of Health and the Ministry of Gender, Labor, and Social Development, which was responsible for child protection; five NGOs working in the field of psychosocial disorders; and UNICEF.

The Core Team carried out an assessment of the psychosocial situation of the conflict-affected population in eight districts of northern Uganda, disseminated the results to the district leaders, and facilitated the affected districts in the development of psychosocial components to be included in District Development Plans. The Core Team developed indicators, as well as a monitoring and evaluation plan, that they then implemented. The Core Team was instrumental in the coordinated safe return and reintegration of abducted children into their communities.

As a result of having mental health in the Health Sector Policy and the Health Sector Strategic Plan, a budget line for mental health was created. Although the allocation to mental health from the Government of Uganda was only 0.7% of the total health budget, having mental health as a budget item made it easier for other funding agencies to support mental health efforts in Uganda.

The African Development Bank (AfDB) provided a loan to the Government for support in the integration of mental health into primary health care. This AfDB assisted project is to provide $17.73 million to mental health efforts in Uganda over a 5-year period. Activities include rehabilitation of Butabika National Referral Psychiatric Hospital, down-sizing it from a 900-bed to a 450-bed hospital, as well as the construction of 6 regional mental health units. The project includes provision of essential mental health medications and support to the training of healthcare workers at all levels of the care system, from training primary healthcare nurses in the recognition and management of common mental disorders, to the training of specialized personnel, such as psychiatrists, psychologists, and psychiatric social workers.[52]

Lessons Learned

It is often thought that mental health is not a priority in low-income countries, or that feasible mental health interventions are not available. This case study, however, demonstrates that mental disorders are of importance in low-income countries, especially those affected by disasters, complex emergencies, and HIV/AIDS. It also demonstrates that countries, even with few resources, can take measures to considerably improve mental health services.

This case study also suggests that it is possible to design and implement a strategy for dealing with mental disorders that builds on an existing healthcare system. As a result of the investments made, resources for mental health are better allocated in Uganda than before, and funds for mental health have moved from the large psychiatric institution to the regional levels, where services are more accessible to the populations that require them.

Nonetheless, there remain great challenges in trying to provide appropriate mental health services in Uganda. These include the need to strengthen information and public education so the population is aware of what constitutes mental disorders, as well as where help can be sought. A further challenge is likely to be sustainability of the established services. The AfDB project provides the infrastructure and the start-up costs; however, the Government of Uganda will have to ensure that recurrent costs for staff, maintenance of equipment and infrastructure, referral and supervision, and other inputs such as drugs are provided for in the long-term.

FUTURE CHALLENGES

The world must face a number of challenges if it is to reduce the burden of non-communicable diseases in low- and middle-income countries. First, the number of people with new cases of non-communicable diseases will grow in low- and middle-income countries as a result of lifestyle changes and the aging of the population. In addition, because non-communicable diseases are chronic, the number of people with these diseases will also rise. The increasing number of people who will be at risk of and living with chronic diseases in low- and middle-income countries will pose a huge challenge to the health of these countries, to their health systems, and to their national finances.

Related to this, a number of low-income countries will have to deal with the challenge of addressing increasing amounts of non-communicable disease simultaneously with having to address substantial burdens of communicable diseases. This will severely tax the managerial, technical, and financial capacity of many developing countries. It will also require greater attention by low-income countries to non-communicable diseases and to improved surveillance of these diseases, as well.

In addition, it will be important to spread as rapidly as possible to low-and middle-income countries the lessons that the high-income countries have already learned about how to address non-communicable diseases in cost-effective ways. This body of evidence, especially for low-cost interventions that have a high payback, needs to be disseminated in low- and middle-income countries as rapidly as possible. Ongoing mechanisms need to be established to ensure, as well, that cost-effective diagnostics and drugs continuously get disseminated as early as possible to low- and middle-income countries.

Having said this, however, it will also be important that low- and middle-income countries take the measures that are known to prevent non-communicable diseases as soon as they can. They should not wait to build the political consensus that they need to undertake a comprehensive approach to reducing tobacco smoking, for example. Nor do they need to wait to do the same for excessive alcohol consumption. Even in the face of undernutrition, a number of countries will need to promote healthier diets and more physical activity for people who are overweight. Some of the low-cost but effective treatments for cardiovascular disease, such as aspirin, can also be promoted.

MAIN MESSAGES

Non-communicable diseases now constitute the largest burden of disease worldwide. In all regions of the world, except Sub-Saharan Africa, the burden of these diseases is greater than the burden of communicable diseases. Cardiovascular disease is the single largest cause of death worldwide. Diabetes, some forms of cancer, and mental disorders are also major causes of disability and death from non-communicable

diseases. In fact, about 14% of the DALYs lost in 2001 were attributable to CVD, about 7% to cancer, 1.3% to diabetes, and about 5% to the four mental disorders discussed earlier.

The leading risk factors for cardiovascular disease are hypertension, obesity, high cholesterol, and tobacco use. A lack of physical activity contributes to CVD and obesity, and the main risk factor for diabetes is obesity. Some cancers are associated with an infectious agent, such as hepatitis B, *h.pylori*, or the human papilloma virus. Other cancers are linked with tobacco use. Little is known about the non-genetic risk factors that are associated with mental disorders.

The costs of non-communicable diseases and the use of tobacco and alcohol abuse are substantial. They have a considerable impact on people in their productive years of life. In addition, mental disorders and diabetes are associated with very large amounts of disability. The costs of trying to prevent the burden of non-communicable diseases include efforts to promote "healthier lifestyles," including a healthy diet and maintaining an appropriate weight and increasing physical activity, while trying to reduce obesity, cigarette consumption, and excessive drinking. The costs of treating non-communicable diseases can be high both because of the high cost of some medical treatments for specific episodes of illness, as well as the need to treat some diseases and conditions for many years. Mental disorders, for example, frequently start early in life and often continue throughout a life. Nonetheless, aspirin and some medicines used for hypertension, for example, are highly cost-effective at dealing with CVD, even in low- and middle-income settings.

The single most important step that countries can take to reduce the burden of non-communicable diseases is to reduce the consumption of tobacco. There is good evidence from high-income and some lower-income countries that taxing cigarettes more heavily, banning smoking from public places, and trying to educate the population about the impact of tobacco on health can all contribute to reducing tobacco consumption.

Reducing the burden of non-communicable diseases will also require that obesity be reduced through healthier diets, fewer calories, increased intake of fruits and green leafy vegetables, and more physical activity. Other measures to reduce obesity can be complemented with food labeling legislation and legislation to encourage the use of healthier ingredients in food products.

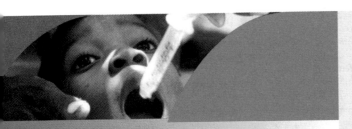

Study Questions

1. How important are non-communicable diseases to the global burden of disease?

2. Why are non-communicable diseases less important to that burden in Sub-Saharan Africa?

3. What are the leading risk factors for cardiovascular disease?

4. What are the most important cancers that affect low-income countries?

5. What are the most important risk factors for cancers?

6. What factors are causing the "epidemic" of diabetes that is occurring worldwide?

7. Why are mental disorders so important to the burden of disease if so few people die of them?

8. What measures have proven effective in reducing the use of tobacco?

9. What lessons of Uganda's approach to mental health concerns are important for other resource-poor countries?

10. What measures have been effective in reducing the abuse of alcohol?

REFERENCES

1. Lopez AD, Mathers CD, Murray CJL. The burden of disease and mortality by condition: data, methods, and results for 2001. In: Lopez AD, Mathers CD, Ezzati M, Jamison DT, Murray CJL, eds. *Global Burden of Disease and Risk Factors*. New York: Oxford University Press; 2006:45–240.

2. Gaziano TA., Srinath Reddy K, Paccaud F, Horton S, Chaturvedi V. Cardiovascular disease. In: Jamison DT, Breman JG, Measham AR, et al., eds. *Disease Control Priorities in Developing Countries*. 2nd ed. New York: Oxford University Press; 2006:649–650.

3. Gaziano TA., Srinath Reddy K, Paccaud F, Horton S, Chaturvedi V. Cardiovascular disease. In: Jamison DT, Breman JG, Measham AR, et al., eds. *Disease Control Priorities in Developing Countries*. 2nd ed. New York: Oxford University Press; 2006:650.

4. National Institutes of Health. Obesity, Physical Activity, and Weight-control Glossary. Available at: Available at: http://win.niddk.nih.gov/publications/glossary/MthruZ.htm. Accessed April 15, 2006.

5. International Diabetes Association. *Diabetes Atlas*. 2nd ed. Brussels: International Diabetes Federation; 2003.

6. Ryerson B, Tierney EF, Thompson TJ, et al. Excess physical limitations among adults with diabetes in the U.S. population, 1997–1999. *Diabetes Care*. 2003;26(1):206–210.

7. Mathers C, Stein C, Fat CMF, et al. *Global Burden of Disease 2000: Version 2 Methods and Results*. Geneva: World Health Organization; 2000.

8. Haffner SM. Epidemiology of type 2 diabetes: risk factors. *Diabetes Care*. 1998;21 Suppl 3:C3–6.

9. Venkat Narayan K, Zhang P, Kanaya AM, et al. Diabetes: the pandemic and potential solutions. In: Jamison DT, Breman JG, Measham AR, et al., eds. *Disease Control Priorities in Developing Countries*. 2nd ed. New York: Oxford University Press; 2006:645–662.

10. Centers for Disease Control and Prevention. Fact Sheet—Schistosomiasis. Available at: http://www.cdc.gov/ncidod/dpd/parasites/schistosomiasis/default.htm. Accessed April 20, 2006.

11. Jamison DT, Breman JG, Measham AR, et al., eds. *Priorities in Health*. Washington, DC: The World Bank; 2006.

12. Lopez AD, Mathers CD, Murray CJL. The burden of disease and mortality by condition: data, methods, and results for 2001. In: Lopez AD, Mathers CD, Ezzati M, Jamison DT, Murray CJL, eds. *Global Burden of Disease and Risk Factors*. New York: Oxford University Press; 2006:158.

13. Lopez AD, Mathers CD, Murray CJL. The burden of disease and mortality by condition: data, methods, and results for 2001. In: Lopez AD, Mathers CD, Ezzati M, Jamison DT, Murray CJL, eds. *Global Burden of Disease and Risk Factors*. New York: Oxford University Press; 2006:128.

14. Lopez AD, Mathers CD, Murray CJL. The burden of disease and mortality by condition: data, methods, and results for 2001. In: Lopez AD, Mathers CD, Ezzati M, Jamison DT, Murray CJL, eds. *Global Burden of Disease and Risk Factors*. New York: Oxford University Press; 2006:230.

15. Hyman S, Chisholm D, Kessler R, Patel V, Whiteford H. Mental disorders. In: Jamison DT, Breman JG, Measham AR, et al., eds. *Disease Control Priorities in Developing Countries*. 2nd ed. New York: Oxford University Press; 2006:605–625.

16. Lopez AD, Mathers CD, Murray CJL. The burden of disease and mortality by condition: data, methods, and results for 2001. In: Lopez AD, Mathers CD, Ezzati M, Jamison DT, Murray CJL, eds. *Global Burden of Disease and Risk Factors*. New York: Oxford University Press; 2006:228–233.

17. Jha P, Chaloupka FJ, Moore J, et al. Tobacco addiction. In: Jamison DT, Breman JG, Measham AR, et al., eds. *Disease Control Priorities in Developing Countries*. 2nd ed. New York: Oxford University Press; 2006:870.

18. Jha P, Chaloupka FJ, Moore J, et al. Tobacco addiction. In: Jamison DT, Breman JG, Measham AR, et al., eds. *Disease Control Priorities in Developing Countries*. 2nd ed. New York: Oxford University Press; 2006:869.

19. Jamison DT, Breman JG, Measham AR, et al., eds. *Priorities in Health*. Washington, DC: The World Bank; 2006.

20. Jamison DT, Breman JG, Measham AR, et al., eds. *Priorities in Health*. Washington, DC: The World Bank; 2006.

21. Rehm J, Chisholm D, Room R, Lopez AD. Alcohol. In: Jamison DT, Breman JG, Measham AR, et al., eds. *Disease Control Priorities in Developing Countries*. 2nd ed. New York: Oxford University Press; 2006:887.

22. Rehm J, Chisholm D, Room R, Lopez AD. Alcohol. In: Jamison DT, Breman JG, Measham AR, et al., eds. *Disease Control Priorities in Developing Countries*. 2nd ed. New York: Oxford University Press; 2006:888.

23. Rehm J, Chisholm D, Room R, Lopez AD. Alcohol. In: Jamison DT, Breman JG, Measham AR, et al., eds. *Disease Control Priorities in Developing Countries*. 2nd ed. New York: Oxford University Press; 2006:889.

24. Rehm J, Chisholm D, Room R, Lopez AD. Alcohol. In: Jamison DT, Breman JG, Measham AR, et al., eds. *Disease Control Priorities in Developing Countries*. 2nd ed. New York: Oxford University Press; 2006:890.

25. Rodgers A, Lawes CM, Gaziano TA, Vos T. The growing burden of risk from high blood pressure, cholesterol, and bodyweight. In: Jamison DT, Breman JG, Measham AR, et al., eds. *Disease Control Priorities in Developing Countries*. 2nd ed. New York: Oxford University Press; 2006:854.

26. World Health Organization. *Investing in Mental Health*. Geneva: World Health Organization; 2003.

27. Lightwoood J, Collins D, Lapsley H, Novotny TE. Estimating the costs of tobacco use. In: Jha P, Chaloupka FJ, eds. *Tobacco Control in Developing Countries*. London: Oxford University Press; 2000:107–153.

28. Chaloupka FJ, Tauras JA, Grossman M. The economics of addiction. In: Jha P, Chaloupka FJ, eds. *Tobacco Control in Developing Countries*. London: Oxford University Press; 2000:107–153.

29. World Health Organization. *Global Status Report on Alcohol 2004*. Geneva: World Health Organization; 2004.

30. Jha P, Chaloupka FJ, Moore J, et al. Tobacco addiction. In: Jamison DT, Breman JG, Measham AR, et al., eds. *Disease Control Priorities in Developing Countries*. 2nd ed. New York: Oxford University Press; 2006:869–885.

31. Jha P, Chaloupka FJ, Moore J, et al. Tobacco addiction. In: Jamison DT, Breman JG, Measham AR, et al., eds. *Disease Control Priorities in Developing Countries*. 2nd ed. New York: Oxford University Press; 2006:876.

32. Jha P, Chaloupka FJ, Moore J, et al. Tobacco addiction. In: Jamison DT, Breman JG, Measham AR, et al., eds. *Disease Control Priorities in Developing Countries*. 2nd ed. New York: Oxford University Press; 2006:881.

33. Jha P, Chaloupka FJ, Moore J, et al. Tobacco addiction. In: Jamison DT, Breman JG, Measham AR, et al., eds. *Disease Control Priorities in Developing Countries*. 2nd ed. New York: Oxford University Press; 2006:893.

34. Rehm J, Chisholm D, Room R, Lopez AD. Alcohol. In: Jamison DT, Breman JG, Measham AR, et al., eds. *Disease Control Priorities in Developing Countries*. 2nd ed. New York: Oxford University Press; 2006:887–906.

35. Rehm J, Chisholm D, Room R, Lopez AD. Alcohol. In: Jamison DT, Breman JG, Measham AR, et al., eds. *Disease Control Priorities in Developing Countries*. 2nd ed. New York: Oxford University Press; 2006:894.

36. Rodgers A, Lawes CM, Gaziano TA, Vos T. The growing burden of risk from high blood pressure, cholesterol, and bodyweight. In: Jamison DT, Breman JG, Measham AR, et al., eds. *Disease Control Priorities in Developing Countries*. 2nd ed. New York: Oxford University Press; 2006:863.

37. Rodgers A, Lawes CM, Gaziano TA, Vos T. The growing burden of risk from high blood pressure, cholesterol, and bodyweight. In: Jamison DT, Breman JG, Measham AR, et al., eds. *Disease Control Priorities in Developing Countries*. 2nd ed. New York: Oxford University Press; 2006:856.

38. Rodgers A, Lawes CM, Gaziano TA, Vos T. The growing burden of risk from high blood pressure, cholesterol, and bodyweight. In: Jamison DT, Breman JG, Measham AR, et al., eds. *Disease Control Priorities in Developing Countries*. 2nd ed. New York: Oxford University Press; 2006:855–856.

39. World Health Organization. *Policies and Managerial Guidelines*. Geneva: National Cancer Control Programme; 2002.

40. Hyman S, Chisholm D, Kessler R, Patel V, Whiteford H. Mental disorders. In: Jamison DT, Breman JG, Measham AR, et al., eds. *Disease Control Priorities in Developing Countries*. 2nd ed. New York: Oxford University Press; 2006:621–622.

41. Hyman S, Chisholm D, Kessler R, Patel V, Whiteford H. Mental disorders. In: Jamison DT, Breman JG, Measham AR, et al., eds. *Disease Control*

Priorities in Developing Countries. 2nd ed. New York: Oxford University Press; 2006:620.

42. Jha P, Chaloupka FJ. The economics of global tobacco control. *BMJ*. 2000;321(7257):358–361.

43. Witold Z. *Evolution of Health in Poland Since 1988*. Warsaw: Marie Sklodowska-Curie Memorial Cancer Center and Institute of Oncology, Department of Epidemiology and Cancer Prevention; 1998.

44. Zatonski W. Democracy and health: tobacco control in Poland. In: de Beyer J, Brigden LW, eds. *Tobacco Control Policy, Strategies, Successes and Setbacks*. Washington, DC: The World Bank and International Development Research Center; 2003:97–119.

45. Malan M, Leaver R. Political Change in South Africa: New Tobacco Control and Public Health Policies. In: deBeyer J, Waverly Brigden LW, eds. *Tobacco Control Policy: Strategy, Success, and Setbacks*. Washington, DC: The World Bank and International Development Research Center; 2003.

46. World Health Organization. *Global Initiative for the Prevention of Avoidable Blindness*. Geneva: World Health Organization; 1997. WHO/PBL/97.61.

47. Lopez AD, Mathers CD, Murray CJL. The burden of disease and mortality by condition: data, methods, and results for 2001. In: Lopez AD, Mathers CD, Ezzati M, Jamison DT, Murray CJL, eds. *Global Burden of Disease and Risk Factors*. New York: Oxford University Press and The World Bank; 2006:180–185.

48. Thomas R, Paul P, Rao GN, Muliyil J, Matahai A. Present status of eye care in India. *Surv Ophthalmol* 2005;50(1):85–101.

49. Bachani D, Gupta GK, Murthy G, Jose R. Visual outcomes after cataract surgery and cataract surgical coverage in India. *Int Ophthamol.* 1999;23(1):49–56.

50. The World Bank. *Cataract Blindness Control Project Implementation Completion Report*. Washington, DC: The World Bank; 2002.

51. Javitt J, Venkataswamy G, Sommer A. The economic and social aspect of restoring sight. In: Henkind P, ed. *ACTA: 24th International Congress of Ophthalmology*. New York: JP Lippincott; 1983:1308–1312.

52. Government of Uganda. *Uganda Health Sector Strategic Plan 1999–2004*: Uganda: Government of Uganda; 1999.

53. Willett WC, Koplan JP, Nugent R, Dusenbury C, Puska P, Gaziano TA. Prevention of Chronic Disease by Means of Diet and Lifestyle Changes. In: Jamison DT, Breman JG, Measham AR, et al., eds. *Disease Control Priorities in Developing Countries*. 2nd ed. New York: Oxford University Press; 2006:833-850.

CHAPTER 13

Unintentional Injuries

LEARNING OBJECTIVES

By the end of this chapter the reader will be able to:

- Define the most important types of unintentional injuries
- Describe the burden of disease related to those injuries
- Discuss how that burden varies by age, sex, region, and type of injury
- Outline the costs and consequences of those injuries
- Review measures that can be taken to address key injury issues in cost-effective ways
- Describe some successful cases of preventing unintentional injuries

VIGNETTES

Juan was 25 years old. He was driving his fifteen-year-old car from Lima, Peru, to a small town in the mountains, where he planned to visit his grandmother. Juan had received only a small amount of driver training. His car was very old, had never been inspected for safety, and had worn tires and poor brakes. The road was very mountainous, did not have good lane markings or signs, and had few safety barriers. As the sun was setting, another car came rapidly around a mountain bend, headed right toward Juan's car. Juan tried to avoid the car but in doing so went off the road. His car slid down the side of the mountain and Juan was killed in the crash.

Mary was 12 years old and lived in a farming community in northern Tanzania. People in her village used fertilizer and pesticide in their agricultural work. They cooked with kerosene stoves. One day, after coming home from school, Mary was thirsty and saw some of her favorite soft drink near the area in which her mother cooked. Mary reached for the drink and began to consume it quickly. As she did so, she realized that her mother was storing in the soft drink bottle the kerosene that she used for cooking. Mary lived far from health services, got very sick that evening, and died of kerosene poisoning before she could get proper medical treatment.

Paitoon was a 70-year-old physician in Bangkok, Thailand. He was still practicing medicine, but was becoming more frail every month. He fancied himself to be a young man and enjoyed fixing things around his house and his office. While standing on a stool in his office one day to repair a broken light, Paitoon fell. Like many people his age who suffer falls, Paitoon broke his hip. Paitoon was hospitalized, had surgery, and could not attend to his patients for several months while he recovered.

Shahnaz was a 26-year-old woman in Lahore, Pakistan. Like almost all lower-income woman in Pakistan, Shahnaz spent much of the day doing chores around the house. She lived in a very small house with a tiny cooking area. While preparing dinner one evening, the sleeve of Shahnaz's outfit dipped into the cooking fire. Before her family could help her, all of Shahnaz's clothing was engulfed in flames. Shahnaz died the next day from burns.

THE IMPORTANCE OF UNINTENTIONAL INJURIES

Unintentional injuries are among the single leading causes of death and DALYs lost worldwide. In 2001, about 3.5 million people died of unintentional injuries.[1] This is about the same number of people who died of respiratory infections worldwide. It was more than the number of people who died of HIV/AIDS, diarrheal diseases, and vaccine preventable diseases of children. It was also more than the number of people who died of maternal and perinatal conditions combined.[2] In addition, unintentional injuries often lead to disability. Thus, while they represent about 6% of all deaths worldwide,[2] they represent almost 8% of the DALYs lost.[3] Although unintentional injuries are often neglected in global health work, they are, in fact, exceptionally important.

This chapter is about unintentional injuries. It first reviews definitions that are commonly used when discussing unintentional injuries. The chapter then reviews the global burden of disease from these injuries and how that burden varies by type of injury, sex, age, and region of the world. After that, the chapter examines the costs and consequences of unintentional injuries. The chapter concludes by examining measures that can be taken to reduce the burden of unintentional injuries and by reviewing some cases of successful injury prevention efforts.

KEY DEFINITIONS

As we begin this chapter, it is important to define the focus of our attention. For the purposes of this chapter, we can define an "injury" as:

> the result of an act that damages, harms, or hurts; unintentional or intentional damage to the body resulting from acute exposure to thermal, mechanical, electrical, or chemical energy or from the absence of such essentials as heat or oxygen.[4]

Some injuries, such as being shot by someone trying to do you harm, are intentional injuries. Unintentional injuries are "that subset of injuries for which there is no evidence of predetermined intent."[5]

Chapter 14 deals with humanitarian emergencies and civil conflict, but it also will discuss briefly some issues related to intentional injury. This chapter, however, will deal only with unintentional injuries, other than occupational injuries.

In focusing on unintentional injuries, this chapter will deal with:

- road traffic accidents
- poisonings
- falls
- fires
- drownings

Since the chapter focuses on the unintentional injuries noted above, it will use the term "injury" to refer to these injuries for the sake of simplicity. Any references to "intentional injuries" will be specified.

THE BURDEN OF UNINTENTIONAL INJURIES

About 3.5 million people died in 2001 of unintentional injuries worldwide, which was about 6% of all deaths in the world that year. In terms of DALYs lost, unintentional injuries that year were almost 8% of the total.[5] Table 13-1 shows the share of deaths globally that can be attributed to unintentional injuries and how that compares with deaths from a number of other causes.

Although injuries have most commonly been thought of as a problem of the developed world, more than 90% of deaths from unintentional injuries in 2001 were in low- and middle-income countries.[6,7] This is another reminder that low- and middle-income countries simultaneously face the multiple burdens of communicable diseases, non-communicable diseases, and injuries.

TABLE 13-1 Deaths from Unintentional Injuries, 2001, Compared to Total Deaths from Group I and Group II Diseases

Region	Group I Deaths (% of all deaths)	Group II Deaths (% of all deaths)	Unintentional Injuries (% of all deaths)
East Asia & Pacific	19%	71%	7%
Europe & Central Asia	6%	84%	7%
Latin America & the Caribbean	22%	67%	6%
Middle East & No. Africa	24%	65%	9%
South Asia Region	43%	47%	7%
Sub-Saharan Africa	71%	21%	5%

Source: Data with permission from The World Bank. Lopez AD, Mathers CD, Murray CJL. The burden of disease and mortality by condition: data, methods, and results for 2001. In: Lopez AD, Mathers CD, Ezzati M, Jamison DT, Murray CJL, eds. *Global Burden of Disease and Risk Factors.* New York: Oxford University Press; 2006:132–167.

TABLE 13-2 Percentage Distribution of Deaths and DALYs from Unintentional Injuries, Low- and Middle-Income Countries, 2001 (in Thousands)

	% of Total Deaths from Unintentional Injuries	% of Total DALYs from Unintentional Injuries
Road Traffic Accidents	33%	28%
Poisonings	10%	6%
Falls	10%	12%
Fires	9%	9%
Drownings	11%	8%
Other Unintentional Injuries	26%	36%

Source: Adapted with permission from The World Bank. Lopez AD, Mathers CD, Murray CJL. The Burden of Disease and Mortality by Condition: Data, Methods, and Results for 2001. In: Lopez AD, Mathers CD, Ezzati M, Jamison DT, Murray CJL, eds. *Global Burden of Disease and Risk Factors.* New York: Oxford University Press; 2006:128-184.

The leading cause of deaths from unintentional injuries in 2001 that were categorized were road traffic injuries. This was followed by drowning, poisonings, falls, and fires. The leading cause of DALYs lost from unintentional injuries was road traffic injuries. This was followed by falls, fires, drownings, and poisonings. The difference in order between deaths and DALYs largely reflects the disability associated with fires and falls.[8] Table 13-2 portrays the percentage distribution for deaths and DALYs of the main categories of unintentional injuries.

The percent of deaths from unintentional injuries in low- and middle-income countries in 2001 was 2.2%—twice as high as that in high-income countries. The rate of deaths from unintentional injuries in the low- and middle-income countries was six times that in high-income countries. Males more commonly suffer from unintentional injuries than females, and about twothirds of the deaths from unintentional injuries were among males.[5] In low- and middle-income countries, men were more likely to die than women of all six categories of unintentional injuries, except fires, as shown in Table 13-3.

Men were also almost three times as likely as women to die in road traffic accidents. They were almost twice as likely to die as women in all other categories of unintentional injury, except fires, for which women were almost twice as likely to die as men.[8]

When the leading causes of death globally are examined by age, we note that only HIV/AIDS kills more men aged 30–44 than are killed by unintentional injuries. Only cancer and cardiovascular disease kill more women every year than die from unintentional injury. Table 13-4 gives a breakdown of deaths from unintentional injuries for men compared to women.

Deaths are only part of the injury story. Although the number of deaths is significant, the number of people who suffer disability annually from an injury is much greater than those who actually die from an injury. As an example, a study of fatal and non-fatal injuries in two states in the United States reported 13,052 deaths from injury but also identified over 2 million injuries for which medical care was sought over the course of the study.[9] In other words, for every person who died from an injury there were approximately 153 people who were injured seriously enough to seek the help of a health professional. Moreover, this figure does not

TABLE 13-3 Death Rates from Unintentional Injuries per 100,000 for Males and Females, Low- and Middle-Income Countries, 2001

	Males	Females
All Unintentional Injuries	75	41
Road Traffic Accidents	28	11
Poisonings	7	4
Falls	8	5
Fires	4	6
Drowning	9	4
Other Unintentional Injuries	19	11

Source: Adapted with permission from The World Bank. Norton R, Hyder AA, Bishai D, Peden M. Unintentional injuries. In: Jamison DT, Breman JG, Measham AR, et al., eds. *Disease Control Priorities in Developing Countries.* 2nd ed. New York: Oxford University Press; 2006:738.

TABLE 13-4 Distribution of Deaths from Unintentional Injuries, Males and Females in Low- and Middle-Income Countries, 2001 (in Thousands)

	Total Deaths from Unintentional Injuries	
	Males	Females
Road Traffic Accidents	781	288
Poisonings	211	117
Falls	199	117
Fires	113	187
Drownings	252	116
Other Unintentional Injuries	539	293

Source: Adapted with permission from The World Bank. Lopez AD, Mathers CD, Murray CJL. The burden of disease and mortality by condition: data, methods, and results for 2001. In: Lopez AD, Mathers CD, Ezzati M, Jamison DT, Murray CJL, eds. *Global Burden of Disease and Risk Factors.* New York: Oxford University Press; 2006:130–131.

include those injuries for which people did not seek medical help, whether due to the minor nature of the problem, lack of access to care, or other unknown reasons.

It is apparent that when disability due to injuries is taken into consideration, as well as mortality, the scope of the problem presented by such injuries is magnified. Moreover, these figures likely underestimate the total impact of injuries around the world. The true burden is likely to be much higher than that based on simple reporting of injuries within the developing world. Indeed, some authorities have questioned the reliability of disability data from lower-income settings where mechanisms to accurately collect and report injury data are lacking and where many injured persons do not seek or do not have access to medical care.[10–12]

When we examine data for unintentional injuries by region, we see some variation. Deaths for unintentional injuries as a share of total deaths in Sub-Saharan Africa are relatively lower than in any other region, probably a reflection of the very high burden of communicable diseases in Sub-Saharan Africa. The share of deaths due to unintentional injuries in the Middle East and North Africa region is much higher than in any other region, largely a reflection of the high rates of motor vehicle deaths in this region. Table 13-5 shows the share of total deaths by region that is composed of unintentional injuries.

Table 13-6 reflects the percentage of total deaths by region that is caused by road traffic accidents.

There is considerable variation in the contribution of road traffic accidents to total deaths in different regions. The lowest rate is in the Europe and Central Asia Region, as anticipated. This largely reflects better-trained drivers, better engineered and maintained roads, and safer cars than in other regions. The highest rate of deaths for unintentional injuries that are caused by road traffic accidents is in the Middle East and North Africa regions. This probably reflects the extensive use of motor vehicles in this region without sufficient attention to driver education, engineering of roads, automobile safety, or emergency medical services.

CHILDHOOD INJURY

Discussion thus far has centered primarily on older adolescents and adults. However, children throughout the world sustain an alarming number of injuries with high levels of attendant death and disability. Moreover, estimates place 98% of childhood injury deaths in the low- and middle-income countries.[11]

Deaths from unintentional injuries for children aged 0–4 in low- and middle-income countries in 2000 were about 2.7% of total deaths. For those 5–14 years of age, these deaths were 3.5% of total deaths. With regard to specific injuries, children younger than five years account for 25% of drowning deaths and 15% of fire-related deaths globally.[7] To cast a slightly different perspective on these figures and the disproportionate occurrence of injuries in the young, children age 0–14 years comprise about 30% of the population but account for 50% of total injury-related DALYs.[11,13]

RISK FACTORS FOR UNINTENTIONAL INJURIES

Numerous reasons are thought to underlie the high prevalence of injuries in young children in the developing world. A partial list of factors includes developmental immaturity relative to the dangers these children face within their environments, the influence of poverty on families' ability to provide adult supervision and child care, and exposure to workplaces with unsafe, hazardous, and developmentally inappropriate machinery.[14–16] In support of this last point, a study in the Philippines found that 60% of working children were exposed to unsafe conditions, and 40% of these had suffered a serious workplace injury.[17]

It might be assumed that as children grow older, they become less susceptible to injury. However, the reality is that as children grow older and better able to maneuver in their environment, the incidence of injuries does not decrease. More developmentally mature young persons tend to roam more widely within their environments and thus encounter more risks and complex situations, which challenge

TABLE 13-5 Percentage of Total Deaths from Unintentional Injuries, by Region, for Low- and Middle-Income Countries, 2001

Region	Percentage of Total Deaths from Unintentional Injuries
East Asia & Pacific	7%
Europe & Central Asia	7%
Latin America & the Caribbean	6%
Middle East & No. Africa	9%
South Asia	7%
Sub-Saharan Africa	5%

Source: Adapted with permission from The World Bank. Lopez AD, Mathers CD, Murray CJL. The burden of disease and mortality by condition: data, methods, and results for 2001. In: Lopez AD, Mathers CD, Ezzati M, Jamison DT, Murray CJL, eds. *Global Burden of Disease and Risk Factors.* New York: Oxford University Press; 2006:126-127.

TABLE 13-6 Percentage of Total Deaths from Road Traffic Accidents, by Region, Low- and Middle- Income Countries, 2001

Region	Percentage of Total Deaths from Road Traffic Accidents
East Asia & Pacific	3%
Europe & Central Asia	1%
Latin America & the Caribbean	3%
Middle East & No. Africa	5%
South Asia	2%
Sub-Saharan Africa	2%

Source: Adapted with permission from The World Bank. Lopez AD, Mathers CD, Murray CJL. The burden of disease and mortality by condition: data, methods, and results for 2001. In: Lopez AD, Mathers CD, Ezzati M, Jamison DT, Murray CJL, eds. *Global Burden of Disease and Risk Factors.* New York: Oxford University Press; 2006:126-167.

their reasoning and abilities to react. Although the incidence of injury does not vary appreciably, the types of injuries sustained do vary, with important implications for injury prevention programs.

The risk factors for falls for young people in low- and middle-income countries appear to be associated with physical activity and also may vary with socioeconomic status.[18] The risk factors for injury from falls for older people are mostly related to age and overall physical condition.[18]

Low income, poor housing, and living in a crowded area are all risk factors for burns. Rural dwellers also suffer higher rates of burns than urban people. Children are more likely to suffer burns than any other age group. In addition, as discussed before, in South Asia and China, females are more likely to be burned than men.[19]

The risk factors for drowning in low- and middle-income countries are consistent with what we would expect. Young children are the most likely age groups to drown and males are more likely to drown than females. Most drownings occur during normal activities that take place near water. This is unlike in high-income countries where most drownings are associated with recreational activities. Children from poorer and larger families probably drown more frequently than other children.[19]

Studies done on poisoning in low- and middle-income countries have shed some light on risk factors. Poisoning is more likely in young boys than young girls. They also tend to be correlated with using nonstandard containers for poisonous goods and storing them within the reach of young children. Lower-income parents who are unable to supervise their children sufficiently around poisons are also more likely to have their children poisoned than better-off parents.[20]

The risk factors for road traffic injuries in low- and middle-income countries that differentiate them from high-income countries are well known. First is the increasing use of motor vehicles in low- and middle-income countries. In addition, in many countries two-wheeled vehicles, which are especially unsafe, are very common. In addition, most low- and middle-income countries pay insufficient attention to road planning, design, engineering, signage, or traffic management. Third, enforcement of speed limits is lax in many low- and middle-income countries and studies done on road traffic accidents show that about half of all such accidents are associated with excessive speed. It is also true in low- and middle-income countries that vehicles are less safe than in high-income countries, that many vehicles will not have safety belts or airbags, and that infant seats for cars are barely known or used. Motorcycle helmets are also used much less than in high-income countries.[21]

THE COSTS AND CONSEQUENCES OF INJURIES

The costs associated with unintentional injuries worldwide are considerable. The economic burden due to such injury includes direct costs such as medical care, hospitalization, rehabilitation, and funeral fees as well as indirect costs such as lost wages, sick leave from work, disability payments, insurance payouts, and costs associated with family care. These costs may be catastrophic for people within certain socioeconomic strata or those without access to sufficient health insurance. In this case, costs are frequently borne by government or private social services. In all cases, however, injuries represent a significant drain on personal and societal resources. The total costs of injuries in Canada during 1993, for example, were estimated to be $14.3 billion Canadian dollars.[22]

The direct costs due to road traffic injuries alone are estimated at 1–2% of the GNP of low- and middle-income countries. The total costs of road traffic injuries globally have been estimated at over $500 billion, with the share borne by the low- and middle-income countries estimated at $65–100 billion. At the regional level, Asia has the highest direct costs attributable to road traffic injuries at $24.5 billion. Africa, the least affected region by cost, still bears a significant burden, with an estimated $3.7 billion annually in total costs.[23,24]

Kenya examined the economic burden due to road traffic injuries and found a rapidly increasing economic burden over a 12-year period from 1984 to 1996. Costs, including health care, administrative expenses, and vehicle and property damage increased from 1.5 billion Kenyan shillings in 1984 to 3.8 billion shillings in 1991, which was equivalent to 5% of GNP. By 1996, injury-related costs had continued to escalate to between 5 and 10 billion Kenyan shillings.[25]

The consequences of unintentional injury are not limited to financial costs. There are significant social consequences for individuals and families that may be associated with such injury. Numerous studies have documented the long-term physical and psychosocial consequences of unintentional injuries. Persisting problems with pain, fatigue, memory problems, and psychosocial functioning are not uncommon in victims of trauma.[26–28] Moreover, these social consequences may be relatively independent of injury severity and reflect the influence of other non-injury variables.[29] Lastly, the psychosocial consequences for families of child injury victims may be significant, with difficulties relating to finances, changes in work-status required to care for injured children, and altered family dynamics.[30]

ADDRESSING KEY INJURY ISSUES

One of the key issues in addressing the burden of injuries is to raise awareness about how to apply rigorous methods of prevention and control to the injury problems. In fact, even among the industrialized countries, the prioritization of injuries as a significant health problem and the application of scientific methods of injury prevention and control are relatively recent phenomena.[11,31] Many public policy makers and public health actors in low- and middle-income countries have failed to appreciate the importance of injuries to the burden of disease or to understand what can be done to prevent unintentional injuries.

In order to design effective prevention and control activities for unintentional injuries, formal surveillance systems are fundamental to obtain reliable information as to numbers and patterns of injury. Although the formal surveillance systems in many developed countries may be inappropriate to developing country settings, minimal standards for injury morbidity and mortality should be implemented in all countries. In this light, the World Health Organization has published guidelines for collecting, coding, and reporting injury data, which have been specifically developed for use in low-resource settings and do not require the use of technology intensive data management systems or specialized training.[32,33]

In addition, it will be important to develop local capacity to analyze injury data and design injury prevention and mitigation programs. Injury prevention and control activities from one setting can not be grafted onto another setting. Rather, planners with an intimate understanding of local knowledge, attitudes, beliefs, and practices are required to design effective interventions for injury prevention in specific settings.

The theoretical foundation of many injury prevention and control efforts is called Haddon's Matrix, and it is widely used in efforts to understand and address injury issues. Haddon's Matrix models the interaction of host, vector, and environment in an injury event. Moreover, it is dynamic and models the events prior to, during, and after an injury.

The example of road traffic injuries provides a useful learning tool for thinking about injuries using Haddon's Matrix and how they can be prevented. The roadway (environment), automobile (vector), and host (human driver and behavior) interact in the moments leading up to a collision, during the collision, and in the moments after the collision.

Measures to prevent unintentional injuries have usually focused on education, enforcement, and engineering in the context of Haddon's Matrix. Recent efforts to reduce road traffic injuries have emphasized safer roads, safer vehicles, and safer systems. They have also paid increasing attention to land use and transport planning.[34] Roads can be made safer from the engineering point of view by paying particular attention to building safety in road designs, improving high risk intersections and routes, providing for slow moving vehicles and pedestrians, improving barriers and median strips, and enhancing lighting. Ghana was able to reduce road traffic injuries by installing speed bumps at selected places, as discussed further later.[35] In countries in which there are many types of vehicles, it would also help to separate those that can travel at high speed from those, like two-wheeled motorized rickshaws, that can only go slowly and that are unsafe in many ways.[36]

Vehicles can be made safer by engineering safety features into them, such as crash protection zones, headrests, seat belts, and daytime running lights. Including daytime running lights on motorcycles in China did reduce injuries.[34] People can be encouraged to use vehicles in safer ways through enforcement of speed limits, reducing the driving of those consuming alcohol, limiting the hours allowed for commercial driving, and enforcing the use of bicycle and motorcycle helmets.[34] Although there is considerable corruption in the police forces of many countries, enforcement of driving laws has helped in a number of settings to reduce road traffic injuries by up to 34%.[34] The introduction of mandatory seat belt and child restraint laws have been associated in high-income countries with a reduction in deaths and injuries by 25%.[37]

Few developing countries have taken measures to deal with poisonings. However, South Africa carried out a program in which child-proof containers were given to families for free. This program was associated with a cost-effective reduction in child poisonings and deaths.[38] It appears that to reduce poisonings in low- and middle-income countries, it is important to educate families to store poisons away from other household goods and out of the reach of children, to store them in appropriate and marked containers, and to enforce rules that prohibit the sale of poisons in unmarked and inappropriate containers.[39]

It is not easy to prevent falls by older people. It appears, however, that steps that have been taken in high-income countries to address such falls have included working with the elderly to improve their balance and modifying their home environment to reduce risks.[37] In low- and many middle-income countries, it may be that the only cost effective measure that could be taken to reduce falls among the elderly would be to provide community-based education to families about the risks of falls to their elderly relatives and about measures that are appropriate in that cultural context to reducing those risks.

Few efforts at reducing childhood injuries from falls have taken place in a systematic way in low- or middle-income countries. Here, too, it may be that the most reasonable step initially is community-based education of families about the risks of falling and what can be done to reduce those risks. Of course, if schools do have play equipment, it will be valu-able to design that equipment in a way that reduces injury if children fall from it. There is also little evidence from developing countries about what might be done in cost-effective ways to reduce drownings. Perhaps on this front, as well, one has to start with community-based information efforts about increased parental and older sibling supervision and with obvious measures, such as covering wells.[40] Not unexpectedly, there is also very little data on effective measures to reduce burns in low- and middle-income countries, despite their importance both generally and especially for women. Separate from the special circumstances of "dowry deaths," it appears that, for this, too, community-based efforts at behavior change must be the starting point for improved action.[41]

EMERGENCY MEDICAL SERVICES

In low- and many middle-income countries, unintentional injuries will remain an important component of the burden of disease for some time. In addition, that burden may grow in both absolute and relative importance as some societies witness economic growth and increasing motorization of transport. Thus, even low-income countries should examine investments in low-cost but effective ways of improving emergency medical services in their country. As discussed in Chapter 9 on women's health, one important measure would be to arrange for emergency transport. This could be in special vehicles made for low-income or rural communities or it could be advance arrangements with the owner of available transport. In addition, one could train members of the community who frequently come in contact with road accidents, such as truck drivers, in how to provide first aid and transport to accident victims. This was done with some important successes, for example, in Ghana.[42] Low-income countries could also begin to invest in better training of healthcare personnel who work in emergency services. They could do the same in emergency transport services based in selected locations known to the public, for example, so that the emergency transport could be hailed quickly, even in environments in which most people would not have a telephone.[43]

CASE STUDIES

Two very brief cases are presented below about efforts that countries have undertaken to reduce the burden of morbidity, disability, and death linked with road traffic accidents. The first concerns the use of speed bumps in Ghana, which were meant to slow drivers down and thereby reduce accidents. The second concerns the use of a mandatory motorcycle helmet law in Taiwan. Both appear to have produced substantial gains in health at relatively low cost, as other countries might wish to do, as well.

Motorcycle Helmet Use in Taiwan

Helmet use for moped and motorcycle riders can help to protect them from death and serious injury. Worldwide, head injuries sustained by a rider are the principal cause of death in riders after a road accident. Yet, the risk of injury if a rider wears a helmet is only one third the risk of those who do not wear a helmet. Nevertheless, unless a country has a law requiring helmet use, riders will most likely not use one. In addition, helmet use interventions in developing countries must be "sensitive to local manufacturing capabilities, cost, and comfort for local climates" in order to provide local governments with the means to legislate regulatory laws that are easily enforced in the community.[44]

In Taiwan, more than 60% of all motor vehicles registered in the late 1990s were motorcycles. As the number of motorcycles has increased, the incidence of motorcycle road traffic injuries has risen. Moreover, nearly 80% of motor vehicle fatalities in Taiwan, most of which involve motorcycle riders, have resulted from serious head injuries.[45]

In 1994 Taipei City began a 6-month pilot program in the use of motorcycle helmets. This resulted in increasing helmet use from 21% to 79% of motorcycle riders in only 5 months. It also reduced injuries and fatalities by 33% and 56%, respectively. However, since the intervention was not linked with a mandatory helmet use law, this was a short-lived success that ended soon after it began.[45]

Three years later, Taiwan passed a nation-wide law regulating motorcycle helmet use for all riders. In Taipei City, the law was preceded by a 6-month information campaign that was meant to inform residents on the benefits of helmet use. Within 2 months, helmet use was nearly 96% nationally with greater use in Taipei City than in other counties, partly due to greater law enforcement. Furthermore, head injuries decreased by 33% and the severity of these injuries also decreased as indicated by the reduced number of patients with head injuries admitted to intensive care units, as well as those dying or being in a vegetative state following their injury. Linked to the helmet law, head injuries in Taiwan dropped from the fourth to the fifth leading cause of death. Associated with the new law, hospital costs decreased by US$3.93 million per month.[45]

As indicated by higher levels of use in Taipei City than in other areas of Taiwan, the passage of a law requiring helmet use is not sufficient to ensure that it will produce the intended benefits. Rather, it is also important that an education campaign be oriented toward getting motorcycle riders to wear their helmets and that the laws requiring helmet use be enforced.

Rumble Strips and Speed Bumps in Ghana

In 2000, speeding contributed to over 50% of all motor vehicle accidents in Ghana. In addition, as in other countries, many of those injured as a result of these accidents were pedestrians or passengers in vehicles who had no seat belts or were not using them. Studies in developed countries demonstrate that reducing speed by 1 km/hr results in a 3% reduction in crashes and a higher likelihood of survival if hit by a car. In this light, the government of Ghana decided to put rumble strips and speed bumps at road intersections which had proved to be dangerous.[46]

The Ghanaian authorities first located accident hot spots on the main highway between Accra and Kumasi and installed rumble strips along the highest risk area, the Suhum Junction. In less than a year, this public health measure resulted in a 35% decrease in the number of motor vehicle crashes and a 55% reduction in related fatalities. The cost of laying rumble strips was US$20,900, compared to an estimated US$100,000 to redesign lanes or US$180,000 to construct a physical division to separate pedestrians from vehicles.[46]

As noted earlier in the chapter, there are other cost-effective measures that countries can take to reduce the burden of road traffic injuries. Nonetheless, it appears that even relatively poor countries, such as Ghana, can avert a considerable toll of injuries, disability, and death from road traffic injuries through the construction of very low-cost speed bumps and rumble strips in selected locations.

FUTURE CHALLENGES

The fact that there is so little data in this chapter that comes from low- and middle-income countries indicates that one important challenge for reducing the burden of unintentional injuries will be to focus additional attention on this topic within these countries. It is too large a source of deaths and disabilities to ignore, even in the face of continuing communicable diseases and a growing burden of non-communicable diseases.

There is increasing information about what works in cost-effective ways to reduce the burden of injury in high-income countries and this can serve as a starting point for adapting this learning to other settings. It will be important for selected low- and middle-income countries to carry out pilot schemes in preventing injury, especially from road traffic accidents, and then to expand them more broadly as they learn how to make them work effectively in different settings.

As low- and middle-income countries develop economically and become more motorized, it will be valuable for them to engineer safety into their newer investments in road transportation. Insufficient attention has been paid by many countries in enhancing their people's knowledge of good public health practice and it will be important that they increase their efforts significantly to provide information and education to the public about key areas of injury prevention. Although governance is weak in many countries, they can already begin to selectively enforce laws concerning road safety that can have a high return with little effort, such as encouraging the use of motorcycle helmets. As governance improves and people have more knowledge of road safety and trust that enforcement of laws will be honest, the government can pay more attention to enforcing other regulations affecting road safety. The challenge of reducing injuries from falls, burns, and drowning will depend, as seen in the last section of this chapter, almost completely on informing and educating the public in a community-based manner.

MAIN MESSAGES

Unintentional injuries are an important cause of deaths and DALYs lost in all regions of the world. In 2001, about 3.5 million people died of such injuries. In addition, these injuries are major causes of disability, with many people being disabled by injuries, even if they do not die from them. The rate of deaths from unintentional injuries is twice as high in low- and middle-income countries as it is in high-income countries.

The leading cause of both deaths and DALYs lost from unintentional injuries is road traffic accidents. This is followed by deaths from drowning, poisoning, falls, and fires. Men are almost three times as likely to die in road traffic accidents as women. However, women die more frequently in fires than men do. Deaths from road traffic accidents as a share of total deaths is particularly high in the Middle East and North Africa Region, compared to other regions. Unintentional injuries are an important source of deaths for young children, who account for 25% of drowning deaths and 15% of fire-related deaths globally.

The risk factors for road traffic accidents revolve around "education, enforcement, and engineering." The risk factors of other leading causes of unintentional injuries relate largely to lower socioeconomic status, inadequate supervision of children, a failure to store poisons safely, and household cooking arrangements that pay insufficient attention to fire hazards in areas that tend to be crowded and hazardous themselves.

Although there have been few studies of the economic costs of unintentional injuries in low- and middle-income countries, estimates of such costs have ranged from 1–2% of GNP. The social costs of dealing with the disabilities caused by accidents can also be very high.

There is increasing evidence from high-income countries of measures that can be taken to improve operator safety, build safety into vehicles, make plans for land use and traffic, and to enforce key traffic rules. These measures can selectively be implemented in low- and middle-income countries and adapted to their local settings. Reducing the burden of road traffic injuries and other injuries will require enhancing community-based approaches to providing information about how the community can reduce risk factors for such injuries.

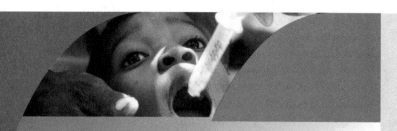

Study Questions

1. How important are unintentional injuries to the global burden of disease?

2. What unintentional injuries cause the most deaths?

3. How does the rate of death from road traffic accidents vary by region and why?

4. What are the most important unintentional injuries that affect children?

5. Do men and women suffer from unintentional injuries at the same rates? Why or why not?

6. What are the risk factors for road traffic accidents?

7. What are the risk factors for drownings?

8. What are the key risk factors for burning, and how do they vary by region?

9. What is Haddon's Matrix, and how would you apply it to analyze accidents?

10. What are the most cost-effective steps that low- and middle-income countries can take to reduce the burden of road traffic accidents on health?

REFERENCES

1. Lopez AD, Mathers CD, Murray CJL. The burden of disease and mortality by condition: data, methods, and results for 2001. In: Lopez AD, Mathers CD, Ezzati M, Jamison DT, Murray CJL, eds. *Global Burden of Disease and Risk Factors.* New York: Oxford University Press; 2006:130.

2. Lopez AD, Mathers CD, Murray CJL. The burden of disease and mortality by condition: data, methods, and results for 2001. In: Lopez AD, Mathers CD, Ezzati M, Jamison DT, Murray CJL, eds. *Global Burden of Disease and Risk Factors.* New York: Oxford University Press; 2006:126–130.

3. Lopez AD, Mathers CD, Murray CJL. The burden of disease and mortality by condition: data, methods, and results for 2001. In: Lopez AD, Mathers CD, Ezzati M, Jamison DT, Murray CJL, eds. *Global Burden of Disease and Risk Factors.* New York: Oxford University Press; 2006:228–232.

4. Trauma System Agenda for the Future: Glossary. Available at: http://www.nhtsa.dot.gov/people/injury/ems/emstraumasystem03/glossary.htm. Accessed June 23, 2006.

5. Norton R, Hyder AA, Bishai D, Peden M. Unintentional injuries. In: Jamison DT, Breman JG, Measham AR, et al., eds. *Disease Control Priorities in Developing Countries.* 2nd ed. New York: Oxford University Press; 2006:737.

6. Peden M, McGee K, Krug E. *The Injury Chart Book: A Graphical Overview of the Global Burden of Injuries.* Geneva, Switzerland: World Health Organization; 2002b.

7. Razzak J, Sasser S, Kellermann A. Injury prevention and other international public health initiatives. *Emerg Med Clin N Am.* 2005;23:85–98.

8. Norton R, Hyder AA, Bishai D, Peden M. Unintentional injuries. In: Jamison DT, Breman JG, Measham AR, et al., eds. *Disease Control Priorities in Developing Countries.* 2nd ed. New York: Oxford University Press; 2006:738.

9. Wadman M, Muelleman R, Coto J, et al. The pyramid of injury: using ecodes to accurately describe the burden of injury. *Ann Emergency Med.* 2003;42:468–478.

10. Bangdiwala S, Anzola-Perez E, Rommer C, et al. The incidence of injuries in young people: I. Methodology and results of a collaborative study in Brazil, Chile, Cuba, and Venezuela. *Int J Epidemiol.* 1990;19:115–124.

11. Bartlett S. The problem of children's injuries in low-income countries: a review. *Health Policy Plan.* 2002;17(1):1–13.

12. Mohan D. Injuries in less industrialized countries: what do we know? *Inj Prev.* 1997;3:241–242.

13. Lopez AD, Mathers CD, Murray CJL. The burden of disease and mortality by condition: data, methods, and results for 2001. In: Lopez AD, Mathers CD, Ezzati M, Jamison DT, Murray CJL, eds. *Global Burden of Disease and Risk Factors.* New York: Oxford University Press; 2006:45–240.

14. Jordan J, Valdez-Lazo F. Education on safety and risk. In: Manciaux M, Romer C, eds. *Accidents in Childhood and Adolescence: The Role of Research.* Geneva: World Health Organization; 1991.

15. Ljungblom B-A, Köhler L. Child development and behavior in traffic. In: Manciaux M, Romer CJ, eds. *Accidents in Childhood and Adolescence: The Role of Research.* Geneva: World Health Organization; 1991.

16. Leflamme L, Diderichsen F. Social differences in traffic injury risk in childhood and youth—a literature review and a research agenda. *Inj Prev.* 2000;6:293–298.

17. ILO. *Child Labour: Targeting the Intolerable.* Geneva: International Labour Office; 1996.

18. Norton R, Hyder AA, Bishai D, Peden M. Unintentional injuries. In: Jamison DT, Breman JG, Measham AR, et al., eds. *Disease Control Priorities in Developing Countries.* 2nd ed. New York: Oxford University Press; 2006:740–741.

19. Norton R, Hyder AA, Bishai D, Peden M. Unintentional injuries. In: Jamison DT, Breman JG, Measham AR, et al., eds. *Disease Control Priorities in Developing Countries.* 2nd ed. New York: Oxford University Press; 2006:741.

20. Norton R, Hyder AA, Bishai D, Peden M. Unintentional injuries. In: Jamison DT, Breman JG, Measham AR, et al., eds. *Disease Control Priorities in Developing Countries.* 2nd ed. New York: Oxford University Press; 2006:740.

21. Norton R, Hyder AA, Bishai D, Peden M. Unintentional injuries. In: Jamison DT, Breman JG, Measham AR, et al., eds. *Disease Control Priorities in Developing Countries.* 2nd ed. New York: Oxford University Press; 2006:739–740.

22. Ministry of Health—Canada. *Economic Burden of Illness in Canada.* Ottawa, Ontario: Canadian Public Health Association; 1993.

23. Hoffman K, Primack A, Keusch G, Hrynkow S. Addressing the growing burden of trauma and injury in low- and middle-income countries. *Am J Public Health.* 2005;95:13–17.

24. Jacobs G, Aaron-Thomas A, Astrop A. *Estimating Global Road Fatalities.* London: Transport Research Laboratory; 2000.

25. Odero W, Meleckidzedeck K, Heda P. Road traffic injuries in Kenya: magnitude, causes and status of intervention. *Inj Control Safe Promot.* 2003;10(1–2):53–61.

26. Depalma J, Fedorka P, Simko L. Quality of life experienced by severely injured trauma survivors. *AACN Clinical Issues.* 2003;14(1):54–63.

27. van der Sluis C, Eisma W, Groothoff J, ten Duis H. Long-term physical, psychological and social consequences of severe injuries. *Inj* 1998;29(4):281–285.

28. Landsman I, Baum C, Arnkoff D, et al. The psychosocial consequences of traumatic injury. *Behav Med.* 1990;13(6):561–581.

29. Mayou R, Bryant B. Outcome in consecutive emergency department attenders following a road traffic accident. *Brit J Psychiatry.* 2001;179:528–534.

30. Osberg J, Khan P, Rowe K, Brooke M. Pediatric trauma: impact on work and family finances. *Pediatrics.* 1996;98(5):890–897.

31. Haddon W. The changing approach to epidemiology, prevention, and amelioration of trauma: the transition to approaches etiologically rather than descriptively based. *Inj Prev.* 1999;5:231–235.

32. Holder Y, Peden M, Krug E, et al. *Injury Surveillance Guidelines.* Geneva: World Health Organization; 2001.

33. McGee K, Peden M, Waxweiler R, et al. Injury surveillance. *Inj Control Safe Promot.* 2003;10:105–108.

34. Norton R, Hyder AA, Bishai D, Peden M. Unintentional injuries. In: Jamison DT, Breman JG, Measham AR, et al., eds. *Disease Control Priorities in Developing Countries.* 2nd ed. New York: Oxford University Press; 2006:742–743.

35. Norton R, Hyder AA, Bishai D, Peden M. Unintentional injuries. In: Jamison DT, Breman JG, Measham AR, et al., eds. *Disease Control Priorities in Developing Countries.* 2nd ed. New York: Oxford University Press; 2006:746.

36. Norton R, Hyder AA, Bishai D, Peden M. Unintentional injuries. In: Jamison DT, Breman JG, Measham AR, et al., eds. *Disease Control Priorities in Developing Countries.* 2nd ed. New York: Oxford University Press; 2006:742–750.

37. Norton R, Hyder AA, Bishai D, Peden M. Unintentional injuries. In: Jamison DT, Breman JG, Measham AR, et al., eds. *Disease Control Priorities in Developing Countries.* 2nd ed. New York: Oxford University Press; 2006:744.

38. Krug E, Sharma G, Lozano R. The global burden of injuries. *Am J Public Health.* 2000;90:523–526.

39. Norton R, Hyder AA, Bishai D, Peden M. Unintentional injuries. In: Jamison DT, Breman JG, Measham AR, et al., eds. *Disease Control Priorities in Developing Countries.* 2nd ed. New York: Oxford University Press; 2006:747–748.

40. Norton R, Hyder AA, Bishai D, Peden M. Unintentional injuries. In: Jamison DT, Breman JG, Measham AR, et al., eds. *Disease Control Priorities in Developing Countries.* 2nd ed. New York: Oxford University Press and World Bank; 2006:745.

41. Norton R, Hyder AA, Bishai D, Peden M. Unintentional injuries. In: Jamison DT, Breman JG, Measham AR, et al., eds. *Disease Control Priorities in Developing Countries.* 2nd ed. New York: Oxford University Press and World Bank; 2006:744–745.

42. Mock C, Arreola-Risa C, Quansah R. Strengthening care for injured persons in less developed countries: a case study of Ghana and Mexico. *Inj Control Saf Promot.* 2003;10(1–2):45–51.

43. Kobusingye OC, Hyder AA, Bishai D, Joshipura ERH, Mock C. Emergency Medical Services. In: Jamison DT, Breman JG, Measham AR, et al., eds. *Disease Control Priorities in Developing Countries.* 2nd ed. New York: Oxford University Press; 2006:1265.

44. World Health Organization and The World Bank. World Report on Road Traffic Injury Prevention. Available at: http://www.who.int/world-health-day/2004/infomaterials/world_report/en/. Accessed February 25, 2007.

45. Chiu WT, Kuo CY, Hung CC, Chen M. The effect of the Taiwan motorcycle law on head injuries. *Am J Public Health.* 2004;90(5):793–796.

46. Afukaar FK. Speed control in developing countries: issues, challanges and opportunities in reducing road traffic injuries. *Inj Control Saf Promot.* 2003;10(1–2):77–81.

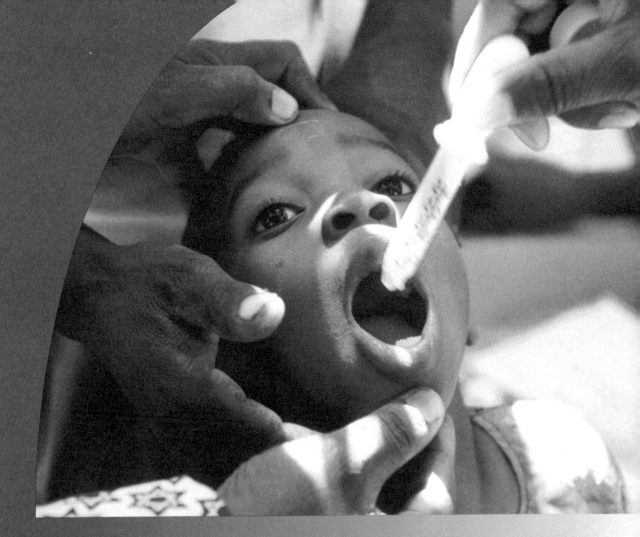

PART IV

Working Together to Improve Global Health

Natural Disasters and Complex Humanitarian Emergencies

VIGNETTES

Javad lived in the Pakistani province of Kashmir when the earthquake hit. All the buildings in his village were destroyed. Hundreds of people in the village were killed, mostly a result of being buried in the rubble. Many other people were badly injured from rubble falling on them. Their injuries were overwhelmingly orthopedic in nature. As the earthquake destroyed the village, it also destroyed wells, a health center, and roads leading to and from the village. Javad feared that many of those injured would soon die.

Samuel was living in the Eastern part of Sierra Leone when the war started. He did all that he could to protect his family, but it was not enough. In the first year of the conflict, as he and his family were getting ready to flee, a band of armed men stormed the village. As Samuel had heard they would do, they used machetes to kill or take limbs off of many village people. They also raped a large number of women. In addition, they kidnapped some of the children in hopes of making them into sex slaves or soldiers.

As the civil war spread in Rwanda, Sarah and her family fled across the border to what was fast becoming a large refugee camp in Zaire, later called the Democratic Republic of Congo. Although the camp workers did what they could to help the refugees, the circumstances at the camp were not good. There was little shelter, water, or food. In addition, a cholera epidemic went through the camp not long after Sarah's arrival there. It hit the camp especially hard and led to a large number of deaths.

A number of international organizations rushed staff to refugee camps, just across the border from intense fighting. Some of the agencies involved had long experience doing such work and had clear guidelines for their staff concerning relief efforts. Other agencies, however, were not so experienced in this work. They brought to the camps medicine that was not appropriate for the health conditions they found and food to which the local people were completely unaccustomed. Although it would have been most efficient if all of the aid agencies worked together, they did not. Many of them had their own way of working and wanted the local government to do it their way.

THE IMPORTANCE OF NATURAL DISASTERS AND COMPLEX EMERGENCIES TO GLOBAL HEALTH

Complex emergencies and natural disasters have a significant impact on global health. They can lead to increased death, illness, and disability and the economic costs of their health impacts can also be very large. Measures can be taken in cost-effective ways, however, to reduce the costs of disasters and conflicts and to address the major health problems that relate to them. These measures would be most effective if those involved in disaster relief would work together according to agreed standards that focused on the most important priorities for action.

This chapter will review the relationships between natural disasters and health and complex humanitarian emergencies (CHEs) and health. The chapter will begin by introducing you to some key concepts and definitions that relate to these topics. The chapter will then review the incidence of natural disasters and CHEs. Following that, the chapter will review their main health impacts. Lastly, the chapter will examine measures that can be taken to prevent and address some of their effects on health in cost-effective ways.

KEY TERMS

Understanding the health impacts of natural disasters and complex humanitarian emergencies requires an intro-

duction to several terms and concepts that are examined briefly here.

A disaster is "any occurrence that causes damage, ecological destruction, loss of human lives, or deterioration of health and health services on a scale sufficient to warrant an extraordinary response from outside the affected community area."[1] Another way to think of this would be as "an occurrence, either natural or man made, that causes human suffering and creates human needs that victims can not alleviate without assistance."[2] Some disasters are natural. These include, for example, the results of floods, volcanoes, and earthquakes. Some, however, are man-made, such as the cloud of poisonous gas that rained over the town of Bhopal, India, in 1984, as a result of an industrial accident. Some disasters are rapid-onset, such as an earthquake, while others are slow-onset, such as a drought or famine. Although the long-term effects of these natural and man-made disasters can be substantial, they are often characterized by an initial event and then its aftereffects. Some examples of recent natural disasters that caused a significant loss of life are listed in Table 14-1.

In response to the large number of civil conflicts that have taken place, the term "complex emergency" or "complex humanitarian emergency" has been established. A complex emergency can be defined as a "complex, multi-party, intra-state conflict resulting in a humanitarian disaster which might constitute multi-dimensional risks or threats to regional and international security. Frequently within such conflicts, state institutions collapse, law and order break down, banditry and chaos prevail, and portions of the civilian population migrate."[3] CHEs have also been described as: "situations affecting large civilian populations which usually involve a combination of factors, including war or civil strife, food shortages, and population displacement, resulting in significant excess mortality."[4]

Such emergencies include war and civil conflict. They usually affect large numbers of people and often include severe impacts on the availability of food, water, and shelter. Linked to these phenomena and the displacement of people that often go with them, complex humanitarian emergencies usually result in considerable excess mortality, compared to what would be the case without such an emergency.[5] Some of the better known complex humanitarian emergencies are listed in Table 14-2.

Complex emergencies create "refugees." Under international law, a refugee is a person who is outside his/her country of nationality or habitual residence; has a well-founded fear of persecution because of his/her race, religion, nationality, membership in a particular social group or political

---

TABLE 14-1 Selected Natural Disasters, 2004 and 2005

2004

March—Typhoon Gafilo, with 160-mile-per-hour winds, kills 295 people in Madagascar

May—Flooding and mudslides from heavy rains in the Dominican Republic and Haiti kill 3000 people

June—Monsoon floods in Bangladesh, India, and Nepal leave more than 5 million people homeless and kill 1800

December—Tsunamis after a 9.0 magnitude earthquake kill more than 225,000 people in India, Indonesia, Sri Lanka, and Thailand

2005

February—Flooding from snow and rain killed 460 people in Pakistan with thousands of people missing

March—An 8.7 magnitude earthquake in Indonesia killed more than 1300 people

July—The heaviest rains in Indian history killed more than 1000 people

July—Famine stemming from drought and locusts put more than 3.6 million people at risk of starvation in Niger

August—Hurricane Katrina kills 1800 people in the United States

October—Rains from Hurricane Stan killed more than 2000 people in Central America and caused many people to evacuate their homes

Source: Data from Infoplease. World Disasters—2004 and 2005 Disasters. Available at: http://www.infoplease.com/ipa/A0001437.html. Accessed February 25, 2007.

opinion; and is unable or unwilling to avail himself/herself of the protection of that country, or to return there, for fear of persecution. They are a subgroup of the broader category of displaced persons.[6] It is important to note that there are a number of international conventions that define refugees and that accord them rights according to international law, as well. Table 14-3 notes a number of countries with significant refugee populations and the countries they fled. A United Nations Agency, the United Nations High Commissioner for Refugees (UNHCR), is responsible for protecting the rights of refugees.

Some of the people who flee or are forced to migrate during a disaster or complex humanitarian emergency leave their homes but stay in the country in which they were living.

These are called internally displaced people (IDP). These are more formally defined as "someone who has been forced to leave their home for reasons such as religious or political persecution or war, but has not crossed an international border."[7] The term is a subset of the more general "displaced person." There is no legal definition of internally displaced person, as there is for refugee, but the thumbnail rule is that "if the person in question would be eligible for refugee status if he or she crossed an international border then the IDP label is applicable."[7] Table 14-4 shows selected examples of countries with large numbers of internally displaced persons. It is important to note that the legal status of IDPs is not as well defined as that for refugees.[8] It is also important to understand that, unlike the case for refugees, no agency or organization is responsible for IDPs. Rather, their own government is responsible for them, but that government is often part of the problem as to why these people are fleeing.

One of the indicators of significance of the health impact of a complex humanitarian emergency is the "crude mortality rate." This is the proportion of people who die from a population at risk over a specified period of time.[9] For addressing CHEs, the crude mortality rate is generally expressed per 10,000 population, per day. The extent to which diseases might spread in a refugee camp depend partly on the "attack rate" of a disease, which is "the proportion of an exposed

---

TABLE 14-2 Selected Complex Humanitarian Emergencies of Importance

Angola—A civil war lasted 27 years and ended in 2002.

Armenia/Azerbaijan—Conflict between the two countries has created almost 250,000 refugees and 600,000 IDPs.

Bosnia and Herzegovina—Between 1992 and 1994, war with various parts of the former Yugoslavia led to more than 100,000 deaths and 1.8 million people displaced.

Burma—Government offensives against a number of ethnic groups have gone on for more than 20 years and produced between 500,000 and 1,000,000 IDPs.

Democratic Republic of Congo—Fighting since the mid-1990s between government forces and rebels have led to more than 2 million displaced people.

Liberia—Civil war from 1990–2004 led to almost 500,000 IDPs and more than 125,000 refugees in Guinea alone.

Nepal—Conflict between the government forces and maoist rebels from 1996 to 2006 has led to 100,000 to 200,000 IDPs.

Rwanda—More than 800,000 people were killed in the 1994 genocide, which also produced more than 2 million refugees who fled to Burundi, what is now the Democratic Republic of Congo, Tanzania, and Uganda.

Sudan—Internal conflicts since the 1980s, including a war with groups in the South and genocide against people in the Darfur region, have displaced 5–6 million people.

Uganda—Rebellion by the Lord's Resistance Army in the North for almost 20 years has led to between 1 and 2 million displaced people.

Source: Data from CIA. The World Fact Book. Available at: http://www.cia.gov/cia/publications/factbook/. Accessed February 25, 2007.

TABLE 14-3 Internally Displaced People—Selected Countries of Importance, 2006

Country	Number of IDPs
Sudan	5,300,000–6,200,000
Colombia	2,900,000–3,400,000
Democratic Republic of Congo	2,330,000
India	600,000
Burma	550,000–1,000,000
Azerbaijan	528,000
Ivory Coast	500,000–800,000
Indonesia	500,000
Liberia	464,000
Algeria	400,000–600,000
Somalia	400,000
Russia	339,000
Bosnia and Herzegovina	309,000

Source: Data from CIA. The World Fact Book. Field Listing Refugees and Internally Displaced People. Available at: http://www.cia.gov/cia/publications/factbook/fields/2194.html. Accessed October 8, 2006.

TABLE 14-4 Selected Refugee Populations and Source of Refugees, 2006

Country	Number of Refugees	Source Countries
Jordan	1,828,000	Palestinian Refugees
Iran	1,040,000	Afghanistan, Iraq
Gaza Strip	990,000	Palestinian Refugees
Pakistan	960,000	Afghanistan
West Bank	700,000	Palestinian Refugees
Tanzania	597,000	Burundi, Democratic Republic of Congo
Syria	446,000	Palestinian Refugees, Iraq
Lebanon	404,000	Palestinian Refugees
China	350,000	Vietnam, North Korea
Serbia	275,000	Croatia, Bosnia, and Herzegovina
Uganda	258,000	Sudan, Rwanda, Democratic Republic of Congo
Chad	255,000	Sudan, Central African Republic
Armenia	235,000	Azerbaijan
Kenya	229,000	Somalia, Ethiopia, Sudan
India	157,000	Tibet/China, Sri Lanka, Afghanistan
Zambia	151,000	Angola, Democratic Republic of Congo, Rwanda
Guinea	141,000	Liberia, Sierra Leone, Ivory Coast
Sudan	139,000	Eritrea, Chad, Uganda, Ethiopia
Ethiopia	125,000	Sudan, Somalia, Eritrea
Thailand	121,000	Myanmar
Nepal	105,000	Bhutan

Source: Data from CIA. The World Fact Book. Field listing refugees and internally displaced people. Available at: http://www.cia.gov/cia/publications/factbook/fields/2194.html. Accessed October 8, 2006.

population at risk who become infected or develop clinical illness during a defined period of time."[3] Finally, it is important to understand "case fatality rate," which is "the number of deaths from a specific disease in a given period, per 100 episodes of the disease in the same period."[10]

THE CHARACTERISTICS OF NATURAL DISASTERS

There are several types of natural disasters. Some of these are related to the weather, including droughts, hurricanes, typhoons, cyclones, and heavy rains. Tsunamis, like the one that occurred in 2004, can also cause extreme devastation, injuries, and death. In addition, earthquakes and volcanoes can have important impacts on the health of various communities. Despite the exceptional nature of the 2004 tsunami and the deaths associated with that, among the natural disasters it is earthquakes that generally kill the most people.

It appears that the number of natural disasters is increasing, affecting larger numbers of people, causing more economic losses than earlier, but causing proportionately fewer deaths than before. In addition, the biggest relative impact of natural disasters is in developing countries. More than 90% of the deaths from these disasters occur in low- and middle-income countries.[11] The relative impact of natural disasters on the poor, of course, is greater than on the better-off because the share of the poorer people's total assets that are lost in these disasters is greater than that lost by higher-income people. Moreover, the poor are often the most vulnerable to losses from natural disasters because they often live in places at risk from such disasters or have housing that can not withstand such shocks.[12]

Natural disasters can cause significant harm to infrastructure, such as water supply and sewage systems, that are needed for safe water and sanitation, and roads that may be needed to transport people requiring health care. Natural disasters can also damage the health infrastructure itself, such as hospitals, health centers, and health clinics. People can die directly as a result of the natural disaster, such as from falling rubble during an earthquake or drowning during a flood. However, they may also die as an indirect result of the disaster because of epidemics linked to the lack of safe water or sanitation, food, or access to health services.[12] In addition, people affected by the disaster could wind up living in camps, which pose a range of health hazards.

THE CHARACTERISTICS OF COMPLEX EMERGENCIES

Over the 10-year period from 1975 to 1985, there were on average about five complex emergencies per year, according to the International Committee of the Red Cross. However, it is estimated that at the end of the 1990s there were about 40 such emergencies per year in countries in which more than 300 million people live.[8] It is also estimated that in 2001 there were more than 14 million refugees and more than 20 million internally displaced people in the world.[13] Although natural disasters have been associated with considerable death and economic loss, the impact of complex emergencies on health over the last decade has been considerably greater than that of natural disasters.

Complex humanitarian emergencies have a number of features that particularly relate to their health impacts. First, these emergencies often go on for long periods of time. The strife in Sudan, for example, has gone on for more than a decade.[14] In addition, these emergencies are increasingly civil wars, as in Bosnia, Liberia, Sierra Leone, Rwanda, and the Democratic Republic of Congo. As a result of the nature of the conflict, it is quite common that one or more of the groups that are fighting will not allow humanitarian assistance to be provided to other groups. In fact, humanitarian workers have increasingly been the targets of those who are fighting, despite what should be their protected status.

During complex emergencies, combatants often intentionally target civilians, as well, for displacement, injury, and death. Many fighters also engage in systematic abuse of human rights, including torture, sexual abuse, and rape "as a weapon of war," as discussed in Chapter 9. Those same fighters often intentionally destroy health facilities. Given the nature of some of the fighting and its impact on civilians, large numbers of people have been displaced by some of these conflicts, as noted above. Sometimes they choose to flee, but sometimes they are forced to flee.[15]

Unfortunately, these are not the only characteristics of complex humanitarian emergencies. The disruption of society often leads to food shortages. Besides the loss of some health facilities, it is also common that the publicly supported health system may break down entirely, as it did, for example, in the civil war in Liberia. Damage may also be done to water supply and sanitation systems.[16] In El Salvador,

for example, the shortage of safe drinking water for the poor was seen as a significant health threat.[14]

It is important to understand that the migration of large numbers of people, some of whom will live in camps, brings with it a number of problems, as well. Migrants carry diseases with them, sometimes into areas that did not previously have that disease. When Ethiopian refugees who were living in Sudan returned home, for example, they brought malaria from Sudan. Diseases can also spread faster among refugee populations than they would normally, given the large number of people living in crowded conditions, often without appropriate hygiene and sanitation. In addition, large numbers of migrants, sometimes suddenly, need care from health systems that were weak before and which may now be almost nonexistent after suffering the effects of civil conflict. Finally, one should note that many factions in civil conflicts use landmines and their health effects on individuals can be devastating.[14]

THE HEALTH BURDEN OF NATURAL DISASTERS

In the 1990s, about 62,000 people per year died on average during natural disasters. There are very few data available on the morbidity and disability associated with natural disasters. The direct and indirect health effects of natural disasters depend on the type of disaster. Earthquakes can kill many people quickly. In addition, they can cause a substantial number of injuries in a very short period of time. In the longer term, earthquake survivors face increased risks of permanent orthopedic disabilities, mental health problems, and possibly an increase in the rates of heart disease and other chronic disease. The indirect effect of earthquakes on health depends on the severity and location of the earthquake and the extent to which it damages infrastructure and forces people out of their homes.[17]

In the popular imagination, people are thought to die from the lava flows of volcanoes. In fact, this is rarely the case. About 90% of the deaths from volcanoes are due to mud and ash or from floods on denuded hillsides affected by the volcano.[18] In addition, volcanoes can harm health by displacing people, rendering water supplies unsafe, and causing mental health problems among the affected population.[18]

Tsunamis take most of their victims immediately by drowning and cause relatively few injuries, compared to the number of deaths.[18] In storms and flooding, most fatalities occur from drowning and few deaths result from trauma or wind-blown objects. These flood-related events generally lead to an increase in diarrheal disease, respiratory infections, and skin diseases. Most of these problems that relate to natural disasters are relatively short-lived, except for drought-related famine. Epidemics do not often spring up as a result of them, except in drought-related famine and when health systems are completely destroyed for long periods of time.

There are few data on the distribution by age and sex of morbidity, disability, and death related to natural disasters. It appears, however, that being very old, very young, or very sick makes one more vulnerable to disasters in which one has to flee for survival. These groups were disproportionately affected by the 1970 tidal wave in Bangladesh and the 2004 Tsunami in Asia. Whether men or women suffer the effects of a natural disaster may depend on when and where it occurs and be most related to the kind of work men or women are doing. Women, however, face considerable risks in the aftermath of natural disasters if housing has been harmed and people are living in camps, as will be discussed further later.[12]

THE HEALTH EFFECTS OF COMPLEX HUMANITARIAN EMERGENCIES

The burden of illness, disability, and death related to complex humanitarian emergencies is large and probably underestimated, given the difficulties of collecting such data. Some of the effects of these CHEs are direct. It has been estimated for, example, that between 320,000 and 420,000 people are killed each year as a direct result of these CHEs.[8] In addition, it is estimated that between 500,000 and 1 million deaths resulted from trauma during the genocide in Rwanda in 1994.[19] It is thought that about 4–13% of the deaths during CHEs in Northern Iraq, Somalia, and the Democratic Republic of Congo were the direct result of trauma.

Other illness, disability, and death, however, come about as an indirect result of the emergencies. These stem from malnutrition, the lack of safe water and sanitation, shortages of food, and breakdowns in health services. They are exacerbated by the crowded and difficult circumstances in which people have to live when they are displaced. One estimate, for example, suggested that almost 1.7 million people more died in a 22-month period of conflict in the Democratic Republic of Congo, than would have died in a "normal" 22-month period in that country.[8]

The burden of deaths related to wars is also hard to estimate. Another estimate suggests that about 200,000 people died in war in 2001 in low- and middle-income countries. Just over 10% of these deaths occurred in the South Asia Region. Almost 70% of these deaths, however, took place in Sub-Saharan Africa.[20] About 6.5 million DALYs were lost in 2001 due to war in low- and middle-income countries. That was about one third as much as was lost due to other forms of violence. It was about two thirds as much as the number

of DALYs lost from all sexually transmitted diseases and about the same as those lost due to maternal sepsis or breast cancer.[20] Other estimates suggest that between 1975 and 1989 more than five million people died in civil conflicts.[21] In terms of deaths from CHEs, some of the most severely affected countries in the last two decades have been the Democratic Republic of Congo, Afghanistan, Burundi, and Angola.[8]

The data on the breakdown of deaths by age in CHEs suggests that child mortality rates early in the CHE are two to three times the rates of adults but that they slowly decline to those of the rest of the population. The data on deaths by sex are limited.[22] About 20% of the non-fatal injuries in the Bosnian conflict were among children. Almost 50% of the deaths in the Democratic Republic of Congo were among women and children younger than 15 years of age.[19] UNICEF estimates that more than 1.5 million children have been killed in war since 1980.[23] In European conflicts, the overwhelming majority of those who died have been men between 19 and 50 years of age.[19]

Causes of Death in CHEs

In the early stages of dealing with large numbers of displaced people in CHEs, most deaths occur from diarrheal diseases, respiratory infections, measles, or malaria.[19,24] Generally, diarrheal diseases are the most common cause of death in refugee situations. Major epidemics of cholera occurred in refugee camps in Malawi, Nepal, and Bangladesh, among others, and the case fatality rates from cholera have ranged from 3–30% in settings such as these. Dysentery, which refers to severe diarrhea caused by an infection in the intestine, has also commonly occurred in such situations over the last 15 years, including in camps in Malawi, Nepal, Bangladesh, and Tanzania. The case fatality rate for dysentery has been highest among the very old and very young, in whom it reaches about 10%.[19,24] In one of the most significant humanitarian crises in the last few decades, tens of thousands of Rwandan refugees poured into the Democratic Republic of Congo during the genocide in Rwanda. Between July and August 1994, 90% of the deaths among the refugees in Goma, Democratic Republic of Congo, were from cholera spread by the contamination of a lake from which the refugees got their water.[19,24]

Measles has also been a major killer in camps for displaced persons. This is especially significant in populations that are malnourished and have not been immunized against measles. As you learned in Chapter 10, the risk of a child dying of measles is increased substantially if the child is vitamin A deficient, as would be the case for many refugees. Up to 30% of the children who get measles in these situations may die from it.[24]

Malaria is also a significant contributor to death in refugee camps. This is especially the case when refugees move from countries in which there is relatively little malaria to places in which it is endemic. The risk of malaria in such cases is highest in Sub-Saharan Africa and a few parts of Asia.[24,25] Acute respiratory infections are also major causes of death in refugee camps. This is to be expected because the camps are crowded, housing is inadequate, and refugees could remain in the camps for many years. Although less common than the problems noted previously, there have also been outbreaks of meningitis in some refugee camps in areas in which that disease is prevalent, such as Malawi, Ethiopia, and Burundi. These outbreaks have generally been contained by mass immunization, as it became clear that there was a risk of epidemic.[26] However, an outbreak in Sudan in 1999 led to almost 2400 deaths.[25] Outbreaks of hepatitis E have occurred in Somalia, Ethiopia, and Kenya. These led to high case fatality rates among pregnant women, in particular.[26]

The populations that are affected by CHEs are generally poor and not well nourished, and nutritional issues are always of grave concern during CHEs, when there may also be problems of food scarcity. In addition, the relationship of infection and malnutrition also poses risks to displaced populations. In CHEs in Sub-Saharan Africa, the rates of acute protein-energy malnutrition during at least the early period of a CHE have been very high, particularly among young children. Reported rates of such malnutrition varied from around 12% among internally displaced Liberians[27] to as high as 80% among internally displaced Somalis.[25] In CHEs in Bosnia and Tajikistan, the elderly were the group that was the worst affected by acute protein-energy malnutrition.[25]

The underlying nutritional status of the refugees or internally displaced people is often poor, and micronutrient deficiencies can also be very important in CHEs. Vitamin A deficiency can be very important among these populations, given their low stores of vitamin A, the fact that some of the diseases most prevalent in camps, such as measles, further deplete the stores they have of vitamin A, and the fact that food rations in camps have historically been deficient in vitamin A. There have also been epidemics of pellagra, which is a deficiency of niacin that causes diarrhea, dermatitis, and mental disorders. One such case affected more than 18,000 Mozambican refugees in Malawi, whose rations in the camp were deficient in niacin. Scurvy, from a lack of vitamin C, has also occurred in a number of settings, such as Ethiopia, Somalia, and Sudan. Iron deficiency anemia has also been a problem in some camps and affects primarily women of childbearing age and young children. It appears that women and children who are in the camps without a male adult are at particular risk of not getting enough food in camps and of suffering acute protein-energy malnutrition and micronutrient deficiencies.[24]

Violence Against Women in CHEs

As discussed in Chapter 9 on women's health, the security conditions during CHEs put women at considerable risk of sexual violence. Rape may be used as a "weapon of war." In addition, the chaos and economic distresses of conflict situations place women at risk of sexual violence and sometimes force them to "trade" sex for food or money, what people call "survival sex." Such women are often very young.

The data on sexual violence against women during CHEs are not good. However, some recent data suggest that the rates of violence against women are very high in these circumstances. A survey carried out in East Timor indicated that 23% of the women surveyed after the crisis there reported that they had been sexually assaulted. 15% of the women in Kosovo who were surveyed reported sexual violence against them during the conflict period. It is estimated that between 50,000 and 64,000 women in Sierra Leone were sexually assaulted during the conflict there, and 25% of Azerbaijani women reported sexual violence against them during a 3-month period in 2000.[28]

Mental Health

Those who study CHEs agree that they are associated with a range of social and psychological shocks to affected people due to changes in their way of living, their loss of livelihoods, damaged social networks, and physical and mental harm to them, their families, and their friends. Nonetheless, there is considerable disagreement among those working with CHEs about the validity of defining the impact on people affected by CHEs through the framework of a "Western" medical model of mental health.[29,30]

Some studies have focused on post-traumatic stress disorder (PTSD) and shown rates of prevalence for PTSD among adults that ranged from 4.6% among Burmese refugees in Thailand to 37.2% among Cambodian refugees in Thailand. The rate of post-traumatic stress disorder is about 1% in the population of the United States. Similar studies showed rates of depression in Bosnian refugees of 39%, Burmese refugees of almost 42%, and Cambodian refugees of almost 68%. By comparison, one estimate of the baseline rate of depression in the U.S. population is 6.4%.[31]

Other studies have looked at the mental health impacts of CHEs on children and the extent to which they suffer from both post-traumatic stress and depression. The studies that have been done on such populations have been small ones that can not be used to draw major conclusions on this question. However, they suggest that children who have been through conflict situations do suffer from high rates of both PTSD and depression. A survey of 170 adolescent Cambodian refugees, for example, indicated that almost 27% of them suffered from PTSD. A survey of 147 Bosnian children refugees suggested that almost 26% of them suffered from depression.[32]

It should be noted, however, that a number of those involved with the mental health impacts of CHEs believe that the stress placed by some on PTSD is not valid. Rather, they believe that while a small minority of those affected may need psychotropic medication, the most important issue is to help people as rapidly as possible to rebuild their lives and their social networks. This requires a variety of forms of social assistance and help in reuniting families, finding families a place to live, rebuilding social networks, and restoring livelihoods.[22,29,30]

ADDRESSING THE HEALTH EFFECTS OF NATURAL DISASTERS

The health effects of rapid-onset natural disasters occur in phases, starting with the immediate impact of the event and then continuing for some time until displaced people can be resettled. It is very important that the health situation be assessed immediately after the disaster has occurred. This assessment will set the basis for the initial relief effort. At the same time, care must begin of those injured in the disaster. Once the immediate trauma cases are taken care of, relief workers and health service providers can turn their attention to other injured people who are in need of early care and treatment. This would include urgent psychological problems. In the earliest stages of the disaster, some important public health functions also need to be carried out, including the establishment of continuous disease surveillance among the affected populations and provision of water, shelter, and food.[18]

Many countries do not have all of the resources needed to cope with the health impacts of the disaster, and they will depend on assistance from other countries to address their health problems. Unfortunately, there have been many instances when such help was poorly coordinated and did not effectively match the conditions on the ground. It has become clear over time, however, that to be most helpful in addressing the impact of natural disasters, external assistance will have to:

- Include all of the external partners
- Be based on a cooperative relationship among the partners

- Have partners working in ways that are complementary to each other
- Be evidence-based and transparent
- Involve the affected communities[33]

In some respects, it is easier to predict places that are at risk of natural disasters than it is to predict where CHEs will occur. There are certain countries that are vulnerable to earthquakes, volcanoes, hurricanes, typhoons, and flooding during major rains. In this light, much can be done to prepare for natural disasters and to reduce their health impact. Disaster preparedness plans can be formulated to:

- Identify vulnerabilities
- Develop scenarios of what might happen and its likelihood
- Outline the role that different actors will play in the event of an emergency
- Train first responders and managers to deal with such emergencies[34]

It is also possible when constructing water systems and hospitals, for example, to take measures that will make them less vulnerable to damage during natural disasters.

Given the way that the health impacts of natural disasters unfurl, what would be the most cost-effective ways for external partners to help in addressing the disaster? There are at least several lessons that have emerged on this front. First, although many countries send search and rescue teams to assist the victims of natural disasters, the efforts of such teams are not cost-effective. Most people who are freed from the rubble of an earthquake, for example, are saved by people in their own community immediately after the event. By the time foreign search and rescue teams arrive, most victims of falling rubble will already have been saved or will be dead. It cost about $500,000 for the United States search and rescue team to carry out its work after an earthquake in Armenia in 1988, but they were only able to save two people.[35]

It is also common that countries will send field hospitals to disaster areas. The cost of each hospital is about $1 million, and they generally arrive two to five days after the initial event. Unfortunately, by the time they arrive, they are of little value in addressing the most urgent trauma cases. It appears to be more cost-effective to have fewer field hospitals but to have a few that will remain in place for some time, in addition to building some temporary but durable buildings that can also serve as hospitals.[35]

Countries send different kinds of goods to disaster-affected places. Unfortunately, these goods can be inappropriate to the needs of the problem. This has often been the case, for example, for drugs. Better results occur when the impacted country clearly indicates what it needs and other countries send only those goods. Large camps of tents are often established after natural disasters. This is generally also not a cost-effective approach to helping the affected community to rebuild. Providing cash or building materials to affected families allows them to rebuild as quickly as possible, in a manner in line with their cultural preferences. The lack of income, even beyond the cost of rebuilding their home, can be a major impediment to the reconstruction of affected areas. Although it must be managed carefully to avoid abuse, cash assistance to families appears to be a cost-effective way of helping communities rebuild.[35]

ADDRESSING THE HEALTH EFFECTS OF COMPLEX HUMANITARIAN EMERGENCIES

It is difficult to take measures that can prevent complex humanitarian emergencies from occurring and harming human health because these emergencies so often relate to civil conflict. Thus, the key to avoiding such problems lies in the political realm and in the avoidance of conflict, rather than by taking measures that are directly health related. "Primary prevention in such circumstances, therefore, means stopping the violence."[36]

However, if such conflicts continue to occur, are there measures of "secondary prevention" that can be taken to detect health-related problems as early as possible and take actions to mitigate them? To a large extent, the early warning systems that exist for natural disasters do not exist for political disasters. Although some groups do carry out analyses of political vulnerability in countries, corruption, and the risk of political instability, these analyses are not used to prepare contingency plans for civil conflict.

Given the extent of conflict, however, it would be prudent if organizations, countries, and international bodies would cooperatively establish contingency plans for areas of likely conflict. It would also be prudent to stage near such areas the materials needed to address displacement and health problems that would occur if conflict breaks out. This would be similar to what is done for disaster preparedness in some places, such as those regularly exposed to hurricanes.[37] You read earlier that complex humanitarian emergencies are characterized by:

- Potentially massive displacement of people
- The likelihood that these displaced people will live in camps for some time
- The need in those camps for adequate shelter, safe water, sanitation, and food

- The importance of security in the camps, especially for women
- The need to address early in the crisis the potentially worst health threats, which are malnutrition, diarrhea, measles, pneumonia, and malaria
- The need to avoid other epidemic diseases, such as cholera and meningitis
- The need as one moves away from the emergency phase of a CHE to dealing with longer-term mental health issues, primary health care, TB, and some non-communicable diseases

Some of the most important measures that can be taken to address these points are discussed briefly hereafter. As you review these, it is important to keep in mind that the aim of these efforts is to establish a safe and healthy environment, treat urgent health problems and prevent epidemics, and then to address less urgent needs and establish a basis for longer-term health services among the displaced people.[38]

Assessment and Surveillance

As with natural disasters, among the first things that needs to be done during the emergency phase of a CHE is to carry out an assessment of the displaced population and establish a system for disease surveillance. Such an assessment would try to immediately gather information on the number of people who are displaced, their age and sex, their ethnic and social backgrounds, and their state of health and nutrition. Although it is difficult to get this information in the chaotic moments of an emergency, it is impossible to rationally plan services for displaced people without this information.

There are a number of health indicators that guide services in CHEs and a surveillance system needs to be established at the start of the emergency phase of a CHE. Given the difficulties of the emergency, the surveillance system must be simple but still give a robust sense of the health of the affected community. Given the importance of nutrition and the likelihood that a large part of the population will be undernourished, it is essential that the weight for height of all children younger than 5 be checked.[39] It is also important to have surveillance for diseases that cause epidemics among displaced persons, such as measles, cholera, and meningitis.

In general, the daily crude mortality rate is used as an indicator of the health of the affected group and one goal is to keep that rate below 1 death per 10,000 persons in the population per day. Where the daily rate is twice the normal rate, it signifies that a public health emergency is occurring. Say, for example, that the baseline crude mortality rate for Sub-Saharan Africa is 0.44/10,000 per day. Thus, if the rate in an affected population were to get to 0.88/10,000 per day, it would signal a public health emergency that would require urgent attention. For children younger than five years, the crude mortality rate for Sub-Saharan Africa is 1.14/10,000 per day. The goal in a public health emergency, therefore, would be to keep that rate below about 2.0/10,000 per day.[40] Death rates in a large camp are not always easy to get and sometimes people have resorted to "creative" ways of getting such data, such as daily reports by grave-diggers.

A Safe and Healthy Environment

It is critical in camps and other situations with large numbers of displaced people that efforts be made to ensure that environmental and personal hygiene are maintained. This will be the key to avoiding the potentially serious effect of diarrheal disease. It is recommended that 15 liters of water per person per day should be provided, that people should not have to walk more than 500 meters to a water source, and that people should not have to wait more than 15 minutes to get their water when they get to a source. Of the 15 liters per day that are recommended, about 2.5 to 3 liters are considered the minimum essential for drinking and food. Another 2 to 6 liters are needed for personal hygiene and the remainder is needed for cooking.[41]

Providing appropriate sanitation in situations of displaced people is also very challenging. Ideally, every family would have their own toilet. This, however, is certainly impossible in the acute phase of an emergency. The goal instead is one toilet for every 20 people. These should be segregated by sex to provide the most safety to women. They should not be more than 50 meters from dwellings, but must be carefully situated to avoid contamination of water sources.[41]

Many of the people who have been displaced will be poor people with little education and, often, poor hygiene practices. It is very important in these circumstances that efforts be made to make the community aware of the importance of good hygiene and to see that soap is available to all families and used.

Of course, people will also need shelter. The long-term goal is to help them return as quickly as possible to their homes. In the short term, if possible, the goal is to have families be sheltered temporarily with other families. Nonetheless, it is obvious from the tables shown earlier that many displaced people do end up living in camps, often for very long periods of time. When shelter is needed, the goal is to provide 3.5 square meters of covered area per person, with due attention paid in the construction of the shelter to the safety of women. Whenever possible, local and culturally appropriate building materials should be used. In the short-run, the aim is to get people into covered areas. When the emergency phase has passed, the need to enhance some of the structures can be prioritized.[42]

Food

It is suggested that each adult in a camp should get at least 2000 kilocalories of energy from food per day. Food rations should be distributed by family unit, but special care has to be taken, as noted earlier, to ensure that female-headed households and children without their families get their rations. Vitamin A should be given to all children, and the most severely malnourished children may also need urgent nutrition supplementation.[43]

Disease Control

As suggested earlier, "The primary goals of humanitarian response to disasters are to 1) prevent and reduce excess morbidity and mortality, and 2) promote a return to normalcy."[40] Along these lines, the control of communicable diseases is one of the first priorities in the emergency phase of a disaster, especially a complex humanitarian emergency.

An important priority in the emergency phase of a complex humanitarian emergency is to prevent an epidemic of measles. This starts with vaccinating all children from 6 months to 15 years. Another important priority is to ensure that children up to 5 years get vitamin A. Systems also need to be put in place so that other epidemics that sometimes occur in these situations, such as meningitis and cholera, can be detected and then urgent measures can be taken to address them. Other priorities will include the proper management of diarrhea in children and the appropriate diagnosis and treatment for malaria, in zones where that is prevalent. Of course, health education and hygiene promotion must take place continuously to try to help families prevent the onset of these diseases in the first place.[40]

Unfortunately, preventing the outbreak of communicable diseases is not the only effort that needs to be taken in the emergency phase of a CHE. Measures need to be in place to handle injuries and trauma, first to stabilize people and then to refer them to where they can receive the additional medical help they need. There will almost certainly be pregnant women among the displaced people, and there will be an immediate need for some reproductive health services. This will generally have to focus on the provision of a minimum package of care that would include safe delivery kits, precautions against the transmission of HIV, and transport and referral in case of complications of pregnancy.[40–44]

The care of non-communicable diseases will be a lower priority in emergency situations than addressing communicable diseases. However, some psychiatric problems will require urgent attention and will need to be treated as far as possible with counseling, the continuation of medicines people were taking, and the provision of new medications, if needed. As the emergency recedes, greater attention can be paid to long-term treatment, counseling, and psychosocial support for dealing with mental health problems and the many disruptions that people have faced in their lives.[31] At that time, one can also turn additional attention to ensuring the appropriate medication of people with other non-communicable diseases.

CASE STUDIES

This chapter does not contain any case studies that have been based on careful review of the evidence about specific interventions. However, some comments follow on two CHEs of importance. One concerns the genocide in Rwanda and the plight of Rwandan refugees in Goma, in what is now the Democratic Republic of Congo. The other concerns a major earthquake that hit Pakistan in 2005. Both cases suggest some lessons for enhancing the global response to CHEs in the future.

Rwanda

In mid-July 1994, nearly one million Rwandan Hutus tried to escape persecution from the newly established government of Rwanda that was led by the Tutsis. The border town of Goma, in what is now the Democratic Republic of Congo, situated in the North Kivu region, became the entry point for the majority of the refugees. Many of them settled on Lake Kivu.[45]

Almost 50,000 people died in the first month after the start of the influx, largely as a result of an epidemic of cholera, which was followed by an epidemic of bacillary dysentery. In the first 17 days of the emergency, the average crude mortality rate of Rwandans was 28.1–44.9 per 10,000 per day, compared to the 0.6 per 10,000 per day in pre-war conditions inside Rwanda. This crude mortality rate is the highest by a considerable margin over the rate found in any previous CHE. In addition, in Goma, diarrheal disease affected young children and adults alike, whereas normally young children are much more severely affected than adults.[45]

Humanitarian assessments began in the first week of August, 3 weeks after the initial flow of refugees. Rapid surveys conducted in the three refugee camps of Katale, Kibumba, and Mugunga indicated that diarrheal disease contributed to 90% of deaths, that food shortages were prevalent, especially among female-headed households, and that acute malnutrition afflicted up to 23% of the refugees. In early August, a meningitis epidemic arose.[45]

The circumstances were complicated by the large numbers of people who fled to Goma in such a short period of time. In addition, the lake represented an easy source of water, but one from which disease could be spread. The soil around Goma was very rocky and it made it very difficult to construct an appropriate number of latrines. In addition, Hutu leaders were given control over distribution of relief but this did not provide for the equitable distribution of food that was hoped for.[45]

By early August, the response of the international community was beginning to have the desired effect, under the coordination of the UNHCR. A disease surveillance network was established. An information system was set up for the camps. 5 to 10 liters of safe water per day was distributed. Measles immunization was carried out, vitamin A supplements were distributed, and disease problems were attacked using standard protocols.[45]

Despite the exceptional efforts made by many people to deal with the crisis, the events in Goma highlighted a number of shortcomings of the response. First, there was a general lack of preparedness for dealing with this type of emergency, despite the well-known political instability of Rwanda. Second, the medical teams on the ground did not have the physical infrastructure or the experience needed for a task of this magnitude. Many of these staff, for example, were not as knowledgeable about oral rehydration as they needed to be, even though this is fundamental to treating diarrheal disease. Third, the work of the military forces that joined the effort was not integrated into the planning of the other work.[45]

Although the Goma crisis was exceptional in many ways, it does suggest a number of lessons for enhancing the response to CHEs in the future. These include the need to:

- Establish early warning systems for CHEs
- Prepare in advance for CHEs
- Strengthen the existing non-governmental groups with capability to respond to CHEs

The Earthquake in Pakistan

In early October 2005, Pakistan experienced an earthquake measuring 7.6 on the Richter scale. The epicenter was in Kashmir but the earthquake also devastated the North-West Frontier Province (NWFP). Within a matter of minutes, homes and livelihoods were destroyed, leaving over 3 million people homeless and many individuals buried under the rubble or injured by debris.[46]

It is estimated that 76,000 people, many of whom were children, lost their lives either from instantaneous death, such as severe head injury or internal bleeding, rapid death, such as asphyxia due to dust, or delayed death, such as wound infections. An additional 80,000 people were injured.[46] Moreover, 84% of the infrastructure in Kashmir, including 65% of all previously existing healthcare facilities, failed to withstand the seismic forces and collapsed. Thus, the immediate needs of the population included "winterized shelter, medical care, food and water, and sanitation facilities."[46]

To respond to the earthquake, the government of Pakistan created the Federal Relief Commission (FRC) and the Earthquake Rehabilitation and Reconstruction Authority (ERRA) that offered short- and long-term recovery efforts. Furthermore, a week after the initial earthquake, the government presented a plan for relief that included compensation for survivors. The World Bank, along with the Asian Development Bank, conducted assessments to identify vulnerable groups and areas that might hinder early recovery, such as unsanitary environments. Moreover, the South Asia Earthquake Flash Appeal (SAEFA) was created to receive donations for the recovery effort.

Doctors Without Borders (MSF) was an integral part of the interventions, as it provided emergency relief within a day of the earthquake, given that MSF medical teams were already on the ground in Kashmir. These teams focused initially on hygiene promotion, distributing tents, cookware and mattresses, and treating the injured. They administered 30,000 measles vaccines and later redirected attention to rebuilding medical infrastructure. In NWFP, MSF created hospitals with beds to house patients, as well as developed medical villages that were used to treat the overwhelming number of injured.

Despite national and international efforts to mobilize an effective response, injured individuals flooded hospitals that were still intact but which did not have the personnel or the equipment to respond effectively. Thus, many patients suffered more severe secondary complications due to prolonged waiting for medical treatment, a common characteristic when earthquakes significantly affect the medical system. [46,47]

Furthermore, small, remote villages remained inaccessible because of significant road damage. Given the impending winter, therefore, the Pakistani military, MSF, and UN agencies used helicopters to distribute basic relief. In addition, the government pledged the provision of tents. People inside and outside of Pakistan responded very generously with donations to help those affected by the disaster. However, many of the donations did not fit what was most needed.[46]

Several valuable lessons emerge from the efforts of the government and military of Pakistan and Pakistan's foreign partners to assist in the rescue and recovery from the earthquake. First, buildings in rural areas in seismic zones should be built or designed to decrease human injury. Second, governments should analyze existing risks to their ability to rapidly respond to emergencies and prepare emergency plans in advance that take those risks into account. Third, donations of materials and supplies should be managed carefully so that they fit real needs. Lastly, NGO expertise, like that provided by MSF in Pakistan, can be very helpful in addressing natural disasters, particularly if the involved organizations already have a presence in the affected country.[46,47]

FUTURE CHALLENGES IN MEETING THE HEALTH NEEDS OF DISASTERS

A number of critical challenges confront efforts to address the health effects of natural disasters and complex humanitarian emergencies. One such challenge for the future is how to prevent these from having such negative health impacts. It is difficult in resource-poor settings, many of which are poorly governed, to focus attention on the prevention of disasters and their impacts. Nonetheless, through better mitigation measures, such as water control, greater education of the community about how to deal with disasters, and having a disaster preparedness plan for which people are trained, it should be possible, even for very poor countries, to reduce deaths from natural disasters. If these steps are coupled with the development of standard approaches for dealing with health issues when they do arise and the forward staging of medicines, equipment, and materials near to disaster prone areas, it should be possible to reduce deaths from natural disasters, even in very low-income settings. Bangladesh, which is subject to annual flooding, has reduced the annual deaths from such floods, for example, with a series of the previously mentioned measures.[48]

There has been considerable progress among the international community in the establishment of common standards and protocols for responses to disasters. There remains, however, the need to enhance these further. Ideally, the organizations involved in responding to natural disasters and CHEs will:

- subscribe to a common set of norms, such as the Sphere Project
- have common protocols for dealing with key issues
- train their staff to work with those protocols
- work in close conjunction with the affected communities and local governments[49]

In addition, it is important that responses to disasters focus on cost-effective approaches to the provision of health-care services in emergencies. We have already seen that search and rescue assistance from abroad is not cost-effective. The same is true for most field hospitals. Moreover, many agencies have provided health services in emergencies that did not focus on immediate needs and that could have waited. Morbidity and mortality can be prevented and reduced more quickly if the agencies involved in disaster relief carefully set priorities for action that would be based on the principle of cost-effectiveness analysis, taking appropriate account of concerns for social justice and equity.[24,50,51]

The continued refinement of indicators that can be used to measure performance of services in disasters will be helpful to gauging the performance of local and international relief efforts.[50]

MAIN MESSAGES

Natural disasters and complex humanitarian emergencies are important causes of illness, death, and disability. They affect large numbers of people, have huge economic impact, and their aftereffects can go on for some time. Their biggest relative impact is on the poor, who are generally more vulnerable to the effects of these disasters than are better-off people. Some of these disasters are man-made. Some are slow-onset and some are rapid-onset.

Natural disasters, such as droughts, famines, hurricanes, typhoons, cyclones, and heavy rains have important health impacts. Earthquakes and volcanoes are also natural disasters with large potential effects on health. It appears that the number of natural disasters is increasing but the number of deaths from them is decreasing. More than 90% of deaths from natural disasters occur in low- and middle-income countries.

Some deaths are a direct result of natural disasters. However, the impact of those disasters on water supply and sanitation systems, health services, and availability of food can also, indirectly, lead to many more deaths. There are also special health problems associated with living in camps, which sometimes happen to those who survive natural disasters that displace many people from their homes.

In the late 1990s, there were about 40 CHEs each year. There are probably more than 14 million refugees in the world and more than 20 million internally displaced people. Overall, CHEs are associated with considerably larger health impacts than natural disasters. In addition, they may have an acute phase when large numbers of people flee and they generally go on for long periods of time.

Complex humanitarian emergencies have increasingly been linked to civil conflict. Like natural disasters, they also have direct and indirect impacts on health. They not only take lives directly through war-related trauma, but also they lead to the destruction of infrastructure. The health effects of some of these conflicts have been dramatic, sometimes because civilians have been targeted by combatants. Women are especially vulnerable in CHEs to sexual violence.

In the emergency phase of a CHE when large numbers of displaced persons are coming into camps, there are a number of health risks that have to be addressed. Among the most important are diarrhea, measles, malaria, and pneumonia. Malnutrition is also of exceptional importance. Cholera epidemics can also arise and kill large numbers of people quickly.

Countries at risk can take a number of measures to mitigate vulnerability to damage from natural disasters. This could include preparing a disaster plan, building seawalls and levees, and requiring, for example, that buildings in earthquake prone areas are earthquake proof. It might also be cost-effective to strengthen other infrastructure, such as water supply systems so that they can withstand important threats.

Addressing the health impacts of a natural disaster requires that the health situation be assessed quickly and that urgent cases be handled immediately. Less urgent problems can be handled in the following days, weeks, and months. Long-term support for those psychologically affected by the disaster will also need to be provided in the medium and long term.

The health situation of a CHE also needs to be assessed quickly and continuously. Early attention in dealing with large numbers of displaced people must focus on the environment, shelter, water, and food. The next step is the prevention of disease outbreaks and their treatment if they do occur. Particular attention must be paid to malnutrition, measles, pneumonia, and malaria. Some immediate attention will also have to be paid to a minimum package of reproductive health services and the avoidance of HIV. As the acute phase of the emergency subsides, more attention can be paid to TB, overall primary health care, non-communicable diseases, and longer-term mental health issues.

There has been some important progress in the coordination and standardization of measures to address CHEs and natural disasters. However, there are still gaps in the preparation and training of staff in some organizations. In addition, there has been inadequate attention to the cost-effectiveness of interventions. There is now enough information about the lessons of CHEs and natural disasters that the priority actions that are needed should be clear and organizations active in relief work need to concentrate their efforts on what will prevent the most deaths, disability, and morbidity, at least cost, with due attention to concerns for social justice.

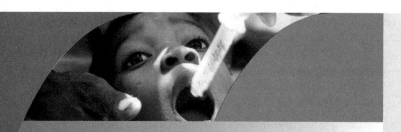

Study Questions

1. How does the annual burden of disease from natural disasters and complex humanitarian emergencies compare with other causes of illness, death, and disability?

2. What is a disaster? A natural disaster? A complex humanitarian emergency?

3. What is an internally displaced person? A refugee? What are the differences between them?

4. What have been some of the most significant natural disasters in the last decade? How many deaths were associated with them? How did people die? How did deaths vary for different types of disasters by age and sex?

5. What countries in Sub-Saharan Africa have been the largest sources of displaced people? What countries in Sub-Saharan Africa have received the largest numbers of refugees?

6. In the early stages of a complex humanitarian emergency, what are likely to be the most significant health concerns for the refugees? How do those health concerns change over time? Who are the most affected by malnutrition, measles, pneumonia, and cholera?

7. In what ways are women especially vulnerable during complex humanitarian emergencies? What problems do they face as a consequence of these vulnerabilities?

8. What are key steps that can be taken to reduce the vulnerability of certain places to the potential health threats of natural disasters?

9. What are key steps that need to be taken within the first few days of people fleeing to a refugee camp? How do those concerns change over time?

10. How can one try to ensure that relief agencies work together around a common framework and that they focus on the most cost-effective activities?

REFERENCES

1. National Highway Transportation Safety Authority. Glossary. Available at: Available at: http://www.nhtsa.dot.gov/people/injury/ems/emstraumasystem03/glossary.htm. Accessed September 29, 2006.

2. Pearson Prentice Hall. Glossary. Available at: http://www.nhtsa.dot.gov/people/injury/ems/emstraumasystem03/glossary.htm. Accessed September 29, 2006.

3. ILSI Risk Science Institute. Food Safety Risk Assesment. Available at: http://www.fsra.net/glossary.html. Accessed October 13, 2006.

4. Burkholder BT, Toole MJ. Evolution of complex disasters. *The Lancet.* 1995(346):1012–1015.

5. Toole MJ, Waldman RJ. The public health aspects of complex emergencies and refugee situations. *Annu Rev Public Health.* 1997;18:285.

6. Wikipedia. Refugee. Available at: http://en.wikipedia.org/wiki/Refugees. Accessed September 29, 2006.

7. Wikipedia. Internally Displaced Person. Available at: http://en.wikipedia.org/wiki/Internally_displaced_person. Accessed September 29, 2006.

8. Brennan RJ, Nandy R. Complex humanitarian emergencies: a major global health challenge. *Emerg Med (Fremantle).* 2001;13(2):149.

9. Last JM. *A Dictionary of Epidemiology.* 4th ed. New York: Oxford University Press; 2001:47.

10. The White Ribbon Alliance. Glossary: Case Fatality Rate. Available at: http://www.whiteribbonalliance.org/Resources/default.cfm?a0=Glossary. Accessed November 9, 2006.

11. de Ville de Goyet C, Zapata Marti R, Osorio C. Natural disaster mitigation and relief. In: Jamison DT, Breman JG, Measham AR, et al., eds. *Disease Control Priorities in Developing Countries.* 2nd ed. New York: Oxford University Press; 2006:1148.

12. de Ville de Goyet C, Zapata Marti R, Osorio C. Natural disaster mitigation and relief. In: Jamison DT, Breman JG, Measham AR, et al., eds. *Disease Control Priorities in Developing Countries.* 2nd ed. New York: Oxford University Press; 2006:1149.

13. Brennan RJ, Nandy R. Complex humanitarian emergencies: a major global health challenge. *Emerg Med (Fremantle).* 2001;13(2):149–150.

14. Hansch S, Burkholder B. When chaos reigns. *Harvard Int Rev.* 1996;18(4):10–14.

15. Brennan RJ, Nandy R. Complex humanitarian emergencies: a major global health challenge. *Emerg Med (Fremantle).* 2001;13(2):148–149.

16. Toole MJ, Waldman RJ. The public health aspects of complex emergencies and refugee situations. *Annu Rev Public Health.* 1997;18:283–312.

17. de Ville de Goyet C, Zapata Marti R, Osorio C. Natural disaster mitigation and relief. In: Jamison DT, Breman JG, Measham AR, et al., eds. *Disease Control Priorities in Developing Countries.* 2nd ed. New York: Oxford University Press; 2006:1149–1150.

18. de Ville de Goyet C, Zapata Marti R, Osorio C. Natural disaster mitigation and relief. In: Jamison DT, Breman JG, Measham AR, et al., eds. *Disease Control Priorities in Developing Countries.* 2nd ed. New York: Oxford University Press; 2006:1150.

19. Brennan RJ, Nandy R. Complex humanitarian emergencies: a major global health challenge. *Emerg Med (Fremantle).* 2001;13(2):151.

20. Lopez AD, Mathers CD, Murray CJL. The burden of disease and mortality by condition: data, methods, and results for 2001. In: Lopez AD, Mathers CD, Ezzati M, Jamison DT, Murray CJL, eds. *Global burden of disease and risk factors.* New York: Oxford University Press; 2006:45–240.

21. Zwi AB, Ugalde A. Political violence in the Third World: a public health issue. *Health Policy Plan.* 1991;6:203–217.

22. Personal communication, Waldman RJ to Skolnik R, March 2007.

23. UN Children's Fund. *The State of the World's Children.* New York: United Nations; 1994.

24. Waldman RJ. Prioritising health care in complex emergencies. *Lancet.* 2001;357(9266):1427–1429.

25. Brennan RJ, Nandy R. Complex humanitarian emergencies: a major global health challenge. *Emerg Med (Fremantle).* 2001;13(2):152.

26. Toole MJ, Waldman RJ. The public health aspects of complex emergencies and refugee situations. *Annu Rev Public Health.* 1997;18:295.

27. Toole MJ, Waldman RJ. The public health aspects of complex emergencies and refugee situations. *Annu Rev Public Health.* 1997;18:297.

28. Marsh M, Purdin S, Navani S. Addressing sexual violence in humanitarian emergencies. *Global Public Health.* 2006;1(2):138.

29. Ager A. Psychosocial needs in complex emergencies. *Lancet.* 2003;360:43–44.

30. Almedom A, Summerfield D. Mental well-being in settings of complex emergency: an overview. *JBiosocial Sci.* 2004;36:381–388.

31. Mollica RF, Cardozo BL, Osofsky HJ, Raphael B, Ager A, Salama P. Mental health in complex emergencies. *Lancet.* 2004;364(9450):2058–2067.

32. Mollica RF, Cardozo BL, Osofsky HJ, Raphael B, Ager A, Salama P. Mental health in complex emergencies. *Lancet.* 2004;364(9450):2061.

33. de Ville de Goyet C, Zapata Marti R, Osorio C. Natural disaster mitigation and relief. In: Jamison DT, Breman JG, Measham AR, et al., eds. *Disease Control Priorities in Developing Countries.* 2nd ed. New York: Oxford University Press; 2006:1154.

34. de Ville de Goyet C, Zapata Marti R, Osorio C. Natural disaster mitigation and relief. In: Jamison DT, Breman JG, Measham AR, et al., eds. *Disease Control Priorities in Developing Countries.* 2nd ed. New York: Oxford University Press; 2006:1155.

35. de Ville de Goyet C, Zapata Marti R, Osorio C. Natural disaster mitigation and relief. In: Jamison DT, Breman JG, Measham AR, et al., eds. *Disease Control Priorities in Developing Countries.* 2nd ed. New York: Oxford University Press; 2006:1157.

36. Toole MJ, Waldman RJ. The public health aspects of complex emergencies and refugee situations. *Annu Rev Public Health.* 1997;18:300.

37. Toole MJ, Waldman RJ. The public health aspects of complex emergencies and refugee situations. *Annu Rev Public Health.* 1997;18:302.

38. Brennan RJ, Nandy R. Complex humanitarian emergencies: a major global health challenge. *Emerg Med (Fremantle).* 2001;13(2):153.

39. Toole MJ, Waldman RJ. The public health aspects of complex emergencies and refugee situations. *Annu Rev Public Health.* 1997;18:296.

40. The Sphere Project. Minimum standards in health services. *The Sphere Handbook 2004: Humanitarian Charter and Minimum Standards in Disaster Response.* Geneva: Oxfam Publishing; 2004:249–312.

41. The Sphere Project. Minimum standards in water supply, sanitation, and hygiene promotion. *The Sphere Handbook 2004: Humanitarian Charter and Minimum Standards in Disaster Response.* Geneva: Oxfam Publishing; 2004:51–102.

42. The Sphere Project. Minimum standards in shelter, settlements, and non-food items. *The Sphere Handbook 2004: Humanitarian Charter and Minimum Standards in Disaster Response.* Geneva: Oxfam Publishing; 2004:203–248.

43. Toole MJ, Waldman RJ. The public health aspects of complex emergencies and refugee situations. *Annu Rev Public Health.* 1997;18:303–304.

44. Krasue SK, Meyers JL, Friedlander E. Improving the availability of emergency obstetric care in conflict-afffected settings. *Global Public Health.* 2006;1(3):229–248.

45. Goma Epidemiology Group. Public health impact of Rwandan refugee crisis: what happened in Goma, Zaire, in July 1994? *Lancet.* 1995 1995;345(8946):339–344.

46. Medicins Sans Frontieres. South Asian Earthquake: 6-month Overview of MSF Operations MSF Response to the Disaster. Available at: http://www.doctorswithoutborders.org/news/2006/04–21–2006.cfm. Accessed February 25, 2007.

47. Noji EK. Earthquakes. In: Noji EK, ed. *The Public Health Consequences of Disasters.* New York: Oxford University Press; 1997.

48. ICDDRB Center for Health and Population Research. Documenting effects of the July–August floods of 2004 and ICDDR,B's response. *Health Sci Bulletin.* 2004;2(3).

49. The Sphere Project. *The Sphere Handbook 2004: Humanitarian Charter and Minimum Standards in Disaster Response.* Geneva: Oxfam Publishing; 2004.

50. Spiegel P, Sheik M, Gotway-Crawford C, Salama P. Health programmes and policies associated with decreased mortality in displaced people in postemergency phase camps: a retrospective study. *Lancet.* 2002;360(9349):1927–1934.

51. de Ville de Goyet C, Zapata Marti R, Osorio C. Natural disaster mitigation and relief. In: Jamison DT, Breman JG, Measham AR, et al., eds. *Disease Control Priorities in Developing Countries.* 2nd ed. New York: Oxford University Press; 2006:1147–1162.

CHAPTER 15

Working Together to Improve Global Health

LEARNING OBJECTIVES

By the end of this chapter the reader will be able to:

- Discuss the value of cooperation in addressing health problems
- Discuss the most important types of cooperative action in global health
- Describe the major organizational actors in global health and their focuses
- Discuss the rationale for the creation of public-private partnerships for health
- Outline the key challenges to enhancing cooperative action in global health

VIGNETTES

The world came close to eradicating polio in 2004. However, in 2005, polio spread from Northern Nigeria to a number of other African countries, due to a failure to immunize children in Northern Nigeria by some groups. By July 2005, polio cases had moved from Africa to Saudi Arabia and Indonesia, and then began appearing in Angola, which had not had a case of polio since 2001. By September 2005, cases appeared in Somalia, which had also been free of polio for several years.[1] Stopping new cases of polio and preventing it from spreading from one country to another requires a global effort to correctly identify polio cases and then immediately carry out special immunization campaigns.

About nine million people worldwide suffer from tuberculosis, which is one of the leading causes of deaths of adults in the developing world. The number of TB cases worldwide, as noted in Chapter 11, has grown with the spread of HIV, and 13% of the deaths of people with AIDS are due to TB.[2] Despite the importance of TB, however, no new drugs for TB have been developed since the 1960s.[3] TB is a disease that largely affects poor people in low- and middle-income countries. These people have little money to spend on drugs and there is minimal economic incentive for pharmaceutical companies to develop new TB drugs. Can actors in global health work together to encourage the development of new drugs for TB and other neglected diseases? What would they have to do to encourage public and private sector investment in such drugs? What would they have to do to ensure investors that if they are able to develop such drugs that there will be a market for them?

Vaccines are among the most cost-effective investments in health. For young children in the developing countries, there are six basic vaccines. There are also other vaccines that would be cost-effective in some countries, including the vaccines for hepatitis B and for Haemophilus influenza type B. Yet, throughout the 1990s there were important gaps in coverage of the six basic vaccines in the poorest countries. In addition, the rate of coverage was actually going down in some countries.[4] Although the hepatitis B vaccine began to be widely used in developed countries in the 1980s, almost 20 years later it is still rarely used in developing countries. The main reasons behind this failure include limited money for immunization, a lack of the infrastructure needed to carry out effective immunization programs, and a lack of political interest in immunization. In 2000, a number of governments, foundations, and individuals established the Global Alliance for Vaccines and Immunization (GAVI), the aim of which is to provide financing and technical assistance to dramatically improve vaccine coverage and the spread of new vaccines. So far, GAVI has been involved in enhancing immunization coverage in a number of low-income countries.[5]

INTRODUCTION

This chapter focuses on how different actors work together to enhance global health. First, it discusses the importance of such cooperation. The chapter then has an extensive review of the key organizational actors in global health activities. Third, the chapter examines the roles in cooperation of different types of organizations. The chapter then outlines how the global health agenda is set and how that agenda has evolved historically. The chapter concludes with an assessment of some of the future challenges to cooperative action and a case study on one of the most successful global health efforts to date.

COOPERATING TO IMPROVE GLOBAL HEALTH[6,7]

There are a number of reasons why different actors cooperate in global health activities and why such cooperation is in everyone's interest. First is the value of cooperating to create consensus around and advocate on behalf of different health causes.[6,7] Although health is an extremely important issue for both individuals and societies, it does not always receive the political, economic, and financial support that it should. A good example of this is the lack of attention by many countries to nutrition, despite the poor nutritional status of their people. The impact of advocacy efforts is likely to be much greater if numerous actors, across organizations and across countries, work together to promote important health causes. This has been evident in the field of HIV, for example, where AIDS activists worldwide have been able to work together to promote the treatment of people who are HIV-positive with anti-retroviral drugs.

The need to share knowledge and to set global standards for health activities are other reasons for cooperation in the global health field. It has become clear from trials of different anti-malarial drugs, for example, that some drug regimens for malaria are more effective than others. This knowledge is especially important because some malaria has become resistant to what has been standard treatment. If lessons like this are to be shared globally, then it is important that technical standards be developed and disseminated by an organization that countries believe is technically sound and internationally representative. As you will read later, helping to define and promulgate such standards is one of the main functions of the World Health Organization.

Another important reason for cooperation to achieve global health aims is the fact that many aspects of global health are "global public goods." Thus, it is only through cooperative efforts that the world can ensure that a sufficient amount of these goods are produced and shared. Individual countries, for example, may not have an interest in reducing pollution generated within their borders that causes health problems in adjacent countries, and it is only through collective action that countries will be able to address such problems. A similar issue arises with respect to efforts to reduce the burden of communicable diseases. Individual countries may have little incentive to take the measures needed to effectively address some communicable diseases, despite the fact that the spread of these diseases does not respect national boundaries. Efforts to deal with them, therefore, require cooperative efforts across countries.

The surveillance of disease also has many aspects of a "global public good" and requires cooperation among many actors to be successful. It is important for all countries to work together to monitor the appearance of diseases and to fashion approaches to dealing with them. Surveillance by individual countries, for example, is not sufficient to stem the spread of disease *across* countries. The global effort to address the SARS problem in 2003 is an excellent example of the need for close collaboration among countries on surveillance.[8]

Cooperation to achieve better global health outcomes can also take place to assist in financing health efforts in poorer countries. There are multiple motivations for this aid. In one case, wealthier countries may contribute out of humanitarian concern for the well being of less fortunate people. Richer countries may also wish to assist in addressing these problems because of "enlightened self-interest." In an age of travel and extensive contacts among people of different countries, governments may be concerned that the health problems of developing countries will endanger their own people if not properly tackled. Many low-income countries, for example, have high burdens of TB but may not have the financial, technical, or institutional resources needed to combat TB effectively. Yet, TB can endanger both their population and that of other countries. Thus, it is in everyone's interest for developed countries to provide financial and technical assistance to developing countries to deal effectively with diseases such as TB.

KEY ACTORS IN GLOBAL HEALTH

Besides governments, there are many different actors involved in global health activities. Some of these are international organizations with a global reach. Others are organizations that work globally but are based in individual countries. Some are public organizations. A number are private and for profit, while others are private but operate on a not-for-profit basis. Foundations are also actively involved in global health activities. Increasingly, there are also organizations that bring the public and private sectors together to work cooperatively on a global health problem. The next section discusses some of the most important organizations that are involved in global health and examples of how they operate in that field.

In considering action on global health, it is valuable to remember that actors may play one or more of several possible roles at a time. They could, for example, engage in advocacy. They could also participate in knowledge sharing and technical assistance. In addition, they might provide financing for health efforts. Table 15-1 lists some of the most important actors in the global health field.

The discussion further examines the nature of these actors and their major contribution to the global health agenda. You should note, however, that this discussion is only introductory. It is meant to outline the stated aims in global health of those organizations. It is beyond the scope of this book to examine such work critically. Considerable information is available for those of you wishing to examine global health actors and cooperation in this field more analytically. [9–12]

Agencies of the United Nations

There are a number of United Nations (UN) agencies that work on health and focus on a specific set of public health concerns. Among the most important are the World Health Organization, the United Nations Children's Fund, the United Nations Fund for Population Activities, and the United Nations Development Program. This section will examine the two UN agencies most involved in health, the World Health Organization and the United Nations Children's Fund.

The World Health Organization

The World Health Organization (WHO) was established in 1948 and is the United Nations agency that is responsible for health. [13] The headquarters of WHO is located in Geneva, Switzerland, and WHO employs about 3500 people, including experts on many health topics. The World Health Organization has offices located in each region of the world,

---

TABLE 15-1 Selected Organizational Actors in Global Health, by Type of Organization

United Nations Agencies
UNAIDS
UNDP
UNFPA
UNICEF
WHO

Multilateral Development Banks
African Development Bank
Asian Development Bank
Inter-American Development Bank
World Bank

Bilateral Development Assistance Agencies
Australian Agency for International Development
Canadian International Development Agency
Danish International Development Agency
Department for International Development of the UK
Dutch Agency for Development Cooperation
United States Agency for International Development

Foundations
The Bill & Melinda Gates Foundation
The Rockefeller Foundation

WHO Related Partnerships
Global Alliance for the Elimination of Leprosy
Roll Back Malaria
Stop TB
Tropical Disease Research Program

Non-Governmental Organizations
CARE
Catholic Relief Services
Doctors Without Borders
OXFAM
Save the Children

Other Special Programs
Global Alliance for Vaccines & Immunization
Global Fund to Fight Against AIDS, TB, & Malaria

Public-Private Partnerships for Health
Global Alliance for TB Drug Development
International AIDS Vaccine Initiative
International Partnership on Microbicides
Malaria Vaccine Initiative

Source: The Author

with special responsibility for work within that geographic area, as shown in Table 15-2. In addition, WHO has a country office in almost all poor countries and in many other countries in which important health efforts or reforms of the health sector are taking place.[13]

The objective of WHO is to promote "the attainment by all peoples of the highest possible level of health."[13] In pursuit of this goal, WHO largely focuses its attention on the following:

- Advocacy and consensus building for various health causes, such as HIV and TB.
- Sharing health knowledge across countries, through studies, reports, conferences, and other forums. The publication of the *World Health Report* on a different topic of global health importance each year is an example of this work.
- Carrying out selected critical public health functions within an international forum, such as the surveillance of epidemics, including influenza, or the outbreak of potentially dangerous diseases, such as Ebola. This also includes, for example, WHO certification of quality standards for the manufacturing of vaccines and pharmaceuticals.
- Setting global standards on key health matters, such as appropriate regimens for drug therapy for leprosy, TB, and HIV.
- Leading the development of international agreements and conventions, such as the Framework Convention on Tobacco Control.
- The provision of technical assistance to its member states, such as helping China to contain the outbreak of SARS or assistance to countries in managing their child vaccine programs.

TABLE 15-2 WHO Regional Offices

Regional Office	Location
The Americas	Washington, DC, USA
Europe	Copenhagen, Denmark
North Africa and the Middle East	Alexandria, Egypt
Sub-Saharan Africa	Harare, Zimbabwe
Southeast Asia	Delhi, India
Western Pacific	Manila, Philippines

Source: Data from World Health Organization. About WHO. Available at: http://www.who.int/about/en/. Accessed on November 3, 2006.

- Serving as the secretariat of a number of cooperative efforts, such as Stop TB, Roll Back Malaria, and the Global Alliance to Eliminate Leprosy.

WHO is primarily a technical agency that engages in advocacy and the sharing of knowledge. Although WHO does have relatively small country budgets to assist in the financing of selected health projects in low- and middle-income countries, it is not a financing agency. Rather, the work that WHO does both globally and in particular countries is largely financed with assistance from the high-income countries.

WHO is governed through its annual World Health Assembly, which sets policy, reviews and approves the budget, and appoints the Director-General of the organization. Voting power at the WHO Health Assembly is based on the principle of "one country–one vote." The overall budget of WHO comes from membership subscriptions and from special donations, again, mostly from better-off countries.

The WHO has helped lead some of the world's most important cooperative efforts in health, including the "Health for All" effort[14] that began with the Declaration of Alma Ata on primary health care. WHO also led the world's smallpox eradication campaign, has played a major role in efforts to expand the coverage of immunization for children in developing countries, and is one of the leaders of the world's global polio eradication program. More recently, WHO has been instrumental in helping to address issues of tobacco control. WHO also leads the global surveillance of disease and has played an active role in work on avian flu, SARS, and other new and emerging diseases, such as the Ebola virus. Additional, more analytical, comments on the work of WHO are cited in the endnotes.[10,11,15,16]

UNICEF

The United Nations Children's Fund was established in 1946 by the UN to respond to the effects of World War II on children in Europe and China. UNICEF is headquartered in New York but has offices in more than 125 countries.[17] The main function of UNICEF is to enhance the health and well being of children. In these efforts, UNICEF has been deeply involved in the promotion of family planning, antenatal care, and safe motherhood practices.

UNICEF is involved in a wide range of activities in support of its mission, including advocacy, knowledge generation and knowledge sharing, and the financing of investments in health. In addition, UNICEF works closely with other development partners such as WHO and the World Bank to help raise the health status of poor women and children globally. UNICEF has carried out significant programs in a number of areas. Traditionally, it has been involved in major ways in nutrition and early childhood development issues, in which it is generally considered the world's leader. Immunization and child survival have also been areas of deep UNICEF involvement. In addition, UNICEF has been a major supporter of primary education, especially for poor girls in low- and middle-income countries. More recently, UNICEF has paid particular attention to child protection, child rights, and HIV/AIDS.[18]

UNICEF has an Executive Board of 36 members who guide all UNICEF work and administration under the leadership of the Executive Director. All of UNICEF's funding is from voluntary contributions; governments provide two thirds of funding while 37 National Committees, consisting of private entities and millions of individuals, raise the remaining third. These National Committees are non-governmental organizations (NGOs) that advocate for children, sell UNICEF products, and fundraise through several well known campaigns, such as "Check out for Children" in grocery stores, "Change for Good" on airplanes, and "Trick or Treat for UNICEF" on Halloween.[19]

UNAIDS

In 1996, six agencies joined forces to launch UNAIDS—the Joint United Nations Program on HIV/AIDS. Today, as shown in Table 15-3, there are 10 co-sponsors for UNAIDS.[20]

UNAIDS is based in Geneva, Switzerland, has offices in more than 70 countries, and is guided by a Program Coordinating Board that consists of 22 representatives from country governments, its co-sponsors, and 5 NGOs.

UNAIDS is the global agency with primary responsibility for dealing with HIV/AIDS. UNAIDS monitors and evaluates the epidemic and the world's response to it. It also advocates on behalf of the epidemic and engages civil society, the private sector, and development partners in the fight against HIV/AIDS. In addition, UNAIDS generates and shares knowledge, sets standards, and mobilizes resources. UNAIDS focuses it attention on the regions of the world most affected by HIV/AIDS, particularly Sub-Saharan Africa.[21]

Another important emphasis of the work of UNAIDS is to assist countries in developing and implementing national AIDS plans. The co-sponsors financially support the preparation of these plans. For instance, in 2002 the World Bank and other UN agencies provided over $1 billion to assist countries with the development and implementation of their national AIDS plans.[22,23] Technical experts from UNAIDS also help countries build their technical and institutional capacity and mobilize resources to fight against HIV/AIDS. UNAIDS, for example, assists countries in preparing applications for fund-

TABLE 15-3 UNAIDS Co-Sponsors

- International Labor Organization
- Office of the United Nations High Commissioner for Refugees
- UNICEF
- United Nations Development Program
- United Nations Educational, Scientific, and Cultural Organization
- United Nations Population Fund
- United Nations Office on Drugs and Crime
- World Bank
- World Food Program
- World Health Organization

Source: UNAIDS. Available at: http://www.unaids.org/en/AboutUNAIDS/Cosponsors_about/default.asp. Accessed November 3, 2006.

ing from the Global Fund to Fight Against AIDS, TB, and Malaria, which is discussed further later.[21]

UNAIDS is engaged in a range of HIV/AIDS activities. First, UNAIDS works with countries to strengthen their surveillance of the epidemic. Second, UNAIDS continues to put an important emphasis on prevention of HIV. Third, UNAIDS is also increasingly involved in efforts to increase the number of HIV-positive people worldwide who are treated with anti-retroviral therapy. UNAIDS has a particular concern for the extent to which the epidemic affects females. In addition, UNAIDS cooperates with others in the search for technologies, such as microbicides and vaccines, that might be able to help halt the epidemic.

Multilateral Development Banks

There are a number of development banks that lend or grant money to developing countries and economies in transition to help promote their economic and social development. These banks are owned by all of their member countries and they are referred to as "multilateral." These institutions have some characteristics of real banks. However, these banks do not function to earn money through their lending operations. Rather, their main focus is to serve as a financial intermediary. Essentially, they channel financial resources from more developed countries and their people through bond sales and grants to help finance development activities in low- and middle-income countries and countries that are making the transition to more open, market-based, economies. All of these banks are involved in work on health, to at least some degree, but the ones most involved are the African Development Bank, the Asian Development Bank, the Inter-American Development Bank, and the World Bank.

Among the multilateral development banks, the World Bank is the largest, has the broadest scope of activities, and is the most involved in health.[24] The World Bank is located in Washington, DC, and is "owned" by more than 180 member countries. The stated aim of the World Bank is to assist countries in improving the lives of their people and reducing poverty. It seeks to do this by helping them to strengthen the management of their economy and to finance investments in selected areas, including agriculture, transport, private sector development, health, and education. The World Bank lends money at reduced rates to countries with per capita incomes above a certain point, lends money interest free to the poorest countries, and also provides grants to some countries for special activities that affect the poor, such as HIV/AIDS. The Bank lends about $20 billion per year and has more than 10,000 staff who work in Washington and in the Bank's offices in a large number of other countries that receive development assistance from the World Bank.[25]

In its health work, the Bank carries out a wide range of functions. It advocates on behalf of important causes, generates and disseminates information and knowledge about key health issues, provides technical assistance to countries, and finances specific investments in health and related work in nutrition and family planning. The World Bank focuses its health work largely on the links between health and poverty. It pays considerable attention to the development of health systems. In public health, the Bank has emphasized nutrition, maternal and child health, HIV/AIDS, malaria, TB, and tobacco control.

The Bank is also a partner in a number of global health initiatives, including GAVI, Stop TB, Roll Back Malaria,

and UNAIDS. In addition, the World Bank has provided financing to other initiatives, such as the International AIDS Vaccine Initiative (IAVI). The Bank over the last few years has provided about $15 billion of financing for its health related work[26] and, until the advent of the Bill & Melinda Gates Foundation, it has been the largest financier of investments in health in resource poor settings. Those interested in a more analytical assessment of the World Bank's work both generally and in health can consult extensive literature on those subjects.

Bilateral Agencies

Another set of organizations that are very actively involved in global health are bilateral agencies. These are mostly the development assistance agencies of developed countries that work directly with developing countries to help them enhance the health of their people. Some of the bilateral development agencies that are most involved in the health sector are shown in Table 15-4.

USAID is the development assistance agency of the U.S. federal government. USAID promotes U.S. foreign policy goals by advancing economic and social development all over the world. USAID works with other governments and with universities, businesses, international agencies, and NGOs to support its development assistance efforts. In the health field, USAID engages in a wide variety of activities, including advocacy for global health, the generation and sharing of knowledge, and the financing of health investments.

USAID is headquartered in Washington, DC, and has regional field offices for Sub-Saharan Africa, Asia and the Near East, Latin America and the Caribbean, and Europe and Eurasia. In addition to these geographic bureaus, USAID has functional bureaus for Economic Growth, Agriculture and Trade, Democracy, Conflict Prevention and Humanitarian Assistance, and Global Health. USAID has offices in many countries, especially poorer countries in Africa, Asia, and Latin America.

USAID's Bureau for Global Health aims to improve health services and enhance the health status of poor and disadvantaged people, particularly in poorer countries. USAID focuses its health work on maternal and child health, HIV/AIDS, other communicable diseases, family planning and reproductive health, nutrition, and health systems. For these purposes, USAID provides grants and technical expertise to other governments, NGOs, and the private sector. In supporting the development of health in other countries, USAID collaborates with other development assistance agencies.[27]

In the 1970s and 1980s, USAID helped support research to develop a number of interventions that are key to saving

TABLE 15-4 Selected Bilateral Development Assistance Agencies Involved in Global Health

Australian Agency for International Development
Canadian International Development Agency
Danish International Development Agency
Department for International Development of the United Kingdom
Dutch Agency for Development Cooperation
United States Agency for International Development

Source: The Author

the lives of poor children in the poorer countries, including oral rehydration therapy, vitamin A supplementation, and immunizations. USAID has also been very supportive of efforts to address malaria, TB, and, most recently, HIV/AIDS. Traditionally, USAID has also been very involved in supporting family planning.

Foundations

Global health has been an area in which foundations have been involved for more than a century. The Rockefeller Foundation[28] and the Ford Foundation[29] have been among the most involved in this field. More recently, the Soros Foundation became involved in health activities in the former Soviet Union. The Soros Foundation[30] focuses largely on the promotion of democracy but became involved in health when it realized the threat that HIV, TB, and drug-resistant TB posed to political and economic stability in this region. Most recently, the Bill & Melinda Gates Foundation has emerged as an extremely important actor in the field of global health. The section below examines the role in global health played by the Rockefeller Foundation, which has historically been the most important foundation involved in health, and the Gates Foundation, which has recently taken the lead in a number of global health areas.

The Rockefeller Foundation

The Rockefeller Foundation is based in New York City and has regional offices in San Francisco, California, Bangkok, Thailand, and Nairobi, Kenya. The foundation aims to "enrich and sustain the lives and livelihoods of poor and excluded people throughout the world."[24] In the health field, the foundation seeks to "reduce avoidable unfair differences in the health status of populations."[28]

The Rockefeller Foundation has focused considerable attention on the development of knowledge and technology that can be applied to addressing the conditions that most affect the health of the poor globally. The Rockefeller Foundation was instrumental in establishing the first schools of public health in the United States and was also deeply involved in the development of a vaccine against yellow fever. The Rockefeller Foundation does finance a small amount of activities in health every year. However, its strength as an organization is the way in which it uses a relatively small amount of money to invest in the generation of knowledge that can make an important difference to the health of the poor globally.

More recently, the Rockefeller Foundation has focused it attention in the health field in three areas. First, the foundation established the framework for developing partnerships between the public and private sector to meet key health needs that had been neglected. In line with this work, the foundation was instrumental in establishing the first and then a number of additional public-private partnerships for health, including the International AIDS Vaccine Initiative, the International Partnership on Microbicides, and the Global Alliance for TB Drug Development. Second, it has tried to help better understand the problems that HIV/AIDS inflicts on families and how they might deal with those problems. Third, the foundation has helped to "strengthen the production, deployment, and empowerment" of key human resources needed for delivering health services in poor countries.[28]

The Bill & Melinda Gates Foundation

The most substantial change in many years in the key actors involved in global health has been the advent of the Bill & Melinda Gates Foundation. The Gates Foundation is based in the United States in Seattle, Washington. The main aims of the foundation in the health field are to help spread known technologies for improving health, such as immunization, to the places where they are most in need. At the same time, the foundation seeks to encourage the development of new technologies that can meet the major health needs of the poor globally. The foundation hopes to meet these aims by "supporting discoveries and inventions essential to solving major global health problems, supporting the development and testing of specific tools and technologies, and helping to ensure that new health interventions and technologies are adopted in the developing world."[31] The foundation has become one of the major financiers of global health efforts. The foundation has an endowment of over $30 billion and it will grow to almost $60 billion with pledged gifts from an American financier.[32] From its establishment in 2002 to 2005, the foundation had provided almost $3.6 billion in grants for health activities.[31]

To a large extent, the foundation has focused its grants in four areas. First, it has paid particular attention to communicable diseases, since they are such an important cause of death for the poor globally. In these areas, it has been particularly involved in financing efforts in AIDS, TB, and malaria. It has supported with major grants, for example, the establishment of AIDS initiatives in Africa and in India, the Global Fund to Fight Against AIDS, TB, and Malaria, the International AIDS Vaccine Initiative, and the International Partnership on Microbicides. Another important area for the foundation is reproductive health, for which it granted $60 million to the Johns Hopkins University to improve reproductive health programs globally.[33] The foundation has also been a major financier of a variety of partnerships and initiatives aimed at key global health problems, including the Vaccine Fund and GAVI to support immunizations, the Global Alliance for Improved Nutrition (GAIN), and an initiative to save the lives of very young children called "Saving Newborn Lives." The foundation gave $750 million to the Vaccine Fund alone. Finally, the foundation has placed major emphasis on encouraging scientific discoveries and their application to the health problems of the poor globally through its program on the "Grand Challenges in Global Health," for which it has provided more than $400 million.[32]

NON-GOVERNMENTAL ORGANIZATIONS

There are thousands of NGOs in the world today that have as one of their primary aims the improvement of the health of poor people in developing countries. Most of these organizations raise money from private sources or receive grants from governments or global health partnerships which they help to invest in activities that address important health issues, such as improving the availability of clean water, strengthening nutrition and immunization programs, or enhancing programs for the treatment of TB and HIV. Some of the organizations are small and focus their attention only on a limited number of activities. Other organizations are very large, comprehensive in the topics they cover, and global in their reach. Some NGOs will be completely secular, while others will be faith-based. Some of the most important NGOs that operate internationally on health are listed in Table 15-5.

Some additional comments are noted later on Save the Children and Doctors Without Borders, which are two of the most important NGOs that work on health globally. These are just two examples of the hundreds of large NGOs and thousands of small NGOs that are involved in health efforts in low- and middle-income countries.

Save the Children

Save the Children was established in 1932 in New York City by a group of people who wanted to help meet the needs of poor people in the Appalachian region of the United States who had been hurt by an economic depression. Today, it is part of an international alliance of related organizations and it one of the largest NGOs in the world. One affiliate of Save the Children is based in the United States in Westport, Connecticut. It is actively involved in relief and development work in a number of areas in health. Save the Children focuses its attention on working with poor families and communities to identify their most important health and development needs. It then addresses these needs in ways that seek to contribute to individual and community self-sufficiency.[34]

Save the Children (U.S.) is involved in efforts to improve health in more than 30 countries, focusing on community-based efforts for poor and disadvantaged people. The health work of Save the Children also pays particular attention to the survival and well being of newborns and children, reproductive health, and HIV/AIDS. "Saving Newborn Lives," as noted earlier, is an initiative of Save the Children that is financed with the assistance of the Bill & Melinda Gates Foundation. This effort tries to identify and disseminate simple approaches to preventing deaths among newborn children.[35] Save the Children is also deeply involved in nutrition through food relief, enhancing agricultural production, and specific investments in nutrition education and food and micronutrient supplementation.

Doctors Without Borders

Doctors Without Borders was founded in 1971 and is based in Brussels, Belgium. It is an umbrella organization made up of affiliated groups in 18 countries.[36] The groups located in Belgium, France, Holland, Spain, and Switzerland carry out health work in more than 80 countries. Doctors Without Borders, usually referred to by its French name, Medicins Sans Frontieres, or by the abbreviation of that name MSF, is best known for its work in humanitarian crises. It has often been involved in the provision of health services following natural disasters, such as earthquakes and hurricanes, or those humanitarian emergencies related to war and famine.[37] MSF, for example, assisted Nicaragua after an earthquake, Ethiopia during a famine, and Somalia after a war. MSF has also been engaged intensively in health services for refugees and displaced people. In addition, when health services have been severely weakened due to war or conflict, MSF often

TABLE 15-5 Selected Non-Governmental Organizations Involved in Global Health

CARE
Catholic Relief Services
Christian Children's Fund
Doctor's Without Borders
OXFAM
Partners in Health
Save the Children
World Vision

Source: The Author

helps to provide health services temporarily, while trying to help rebuild health system capacity. One example of this was in Liberia after its civil war.

MSF is also well known for its commitment to political independence, medical ethics, and human rights. Related to this, MSF has increasingly sought to become a voice in international health policy arenas for the disenfranchised. More recently, MSF has also become very involved with prevention, care, and treatment for HIV/AIDS. In this work, MSF has helped to mobilize international support for anti-retroviral therapy in poor countries and has become a leader in trying to lower the price of those drugs.[37]

PARTNERSHIPS RELATED TO WHO

Some global health problems affect an exceptional number of people in a large number of countries. The costs of addressing these problems are great and the skills needed to combat them are substantial. Most of the resource poor countries can not tackle these problems without aid and no individual development partner can provide enough assistance to help deal effectively with the scale of these problems. Therefore, a number of organizations have decided to work together to help address some of the most important burdens of disease. Some of the partnerships that have ensued are closely related to WHO, as noted in Table 15-6. Two of the most important such partnerships are Stop TB and Roll Back Malaria.

Stop TB

The Global Partnership to Stop TB was established in 2000. It aims to "eliminate TB as a public health problem, and ultimately, to obtain a world free of TB."[38] Stop TB is comprised of a wide array of partners including countries, development agencies, private sector organizations, and NGOs. WHO plays a prominent role in Stop TB, and the secretariat for the partnership is housed at WHO headquarters in Geneva, Switzerland. The primary goal of Stop TB is to ensure that 70% of the people in the world with TB will be diagnosed, that 85% of them will be cured, and that by 2015 the burden of TB disease will be cut in half. The partnership tries to encourage the wider use of effective TB strategies, such as DOTS, including those for dealing with HIV/TB co-infection and drug-resistant TB. It also works to promote the development of new TB diagnostics, drugs, and vaccines. Stop TB engages in advocacy, technical assistance, and helps to mobilize funding for the fight against TB.[2]

Roll Back Malaria

Roll Back Malaria was founded in 1998 by WHO, UNICEF, and the World Bank to advocate for malaria control, to pro-

TABLE 15-6 Selected WHO-Related Partnerships for Global Health

Global Alliance for the Elimination of Leprosy
Global Polio Eradication Campaign
Lymphatic Filariasis Control Program
Roll Back Malaria
Stop TB
Tropical Disease Research Program

Source: The Author

mote the development of better approaches and technologies for malaria containment, and to help finance and spread appropriate malaria control and treatment.[39] The partnership has expanded since then to include a variety of public and private actors in a number of countries. In these activities, they promote appropriate prevention and treatment of malaria. In addition, Roll Back Malaria has established a Malaria Medicines and Supplies Service. This aims at helping resource poor countries better organize and manage the procurement of supplies and medicines needed to manage effective malaria control.[40]

OTHER PARTNERSHIPS AND SPECIAL PROGRAMS

In the last decade, global partners have expressed considerable concern over a number of health issues that affect the poor. One has been the need to strengthen immunization programs for children and for pregnant women. Related to this has been a growing interest in trying to more quickly increase the use of several "newer vaccines" that have been used for some time in better-off countries but have only rarely been provided in poorer countries. In addition to this, there has been a growing fear that the pace of progress against HIV, TB, and malaria has been insufficient and that urgent and bold measures need to be taken to move more forcefully against these diseases. To address immunization more effectively, the Global Alliance for Vaccines and Immunization (GAVI) was established. The Global Fund to Fight Against AIDS, TB, and Malaria ("The Global Fund") was established to make more rapid progress against HIV, TB, and malaria.

GAVI

GAVI is a partnership among public and private sector organizations that was established in 2000.[4] The founding partners of GAVI include WHO, UNICEF, and the World Bank. GAVI is based in Geneva, Switzerland. The Bill & Melinda

Gates Foundation made a major grant to help establish GAVI and provide for its operations. The main aims of GAVI are to improve the ability of health systems to carry out immunization; raise rates of coverage in low-income countries of key vaccines; promote more rapid uptake of underused vaccines, such as hepatitis B, Haemophilus influenzae type B, and yellow fever; speed up the development of other vaccines of importance; and help countries ensure that vaccines are given safely.[41] GAVI has tried to improve global health work through two innovative approaches. The first is to tie its financing to the achievement of goals that are agreed to by the countries that are being helped. The second is to work closely with countries to develop plans to sustain the investments that are being supported. GAVI is an organization that advocates for the importance of immunization, provides technical assistance to countries to enhance their immunization efforts, and finances those efforts.

The Global Fund

The Global Fund to Fight Against AIDS, TB, and Malaria was also established in 2002 and is based in Geneva, Switzerland.[42] The driving force behind the establishment of the Fund was increasing global concern about HIV and a growing recognition among development partners that measures to address the AIDS epidemic had been insufficient. Interest in establishing the Fund was also heightened by the growing attention to global health discussed hereafter, and a special concern for the exceptional burden of HIV, TB, and malaria, especially in Africa.[43]

The Global Fund is a partnership of the public and private sectors and WHO, UNAIDS, and the World Bank are also key partners. The Fund is governed by a Board of Directors that represents governments, international organizations, civil society, and communities affected by AIDS, TB, and malaria. The fund is financed by grants that come largely from developed country governments, but which also come from the private and foundation sector, including the Bill & Melinda Gates Foundation.

The Global Fund is primarily a financing agency but it also engages in advocacy for global health and the three diseases on which it focuses. The main aim of the Fund is to finance proposed investments in these diseases, with an emphasis on AIDS and Africa. It has a particular interest in helping to scale up programs for anti-retroviral therapy against HIV. The Fund has taken innovative approaches to a number of aspects of development assistance for health, including the following:

- It is strictly a financing mechanism and not a technical or implementing agency.

- It seeks to raise funds for investments that will be additional to other funding already available.
- It tries to work on the basis of a national plan that is developed by a group representing diverse national interests, for the use of Global Fund financing.
- It evaluates proposals through an independent review process.
- It tries to operate in a performance-based manner by supporting investments that are meeting their targets and reducing or eliminating support for programs that are not meeting their aims.[42]

In its first two rounds of funding, the Global Fund committed about $1.5 billion to support 154 programs in 93 countries.[44]

Public–Private Partnerships

As interest in global health rose in the mid-1990s, many of the actors in this field increasingly believed that the mechanisms for developing, manufacturing, and distributing new vaccines, drugs, diagnostics, and medical devices needed to alleviate key global health problems were not sufficient. They noted with growing concern, for example, that the vaccine for TB was over 100 years old and that no new TB drugs had been developed for decades. They saw insufficient attention to the development of vaccines against HIV and malaria in both the public and the private sector and fewer firms willing to engage in vaccine development. They also understood that private pharmaceutical firms did not see a profitable market in the development of low-cost diagnostics, vaccines, drugs, or medical devices that could address the major killers of the poor globally. They knew that without changes in the way the market for these products worked that private sector firms would remain on the sidelines.

In the face of these issues, the Rockefeller Foundation encouraged key global health actors to think creatively about how they could spur the more rapid development of products that could attack global health problems in a low cost but effective way. One idea that emerged from this was the notion of organizations that would combine the strengths of public and private organizations in a common quest for better health. They would also seek broader sources of financing for these health ventures; try to tackle intellectual property issues that constrained the availability of affordable diagnostics, drugs, medical devices, and vaccines in poor countries; and see how they could encourage more private sector involvement in the search for these products. In some respects, they were conceived of as venture capital firms that would have a social goal, rather than a goal that was mostly aimed at maximizing profit. Today, there is a wide array of "public–private partnerships for health," or "PPPs," as they are called. The aim of many of these is to develop new products and these are often called Product Development Partnerships. Some of the most important of such partnerships are noted in Table 15-7.

IAVI

Two of the more interesting public-private partnerships for health are the International AIDS Vaccine Initiative (IAVI) and the Institute for One World Health. IAVI was established as a not-for-profit corporation in 1996. It is based in New York City but operates globally and has activities in more than 20 countries. IAVI has three main objectives: to advocate for AIDS vaccines, to help develop programs and policies that would encourage the use of an AIDS vaccine if one were developed, and to engage in research and development of candidate AIDS vaccines.[45] IAVI works with a number of scientific partners under agreements to ensure that if any of the partners does develop an AIDS vaccine with IAVI support, the vaccine "would be made available in developing countries at reasonable prices, would be available in sufficient quantities, and would be made available as soon as it is licensed as safe and effective."[46] IAVI has received financial support from a number of governments; from some private companies, such as Becton Dickinson and Co. (BD); the Rockefeller Foundation; the World Bank; and the Bill & Melinda Gates Foundation.

Institute for One World Health

The Institute for One World Health was founded in the United States in San Francisco, California, in 2000 and is similar in many ways to IAVI.[47] The main aims of this not-for-profit pharmaceutical company are to identify "promising drug development opportunities; take responsibility for shepherding those leads through the complex development process; and, enable the development of drugs that can help to address the diseases that disproportionately affect developing countries."[48] The Institute works in collaboration with a number of universities, hospitals, industry, government, and NGOs. The Institute has received funding from a number of foundations, including the Bill & Melinda Gates Foundation. "By partnering and collaborating with industry and researchers, by securing donated intellectual property, and by utilizing the scientific and intellectual capacity of the developing world," One World Health hopes to deliver "affordable, effective, and appropriate new medicines where they are needed most."[48] The Institute has focused primarily on visceral leishmaniasis, diarrheal disease, malaria, and Chagas disease.[48]

TABLE 15-7 Selected Public-Private Partnerships for Public Health

Global Alliance for TB Drug Development
International AIDS Vaccine Initiative
International Partnership on Microbicides
Malaria Vaccine Initiative
Medicines for Malaria Venture

Source: The Author

Pharmaceutical Firms

In the last decade, international pharmaceutical firms have also engaged in partnerships to try to improve global health at low cost. This has generally been done in one of three ways. First, some firms donate drugs to global health programs. Novartis, for example, donates leprosy drugs to the Global Alliance to Eliminate leprosy, and today no country needs to purchase such drugs.[49] Pfizer and the Edna McConnell Clark Foundation work with the International Trachoma Initiative by donating an antibiotic, azithromycin, to its efforts to reduce trachoma related blindness.[50] Merck donates Ivermectin to the Onchocerciasis Control Program that has been successful in reducing river blindness in Africa.[51] These are only some of the many donation efforts now underway.

In addition, a number of drug companies, including Abbott, Boehringer Ingelheim, Bristol Myers Squibb, Gilead, GSK, and Merck, have agreed to sell anti-retroviral drugs for HIV at greatly discounted prices to developing countries affected by the AIDS epidemic. Some of the drug companies also sponsor programs to address diseases such as HIV in particular countries, such as Merck's support for the national HIV/AIDS control program in Botswana.[52]

The role of the major drug companies in global health is a subject of considerable controversy. There is a serious concern in some members of the global health community, for example, that the approach of the branded drug manufacturers to patents raises the price of drugs beyond what people in low-income countries can afford. Some people also believe that the major manufacturers should be far more generous than they have been in offering their drugs at reduced prices in low- and middle-income countries. Others have expressed concern that these manufacturers have not been open enough in licensing their products to other companies in a way that would reduce their prices in the developing world. The role of pharmaceutical firms in global health is very important, complicated, and controversial and goes considerably beyond the scope of this book.

TRENDS IN GLOBAL HEALTH EFFORTS

The notion of cooperating to improve health globally is not a new one. Rather, different countries have realized for more than 100 years that many health problems could not be solved by individual countries and had to be addressed through collective action across countries.

In the ensuing period, in fact, many actors have cooperated in a variety of health activities. This section examines how the themes of those efforts varied over time. The threat of cholera, for example, led to the first international conference on health in 1851.[53] Numerous international conferences on health followed that and by 1903, the world created The International Commission on Epidemics.[54] In 1909, the International Office of Public Hygiene was set up in Paris and this was followed by the establishment of the League of Nations Health Office in 1920 in Geneva, Switzerland. The International Sanitary Bureau was set up in 1924. The Rockefeller Foundation assisted in financing and providing technical support to the League of Nations Health Office. The early international organizations for health focused their efforts on the surveillance of disease, the provision of global standards for drugs and vaccines, and selected technical advice to countries on key health matters, including medical education.[55]

International efforts in health took a substantial leap forward with the establishment of the United Nations agencies after World War II, including WHO and UNICEF. In the 40 years since then there have been a number of areas of focus for international cooperation on health, as noted hereafter.[15,56,57] Following the establishment of WHO, efforts at international cooperation in health shifted to focus on helping to build capacity for global public health efforts, for health systems development in countries that were newly independent, and in working together to fight disease. Perhaps the greatest single effort at global cooperation in health began in 1966 with the start of the global program to eradicate smallpox. During this period of intensive attention to specific diseases, WHO also led work to combat malaria and other communicable diseases that most affected the poor, such as leprosy,[58] lymphatic filariasis,[59] and onchocerciasis.[60,61]

Historically, another important area of focus for global cooperation has been family planning. Much of the early work on family planning was led by the United States. Over time, the focus on family planning shifted from one that was centered almost exclusively on limiting family size to an approach that centered much more on reproductive

health. This shift was encouraged by and reflected in a series of global conferences on family planning, safe motherhood, reproductive health, and women starting in 1974 in Bucharest, Romania.[62] The 1987 conference on women in Nairobi, Kenya, for example, was used to launch the Safe Motherhood Initiative.[57]

In 1978, the world launched a major effort when it enacted the Alma Ata declaration on primary health care, as mentioned earlier. This declaration noted that health was a fundamental human right and that countries had the obligation to ensure that all people had access to appropriate primary health care. The Alma Ata declaration heralded a new global focus on primary health care and on the health needs of the poor. It also led to much greater attention to the needs for health systems that could deliver primary care and to the importance of taking a community-based approach to the health needs of poor people. The Alma Ata Declaration was linked to the world's efforts to achieve what was called globally "Health for all by the Year 2000."[63]

An immense amount of attention has also been paid to "Child Survival." These efforts focused on what were called the GOBI interventions: growth monitoring, oral rehydration, breast feeding, and immunization. UNICEF was the leader of this effort. USAID was also instrumentally involved in child survival activities, which ultimately became an important focus of attention for the World Bank, WHO, and a variety of bilateral organizations.[64]

As the world moved into the late 1980s and early 1990s, considerable concern arose that despite more than 30 years of global efforts to improve the health of the poor, the unfinished agenda remained very large. Many of those working on health believed that some of the weaknesses stemmed from an approach to health that was too disjointed and that needed to be better grounded in a more systemic view of health that would focus on trying to improve health services more broadly. This led to considerable work being done on "health sector reform." At the same time, the *1993 World Development Report* of the World Bank articulated the need to take an approach to decision making on health investments that would be grounded in cost-effectiveness analysis.[65] This framework for analysis soon became the foundation for actions of a number of key actors in global health.

At about the same time, much greater attention began to be paid, even in low-income countries, to the role of the private sector in health. Development partners also created around this time new ways of working together cooperatively within individual countries. Increasingly, for example, development partners would cooperate and jointly help countries to develop and finance investments in health. In much of the work done prior to this period, many development partners worked individually with a country, often leading to a lack of coordination across that country's health sector efforts.

Toward the mid-1990s, the global health community began to pay considerably more attention to HIV, as well as to other major killers of the poor in resource poor countries, including malaria and TB. Particular attention has been paid to reducing the cost of AIDS drugs and getting more people treated, raising case finding and cure rates for TB by expanding coverage with DOTS, and strengthening malaria control programs through the use of insecticide-treated bed nets, intermittent treatment of pregnant women, and greater use of artemisinin-based combination therapy. There has also been an enormous increase in cooperation through the many health partnerships that have been formed, as noted earlier in the chapter.

SETTING THE GLOBAL HEALTH AGENDA

As we think about how different actors cooperate in global health activities and the themes on which they focus, it is important to consider how global health policies get established. The next section comments briefly on how the overall global health agenda and the agenda for particular global health topics are set. This is another topic that is quite complicated and often the subject of controversy that readers may wish to explore further.

One important activity in setting global health priorities is the World Health Assembly of the World Health Organization.[66] Once each year, ministers of health of WHO member countries meet in Geneva, Switzerland, to consider important global health matters and resolutions proclaiming their interest in and commitment to addressing key health issues. The World Health Assembly has been the foundation for some of the most important global health efforts undertaken, such as the smallpox eradication campaign.

Some important developments in global health have been encouraged by writings, advocacy efforts, and program activities of WHO, multilateral or bilateral development assistance agencies, and some of the important NGOs involved in health. The *1993 World Development Report* of the World Bank focused on health and was widely read and debated around the world. This document set the basis for the next generation of World Bank-assisted health projects in many countries and for important work done by other development organizations and countries in health, as well. Given the importance of World Bank assistance for health to so many countries, the approaches suggested in the *1993 World Development Report* had a major impact on the world's thinking about health in developing countries.

Movement in the policy agenda for global health can also follow significant investments by development partners. This has clearly been the case, for example, as a result of the substantial funds that the Bill & Melinda Gates Foundation has provided to selected global health activities. As noted earlier, the Gates Foundation has focused considerable attention on improving and disseminating technology for improving the health of the poor, as well as selected investments in key health problems, such as HIV. The investments the Gates Foundation has made, for example, in immunization and in the development of AIDS vaccines has considerably raised the world's attention to these matters and placed them more firmly on the global health agenda.

Popular action, often led by NGOs or other advocates for health, can also influence the setting of the global health agenda. In the late 1990s, for example, Professor Jeff Sachs, then of Harvard University, began to be actively involved in speaking and writing about the importance of health to economic and social development. His work attracted attention to health issues and led to considerable international engagement and action on the health of poor people globally. At about the same time, some important NGOs, such as Doctors Without Borders, became major advocates for AIDS treatment and the reduction of the prices of AIDS drugs. Through their advocacy work and efforts to treat people with anti-retroviral drugs, they attracted considerable attention to these topics and had a major impact on the way the world approached them.

Another good example of how an NGO affected the global health agenda is the impact of Partners in Health, an NGO based in the city of Boston in the United States, on the global agenda for TB and for HIV. Largely led by the work of Dr. Paul Farmer and Dr. Jim Kim of Harvard University, Partners in Health tried to develop in Peru and Haiti a model of how one could treat drug-resistant TB and then HIV at an acceptable cost and in a sustainable way. At the time, the prevailing opinion globally was that drugs for these conditions were so expensive that they could not be treated in resource poor settings. The work of Partners in Health helped to shift global efforts toward finding ways to make treatment affordable for all people.[67]

In other respects, one can think of efforts to set the global health agenda as a kind of ongoing meeting around a negotiating table at which important actors in global health are sitting. The organizations most involved in such discussions will generally be WHO, UNICEF, and the World Bank. Selected bilateral development agencies will also participate, such as USAID, the Department for International Development of the UK, and often the Canadian International Development

Agency and the Dutch Development Agency, while AUSAID plays a unique role in some of Asia in the Pacific. Given the importance of AIDS in many ways, UNAIDS is also often involved. The Gates Foundation, the Rockefeller Foundation, and selected NGOs might also be involved. Some other NGOs, such as MSF, may not be present, but through advocacy they do bring their interests to the policy-setting group.

The way in which the agenda is set for specific health topics will be similar to those mentioned previously, but will usually also include actors who have particular interests in the topic at hand. WHO and the World Bank will almost always be involved. The key bilateral agencies will also participate. In addition, the agencies working with the topic under discussion and groups representing people affected by particular conditions increasingly also have inputs to these discussions. If TB is being discussed, for example, then the key NGOs working globally with TB will be involved, as will the TB programs from representative countries. If leprosy is being discussed, then the leprosy programs of some countries will be involved, NGOs working in leprosy will be involved, and groups of people affected by leprosy will also be involved.

FUTURE CHALLENGES

There are a number of challenges to effective collaborative action in global health. First, as discussed in the chapter on communicable diseases, the types of health conditions that the world faces may change and new conditions might develop. Smallpox was once a disease of considerable importance, as was polio. Smallpox was eradicated, and there are very few cases of polio in the world today. In recent years, however, there have been outbreaks of new and emerging diseases, such as Ebola, the avian flu, and SARS. It is possible that there will be a major epidemic of influenza and that other new and emerging diseases will appear in the future. The world will have to be ready, through collaborative efforts, to carry out surveillance, prevention, and treatment of those diseases.

Second, it will be very important for development partners to work together to help countries strengthen their health systems, as well as to try to combat individual diseases. If countries are to be able to meet their most important health needs in a sustainable manner in the future, then they must have health systems that work. In most low-income countries, this will require better management, more appropriate forms of organization, sounder systems for key public health functions, better trained staff at all levels, and a consistent manner of providing financing for health system needs, while helping to cover the costs of health care for the truly poor. Achieving these aims is not as attractive politically as

fighting a specific disease or health problem. Yet, in the long run, a systems approach must be taken to developing health services and different global health actors will have to work together to achieve this, since they are usually only involved in working with a part of the health system of any country.

Another set of future challenges concerns the need to ensure that actors in global health work together to address the knowledge gaps that prevent sufficient progress against health conditions that cause people to be sick too often and to die prematurely, especially poor people in low-income countries. There will continue to be an important need, for example, for increasing our knowledge of the basic science concerning many diseases, including AIDS, TB, and malaria. It will not be possible to develop preventive vaccines for these diseases or better treatment for them, without significant improvements in scientific knowledge. There will also be a need for operational research in global health so that we can learn more about what approaches are effective and efficient. What is the best way, for example, to ensure that people take all of their drugs for HIV or TB? How should a health system in a developing country be organized to ensure that it can operate in a cost-efficient way, while paying sufficient attention to the poor? These questions can only be answered through the generation and sharing of knowledge and experience globally, a process dependent upon cooperation and coordination.

The factors that have encouraged the development of public-private partnerships for health will also continue to challenge the global health community. There are many such partnerships now and it will be very important to learn as quickly as possible which aspects of these partnerships encourage product development in effective and efficient ways and which ones do not. It is also necessary to continue to encourage the development of new and innovative approaches to enabling the development of new diagnostics, vaccines, and therapies that can be affordable in low- and middle-income countries. If any of the public-private partnerships are successful in developing new products, then it will be essential that efforts turn to ensuring that they are used quickly where they are most needed.

The financial needs for addressing global health concerns are very considerable and will continue to have a prominent place on the global health agenda. The multilateral development banks, the bilateral aid agencies, and special programs such as The Global Fund need continuous financing. In addition, some of the important initiatives that have been started, such as the considerable push for treatment against HIV, can not be sustained without many years of additional financing by rich countries, foundations, the private sector, and their partners. The amount of money that is spent on global health is much less than is spent on defense globally. Yet, there are still many risks that donors will develop "aid fatigue" and not have the political will necessary to continue financing global health efforts at the level needed.

It will be important that any development financing for health be as effective as possible. Although the topic of development effectiveness is considerably beyond the scope of this book, Table 15-8 summarizes some of the factors most closely associated with the success of development assistance in health.

There are also a number of important challenges to the way that actors in global health cooperate to assist countries in investing in the health sector. In recent years, development assistance agencies have increasingly tried to cooperate closely in their aid work on specific countries. However, there are always tendencies in development agencies to act independently rather than in coordination with other agencies. Although we should expect these tensions to continue, it is important if development assistance in health is to be effective that agencies work increasingly in a cooperative fashion.

Finally, it will be very important that good leadership in the global health field continues. Different agencies will need to work together in ways that address the challenges noted earlier. New groups and organizations need to join the community of global health actors to continue to inspire innovative and efficient methods of addressing and financing global health needs.

CASE STUDY

Chapter 1 ended with a case study on smallpox, which is widely regarded as one of the great efforts in global cooperation of any kind, but especially in health. It is fitting that one of the last chapters of the book should include a case study of the successful effort to eliminate onchocerciasis in Africa. This case study complements the one in Chapter 5 that addresses the integrated provision of drugs to treat onchocerciasis and vitamin A. More detailed information on this case is available in *Case Studies in Global Health: Millions Saved.*

Background

Onchocerciasis, or river blindness, is a pernicious disease afflicting approximately 18 million people worldwide. More than 99% of its victims are in Sub-Saharan Africa. In the most endemic areas, over a third of the adult population is blind, and infection often approaches 90%.[68] In 11 West African countries in 1974, nearly 2.5 million of the area's 30 million inhabitants were infected with onchocerciasis,

TABLE 15-8 Factors Associated with Positive Outcomes in Development Assistance

- Strong leadership in the host government and in the development partner agencies
- Close collaboration among governments, donors, and non-governmental organizations in the design and implementation of the program
- Household and community participation in the design, implementation, and monitoring of programs
- Simple and flexible technologies and approaches that can be adapted to local conditions and do not require complex skills to operate and maintain
- Approaches that help to strengthen health systems, especially human resources for health
- Consistent, predictable funding

Source: Adapted with permission from The World Bank. Hecht RM, Shah R. Recent trends and innovations in development assistance in health. In: Jamison DT, Breman JG, Measham AR, et al., eds. *Disease Control Priorities in Developing Countries.* 2nd ed. New York: Oxford University Press 2006:246.

and approximately 100,000 were blind. The remaining 19 endemic countries in central and east Africa were home to 60 million people at risk of the disease.

The Intervention

Onchocerciasis is caused by a worm called *Onchocerca volvulus* which enters its human victim through the bite of an infected blackfly. The flies breed in fast-moving waters in fertile riverside regions. Once inside a human, the tiny worm grows to a length of one to two feet and produces millions of microscopic offspring called microfilarie. The constant movement of the microfilarie through the infected person's skin causes torturous itching, lesions, muscle pain, and, in severe cases, blindness. Fertile land is often abandoned for fear of the disease.

Early efforts to control the disease proved ineffective because blackflies cover long distances and cross national borders, rendering unilateral efforts ineffective. An international conference in Tunisia in 1968 concluded that onchocerciasis could not be controlled without regional collaboration and long-term funding of at least 20 years to break the life cycle of the worm. World Bank President Robert McNamara's tour of drought-stricken West Africa in 1972 served as a catalyst to progress. Moved by seeing communities where nearly all the adults were blind and were led by children, McNamara decided to spearhead an international effort against onchocerciasis.[68]

The Onchocerciasis Control Program (OCP), the World Bank's first large-scale health program, was launched in 1974 in conjunction with the WHO, the UN Food and Agriculture Organization (FAO), and UNDP. The program included a significant research budget and set out to eliminate onchocerciasis in 7, and eventually in 11, West African countries.[69] Breeding grounds of blackflies were sprayed with larvicide, and the spraying program was able to persist even through regional conflicts and coups. In the 1980s, a Merck drug called Ivermectin was included as a powerful new weapon against the disease, a single dose of which could effectively paralyze the tiny worms for up to a full year.[70] The drug proved popular because it quickly reduced uncomfortable symptoms and provided protection against other parasites. Merck donated Ivermectin and Dr. William Foege of the Carter Center managed its distribution.

The African Programme for Onchocerciasis Control (APOC) was established in 1995 as a broad international partnership to control the disease throughout Africa and to carry onchocerciasis control to 19 countries in East and Central Africa. These were countries in which long distances and thick forests made spraying difficult. APOC pioneered a system of Community-Directed Treatment with Ivermectin (ComDT) to ensure local participation, reach remote villages, and maintain distribution of the drug after donor funding expires in 2010.[71] ComDT workers are often the only health personnel to reach distant villages, and their access could be used for other health interventions in the future.

The Impact

By 2002, OCP halted transmission of onchocerciasis in 11 West African countries, preventing 600,000 cases of blindness, and protecting 18 million children born in the OCP area from the risk of the disease. About 25 million hectares of arable land—enough to feed an additional 17 million people—is now safe for resettlement.[72] APOC is expanding this success to central and east Africa, where 40,000 cases of blindness are expected to be prevented each year.

Costs and Benefits

OCP operated with an annual cost of less than $1 per protected person. Total commitments from 22 donors amounted to $560 million. The annual return on investment, due mainly to increased agricultural output, was 20%, and it is estimated that $3.7 billion will be generated from improved labor and agricultural productivity.[73] APOC coverage cost even less, at just 11 cents per person. The economic rate of return for the program is 17% for the years 1996 to 2017, and it is estimated that 27 healthy life days will be added per dollar invested.[74]

Lessons Learned

Success in controlling onchocerciasis could not have been attained without a genuinely shared vision among all partners in the program. Commitment among the African governments was critical to coordinating a regional effort across national borders. Long-term commitments from donors, along with Merck's decision to donate Ivermectin indefinitely, were essential elements for the program's sustainability. The participation of a wide range of organizations, such as multilateral institutions, private companies, and local NGOs, allowed for a cost-effective and efficient intervention. The ComDT framework, by emphasizing local ownership and participation, proved a cost-effective and self-sustaining means of delivering drugs to remote populations. The onchocerciasis program proved that effective aid programs, implemented with transparency and accountability, can deliver lasting results.

MAIN MESSAGES

It is very important that key actors work together to address global health problems because they may have effects that go beyond one country, they may be expensive to deal with, and they may require technical and managerial resources larger than some poorer countries can bring to bear on their own. In addition, it is very important that there be global standards in some health fields and these standards need to be broadly developed and widely accepted. Good examples of areas in which it is imperative that different actors work together globally would include efforts to carry out disease surveillance, the global fight for polio eradication, and the standards for some disease control programs, such as TB.

There are many actors in global health and among the most actively involved are WHO, UNICEF, UNAIDS, and the World Bank. Most high-income countries have development assistance organizations and they often play important roles in global health, such as USAID, AUSAID, and DFID. A number of foundations are also deeply involved in global health work and the Bill & Melinda Gates Foundation has become a major actor in global health since the late 1990s. Many NGOs are also very involved in global health efforts and Doctors Without Borders is among the best known of these. These organizations play one of several roles, singly or all together, including advocacy, knowledge generation, technical assistance, or financing.

A relatively new form of organization was created specifically to deal with difficult global health problems, called public-private partnerships for health. These organizations include, among others, the International AIDS Vaccine Initiative and the International Partnership on Microbicides. Essentially, they try to combine the skills and financing of public and private sector organizations, in order to advocate for specific health issues, develop new vaccines, diagnostics, or drugs, and ensure that what they develop will be appropriate to the health needs of poor countries and affordable to them, as well. Some other new organizations, such as GAVI and the Global Fund were established to try to dramatically increase the pace of immunizing children and combating AIDS, TB, and malaria.

The global health community is likely to face many challenges that will continue to require collective action by global health actors. Some of the key challenges will include filling key gaps in knowledge and encouraging public and private sector organizations to develop the diagnostics, vaccines, and drugs needed to address the most important global health issues. They will also include the need for organizations to work together to strengthen health systems, to combat individual diseases, and to try to ensure that critical global health needs have adequate financing.

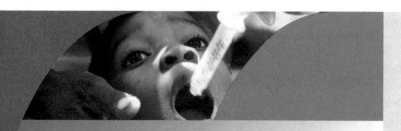

Study Questions

1. What are the most important organizations that work on global health issues?

2. What functions do these organizations play?

3. Why is it important that different actors cooperate to address global health concerns?

4. Name some of the most important successes of cooperative action on global health.

5. What were some of the key factors that led to those successes?

6. What are the lessons of these successes for future global health efforts?

7. What are some of the future challenges that demand continued or strengthened collaboration in global public health?

8. What is a public-private partnership for health and why might they be valuable?

9. Why is cooperative action needed to address problems like onchocerciasis and Guinea worm?

10. How might the world raise the money needed to further address problems like HIV and the need for drug treatment against AIDS?

REFERENCES

1. UNICEF. Polio experts warn of largest epidemic in recent years, as polio hits Darfur: Epidemiologists "alarmed" by continuing spread of virus —warn thousands of children could be paralyzed across west and central Africa. *Joint Press Release.* Available at: http://www.unicef.org/media/media_21872.html. Accessed July 12, 2006.

2. World Health Organization. Tuberculosis: Fact sheet No 104. Available at: http://www.who.int/mediacentre/factsheets/fs104/en/. Accessed July 12, 2006.

3. Global Alliance for TB Drug Development. No R&D in 30 Years. Available at: http://www.tballiance.org/2_3_C_NoRandDin30Years.asp. Accessed July 12, 2006.

4. The GAVI Alliance. GAVI Alliance for Vaccines and Immunization. Available at: http://www.gavialliance.org/. Accessed July 5, 2006.

5. The GAVI Alliance. General Principles for Use of GAVI/Vaccine Fund Resources. Available at: http://www.gavialliance.org/General_Information/About_alliance/GAVI/Principles.php. Accessed July 12, 2006.

6. Merson MH, Black RE, Mills AJ. *International Public Health: Diseases, Programs, Systems, and Policies.* Gaithersburg, MD: Aspen Publishers; 2001.

7. Lele U, Ridker R, Upadhyay J. Health System Capacities in Developing Countries and Global Health Initiatives on Communicable Diseases. Available at: http://www.umalele.org/content/view/85/109/. Accessed July 12, 2006.

8. Heymann DL, Rodier G. Global surveillance, national surveillance, and SARS. *Emerg Infect Dis.* Feb 2004;10(2):173–175.

9. Walt G. Global Cooperation in International Public Health. In: Merson MH, Black RE, Mills AJ, eds. *International Public Health.* Gaithersburg, Maryland: Aspen Publishers; 2001:667–669.

10. Basch P. *Textbook of International Health.* 2nd ed. New York: Oxford University Press; 2001:486–509.

11. Basch P. *Textbook of International Health.* 2nd ed. New York: Oxford University Press; 2001:42–72.

12. Kickbusch I, Buse K. Global influences and global responses: international health at the turn of the twenty-first centery. In: Merson MH, Black RE, Mills AJ, eds. *International Public Health.* Gaithersburg, MD: Aspen Publishers; 2001:701–733.

13. World Health Organization. About WHO. Available at: http://www.who.int/about/en/. Accessed July 12, 2006.

14. World Health Organization. Declaration on Occupational Health for All. Available at: http://www.who.int/occupational_health/publications/declaration/en/index.html. Accessed July 12, 2006.

15. Merson MH, Black RE, Mills AJ. *International Public Health: Diseases, Programs, Systems, and Policies.* Gaithersburg, MD: Aspen Publishers; 2000:667–669.

16. Merson MH, Black RE, Mills AJ. *International Public Health: Diseases, Programs, Systems, and Policies.* Gaithersburg, MD: Aspen Publishers; 2000:701–733.

17. UNICEF. The Structure of UNICEF. Available at: http://www.unicef.org/about/structure/index.html. Accessed July 12, 2006.

18. UNICEF. What We Do. Available at: http://www.unicef.org/whatwedo/index.html. Accessed July 12, 2006.

19. UNICEF. Support UNICEF. Available at: http://www.unicef.org/support/14884.html. Accessed July 12, 2006.

20. Joint United Nations Programme on HIV/AIDS. Cosponsors. Available at: http://www.unaids.org/en/Cosponsors/default.asp. Accessed July 12, 2006.

21. Joint United Nations Programme on HIV/AIDS. Focus Areas. Available at: http://www.unaids.org/en/Coordination/FocusAreas/default.asp. Accessed July 12, 2006.

22. UNAIDS. United Nations Joint Programme on HIV/AIDS. Available at: http://www.unaids.org/en/. Accessed July 5, 2006.

23. The World Bank. *World Bank Annual Report 2002.* Washington, DC: The World Bank; 2002.

24. Health, Nutrition, & Population. Available at: http://www.worldbank.org/html/extdr/hnp/hnp.htm. Accessed July 6, 2006.

25. World Bank. Working for a World Free of Poverty. Available at: http://siteresources.worldbank.org/EXTABOUTUS/Resources/wbgroupbrochure-en.pdf. Accessed July 12, 2006.

26. The World Bank. The World Bank Lending by Theme and Sector. *The World Bank Annual Report 2005.* Washington, DC: The World Bank; 2005.

27. USAID. Health: Overview. Available at: http://www.usaid.gov/our_work/global_health/. Accessed July 12, 2006.

28. The Rockefeller Foundation. Available at: http://www.rockfound.org/. Accessed July 6, 2006.

29. Ford Foundation. Available at: http://www.fordfound.org/. Accessed July 6, 2006.

30. The Soros Foundation. Available at: http://www.soros.org/. Accessed July 6, 2006.

31. Bill & Melinda Gates Foundation. Available at: http://www.gatesfoundation.org/default.htm. Accessed June 9, 2006.

32. Bill & Melinda Gates Foundation. About Us. Available at: http://www.gatesfoundation.org/AboutUs/. Accessed June 9, 2006.

33. Bill & Melinda Gates Foundation. Global Health Program Fact Sheet. Available at: http://www.gatesfoundation.org/GlobalHealth/RelatedInfo/GlobalHealthFactSheet-021201.htm. Accessed July 12, 2006.

34. Save the Children. Mission and Strategy. Available at: http://www.savethechildren.org/mission/index.asp. Accessed July 12, 2006.

35. Save the Children. Save the Children Receives $60 Million Grant from the Bill & Melinda Gates Foundation to Save Newborn Lives Globally. Available at: http://www.savethechildren.org/news/releases/release_120205.asp. Accessed July 12, 2006.

36. Doctors Without Borders. Available at: http://www.doctorswithoutborders.org/. Accessed July 15, 2006.

37. Doctors Without Borders. About Us. Available at: http://www.doctorswithoutborders.org/aboutus/index.cfm. Accessed July 12, 2006.

38. World Health Organization. The Stop TB Department. Available at: http://www.who.int/tb/about/en/. Accessed July 12, 2006.

39. Roll Back Malaria Global Partnership. Available at: http://rbm.who.int/. Accessed July 15, 2006.

40. Roll Back Malaria Global Partnership. What is MMSS? Available at: http://rbm.who.int/mmss/. Accessed July 13, 2006.

41. The GAVI Alliance. Progress and Challenges 2004. Available at: http://www.gavialliance.org/General_Information/About_alliance/pandc2004_index.php. Accessed July 12, 2006.

42. The Global Fund. The Global Fund to Fight AIDS, Tuberculosis, and Malaria. Available at: http://www.theglobalfund.org/en/. Accessed July 6, 2006.

43. The Global Fund. The Global Fund to Fight AIDS, Tuberculosis, and Malaria. History of the Fund in Detail. Available at: http://www.theglobalfund.org/en/about/road/history/default.asp. Accessed July 6, 2006.

44. The Global Fund. The Global Fund to Fight AIDS, Tuberculosis, and Malaria. How the Fund Works. Available at: http://www.theglobalfund.org/en/about/how/. Accessed July 6, 2006.

45. International AIDS Vaccine Initiative. About IAVI. Available at: http://www.iavi.org/viewpage.cfm?aid=24. Accessed July 12, 2006.

46. International AIDS Vaccine Initiative. IAVI's Intellectual Property Agreements for AIDS Vaccine Development. Available at: http://www.iavi.org/viewpage.cfm?aid=40. Accessed July 12, 2006.

47. Institute for One World Health. History: A nonprofit pharmaceutical company is born. Available at: http://www.oneworldhealth.org/about/history.php. Accessed

48. Institute for One World Health. Extraordinary Opportunities, Inspired Solutions. Available at: http://oneworldhealth.org/business/index.php. Accessed July 12, 2006.

49. International Federation of Pharmceutical Manufacturers & Associations. Global Alliance to Eliminate Leprosy. Available at: http://www.ifpma.org/Health/other_infect/health_lep.aspx. Accessed July 12, 2006.

50. National Institutes of Health. A Leading Cause of Blindness May Be Controlled by Simple Course of Oral Antibiotic. Available at: http://www3.niaid.nih.gov/news/newsreleases/1999/trachoma.htm. Accessed July 12, 2006.

51. Benton B. The Onchocerciasis (Riverblindness) Programs: Visionary Partnerships. Available at: http://www.worldbank.org/afr/findings/english/find174.htm. Accessed July 12, 2006.

52. African Comprehensive HIV/AIDS Partnerships. Available at: http://www.achap.org/. Accessed July 12, 2006.

53. Basch P. *Textbook of International Health*. 2nd ed. New York: Oxford University Press; 2001:38–39.

54. Basch P. *Textbook of International Health*. 2nd ed. New York: Oxford University Press; 2001:43.

55. Basch P. *Textbook of International Health*. 2nd ed. New York: Oxford University Press; 2001:45.

56. Basch P. *Textbook of International Health*. 2nd ed. New York: Oxford University Press; 2001:47–70.

57. Whaley RF, Hashim TJ. *A Textbook of World Health: A Practical Guide to Global Health Care*. New York: Parthenon Pub. Group; 1994:187–199.

58. World Health Organization. Fact Sheet No 101: Leprosy. Available at: http://www.who.int/mediacentre/factsheets/fs101/en/. Accessed July 7, 2006.

59. World Health Organization. Fact Sheet No 102: Lymphatic Filariasis. Available at: http://www.who.int/mediacentre/factsheets/fs102/en/. Accessed July 7, 2006.

60. World Health Organization. Onchocerciasis. Available at: http://www.who.int/topics/onchocerciasis/en/. Accessed July 7, 2006.

61. Whaley RF, Hashim TJ. *A Textbook of World Health: A Practical Guide to Global Health Care*. New York: Parthenon Pub. Group; 1994:197.

62. Bruce FC. Highlights From the National Summit on Safe Motherhood: Investing in the Health of Women. *Maternal Child Health J.* 2002 2002;6(1):67–69.

63. WHO. Declaration of Alma-Ata. *International Conference on Primary Health Care*. Alma-Ata, USSR: WHO; 1978.

64. Merson MH, Black RE, Mills AJ. *International Public Health: Diseases, Programs, Systems, and Policies*. Gaithersburg, MD: Aspen Publishers; 2000:682.

65. The World Bank. *World Development Report 1993*. New York: The World Bank, Oxford University Press; 1993:25–29.

66. World Health Organization. Fifty-eighth World Health Assembly. Available at: http://www.who.int/mediacentre/events/2005/wha58/en/. Accessed July 7, 2006.

67. Kidder T. *Mountains Beyond Mountains*. New York: Random House; 2003.

68. Benton B, Bump J, Seketeli A, Liese B. Partnership and promise: evolution of the african river blindness campaigns. *Ann Trop Med Parasitol.* 2002;96(suppl 1):S5–S14.

69. Laolu A. Victory over river blindness. *Africa Recovery*. 2003;17(1):6.

70. The Story of Mectizan®. Available at: http://www.merck.com/about/cr/mectizan/ Accessed August 6, 2004.

71. Amazigo U, Brieger W, Katabarwa M, et al. The challenges of community-directed treatment with Ivermectin (CDTI) within the African Programme for Onchocerciasis Control (APOC). *Ann Trop Med Parasitol.* 2002;96(1):S41–S58.

72. The World Bank. Defeating Onchocerciasis in Africa. Available at: http://www.worldbank.org/operations/licus/defeatingoncho.pdf. Accessed October 1, 2003.

73. Hopkins D, Richards F. Visionary campaign: eliminating river blindness. *Med Health Ann.* 1997:8–23.

74. Benton B. Economic impact of onchocerciasis control through the African Programme for Onchocerciasis Control: an overview. *Ann Trop Med Parasitol.* 1998;92(supplement 1):S33–S39.

Science, Technology, and Global Health

VIGNETTES

Juan lived in the highlands of Peru. He had tuberculosis. He was being treated at a local TB clinic. He had to take 4 drugs for the first 2 months of his treatment and 2 drugs for 4 months after that. Juan felt better within weeks of starting his drugs and struggled to take the remaining pills because there were so many to take and he had to take them for so long.

Wezi lived in Bostwana. About 24% of the adults there are HIV-positive.[1] Bostwana has made some progress in preventing the spread of HIV by promoting delayed sexual debut, reduction in the number of sexual partners, and correct and consistent condom use. Nonetheless, new infections are still occurring. Many people believe that stemming transmission of HIV in countries like Botswana will depend on the discovery of a safe, effective, and affordable HIV vaccine.

Mei-Ling was 4 years old and lived in the West of China. Like so many children in her region, Mei-Ling was infected with hookworms. The community had a de-worming program and every 6 months Mei-Ling was given medicine to get rid of the worms. This medicine was generally safe and effective. However, it had to be given twice a year and there was some indication that the hookworms were becoming resistant to it.

David was 7 years old and lived in the eastern part of Kenya. He had a high fever and chills and his mother took him to the local health clinic. The nurse there examined David, decided he had malaria, and prescribed anti-malarial medicine. This was the third time in a year that David had malaria. A safe, effective, and affordable malaria vaccine would have prevented him from getting malaria, being sick so often, missing so much school, and spending so much money on medical care.

INTRODUCTION

Scientific and technological progress has contributed substantially to improvements in human health. Such progress has included, for example, vaccines for a number of potential killers; a variety of drugs, such as penicillin; and safer and more effective family planning devices.

In fact, some scientific and technological discoveries have been of exceptional importance to public health. The discovery of the smallpox vaccine led to the first important efforts at vaccination, and ultimately to the eradication of smallpox. Jonas Salk's discovery of the polio vaccine began to eliminate the scourge of polio from many societies and this work was advanced further by Albert Sabin's work on the oral polio vaccine. It is difficult to imagine living in a world without antibiotics, but they only emerged just before World War II.

The enhancement of medical devices has also had an important impact on public health. The invention of the bifurcated needle, as you read earlier, was instrumental in enhancing the effectiveness of the smallpox eradication campaign. The intraocular lens for cataracts has provided a very low-cost tool for improving visual acuity, as you read about in Chapter 12.

The purpose of this chapter is to examine how science and technology could assist in speeding the development and dissemination of new products that could address the largest burdens of disease in low- and middle-income countries. First, the chapter will examine the characteristics that such products need to have if they are to have the desired impact. Next, the chapter will review the extent to which some existing diagnostics, vaccines, and drugs possess those traits. The chapter will then discuss the potential of science and technology to develop products in selected areas of importance and review the constraints to product development. Lastly, the chapter will examine mechanisms to assist in overcoming those constraints and three case studies as examples of efforts at the development and dissemination of new products.

As you read this chapter, it is very important that you keep several things in mind. First, you should remember, as noted continuously in the book, that there are very substantial gains in health that could be obtained from the effective implementation of existing technologies. There are, for example, a number of low-cost but highly effective interventions that are well-known but not widely enough used, including:

- Reducing maternal disability and deaths by better identification of complications, speedy transport to the hospital, and appropriate emergency obstetric care

- Reducing neonatal deaths by training birth attendants in resuscitation and the provision of antibiotics and by keeping the baby warm
- Reducing young child deaths by expanding coverage with the six basic antigens
- Reducing infant morbidity and mortality by promoting exclusive breastfeeding for 6 months
- Reducing morbidity and mortality from TB by expanding case finding and cure rates using DOTS as the approach to treatment

In addition, we must remember that better hygiene practices do not require the development of any new products and could substantially improve health.

As you read this chapter, it is also important to keep in mind that the development of new products will not be a "quick fix." Rather, while supporting the continued search for scientific and technical progress, it is critical to continue to focus on the underlying sources of ill health in low- and middle-income countries. These include poverty, the lack of education, the lack of political interest in the health of the poor, and the place of some minority groups and women in society. Enhancement in basic infrastructure, water, and sanitation will also be critical in many settings to sustainable improvements in health.[2]

Finally, you should note that this chapter focuses on a very narrow range of the scientific and technological matters that concern global health. It does not examine research or operational research. Nor does it review, beyond two of the case studies, measures to enhance the availability of existing technology, some of which has been covered elsewhere in the book. Rather, this chapter looks almost exclusively at new product development, the constraints to it, and what might be done to speed up the process.

THE NEED FOR NEW PRODUCTS

As we think about the characteristics of diagnostics, drugs, vaccines, and medical devices that could most effectively and efficiently address the critical health problems of the developing world, we need to keep several points in mind. First, the most important target groups for these products are poor people in low- and middle-income countries. Their financial resources are limited and the countries in which they live, particularly low-income countries, spend very little on health. Second, the quality of care in many countries is low and injection safety is often poor. Third, many low- and middle-income countries have health systems that are poorly organized and can not effectively manage logistics. Transport and storage of goods is weak and electricity for keeping goods cool is often limited, as well.

TABLE 16-1 Some Ideal Characteristics of Diagnostics, Vaccines, and Delivery Devices

Diagnostics—Affordable; specific and sensitive; provides quick and easy-to-interpret results; easy to store and transport; heat stable

Vaccines—Affordable; safe and effective; requires few doses; confers lifelong immunity; easy to transport and store; heat stable

Drugs—Affordable; safe, and effective; not easy for pathogens to become resistant to; requires small doses over a limited period; easy to store and transport; heat stable

Delivery devices—Affordable, safe, and effective; not invasive; easy to transport and store; heat stable

Source: The Author

In this light, what would be some of the ideal characteristics of diagnostics, drugs, vaccines, and medical delivery devices intended to help address the most critical burdens of disease in low- and middle-income countries? The most important of these characteristics are shown in Table 16-1.

As you can see in the table, it is important that diagnostics be specific, sensitive, easy to use, and non-invasive. Ideally, diagnostic tests could be done quickly by relatively untrained workers and would rapidly produce easy-to-read results, as well. They would also be easy to transport, heat stable, not require refrigeration, and inexpensive.

Much the same would be true for the "ideal" drugs. These drugs would be safe, effective, and inexpensive. They could also be used for many years without becoming susceptible to resistance. In addition, the number of pills that patients would have to take would be limited and they would not have to take them for very long.

Vaccines to meet the most important health needs in the developing world would also be safe, effective, and inexpensive. They would be easy to transport and store, would be heat stable, and would not require refrigeration. The ideal vaccines would be an inexpensive combination of many antigens and only one dose would confer lifelong immunity against a number of diseases.

The present state of key products does not meet the "ideals" noted above. Presently, for example, a child receiving full coverage of the six basic antigens would require five contacts with the health system to get all of these vaccines.[3] Could vaccines be developed that combine required antigens in such a way that only a few contacts would be needed between the health system and patients?

You read earlier about the cultural preference in many societies for injections, despite problems with injection safety. Could vaccines be delivered in non-invasive ways, such as sprays, air injectors, and skin patches that would be safe, effective, heat stable, easy to transport, and not very costly?

There is a vaccine for tuberculosis and drugs that are effective against tuberculosis, as well. However, the effectiveness of the TB vaccine against adult pulmonary TB is "variable."[4] In addition, the drugs that are used to treat TB require a large pill burden and TB bacteria are increasingly becoming resistant to some of them.[5] What is needed to develop new drugs for TB that could make treatment shorter and easier? Is it possible to develop a safe and effective TB vaccine?

Artemisinin-based combination therapy is effective against malaria that is resistant to chloroquine. However, the cost per treatment with this drug, even at globally negotiated prices, is about 90 cents for the treatment of a child and

about $1.50 for the treatment of an adult. This is about 15 times the cost per treatment with chloroquine.[6] In addition, while the search for a malaria vaccine has gone on for many years, there is still no approved vaccine for malaria. What would it take to develop additional low-cost and highly effective malaria drugs? What can encourage the development of a safe and effective malaria vaccine?

Drugs for HIV can control the virus for most people but can not cure them. In addition, people develop resistance to those drugs and some of them have serious side effects. Moreover, there is still no preventive or therapeutic vaccine for HIV. How can the world encourage the development of safer and more effective AIDS drugs, an HIV vaccine, and mechanisms by which women could protect themselves better from the risk of HIV, such as microbicides?

The scientific and technological gaps indicated above also apply to some of the "other neglected diseases." Despite the ubiquity of hookworm, there is no vaccine for hookworm, the drug has to be administered regularly, and resistance to the drug is increasing. Can a vaccine be developed for hookworm and some of the other parasitic diseases?

THE POTENTIAL OF SCIENCE AND TECHNOLOGY

Scientific progress has led to a number of areas in which science could be harnessed to address some of the gaps noted in the previous section and to improve human health. Four such areas of science, as examples, are noted below.

Sequencing the genomes of important pathogens will help scientists understand better why those pathogens cause disease, how they develop resistance, and what drugs can best fight them, while reducing the onset of resistance. The genomes have now been sequenced for about 100 microbial species.[7] The speed with which the SARs virus was sequenced is an indication of the speed with which this can be done, if sufficient priority is given to this work.[8] The sequencing of the mosquito genome may allow scientists to engineer mosquitoes so that they can not carry malaria and other diseases, such as lymphatic filariasis.[9]

Improvements in information technology, chemistry, and robotics, as well as in genetic and molecular epidemiology will also facilitate the development of new and better drugs. These tools will allow scientists to understand better the nature of disease. They will also enable scientists to more quickly try different chemical compounds to address those pathogens.[7]

In addition, a number of technologies exist that can assist in the design and manufacture of new and improved vaccines.[7] The use of recombinant DNA technology, for example, helped an Indian vaccine company to reduce the cost of hepatitis B vaccine from about $8 to 50 cents.[9] DNA technology should also be very helpful to the development of drugs.[9]

Genetic modification of plants is a controversial subject, because, among other things, there are concerns over the environmental and health risks associated with them. Yet, it is possible to engineer plants that can carry higher levels of certain nutrients, such as vitamin A, while being very resistant to disease.[10] In addition, plants can be modified genetically so that they can produce "edible vaccines." The most advanced such work is for a vaccine for hepatitis B, but work is underway for other vaccines, as well.[10]

In fact, there is an increasing understanding of the promise of science and technology for improving global health. In one study, the views of 28 experts were sought about the "major biotechnologies that can help improve health in developing countries in the next 5 to 10 years."[11] In particular, these scientists were polled about the extent to which technologies would:

- Improve health
- Be affordable and appropriate to the circumstances of developing countries
- Address the most pressing health needs
- Be developed in the next 5 to 10 years
- Advance knowledge
- Have important indirect benefits[11]

They were also asked how they would use science and technology to achieve these aims. As the highest priority, these scientists would use biotechnology to develop new diagnostics, vaccines, and drugs, in that order. They would use technology to improve the environment, including water and sanitation. The scientists also put a high premium on the development of products that can help empower women to protect themselves against sexually transmitted diseases, including HIV, such as microbicides.[11]

Another manifestation of the use of science and technology to improve global health is the Grand Challenges to Global Health that was launched in 2003 by the Bill & Melinda Gates Foundation, in conjunction with the United States National Institutes of Health, the Canadian Institute of Health Research, and the Welcome Trust.[12]

Some of the most important areas of scientific advances supported by this scheme include:

- Improvement of childhood vaccines
- Creation of new vaccines
- Control of disease-transmitting insects
- Improvement of nutrition
- Curing latent and chronic infection[12]

The first awards under the Grand Challenges Scheme were made in 2004. A number of projects that have been funded aim to improve vaccines. One of the projects, for example, seeks to develop a vaccine that can prevent pertussis with a single dose, instead of the three doses needed now. Another project will try to develop a vaccine against pneumococcus that can be given in a single dose, instead of the four doses of the present vaccine. Several projects will try to make vaccines more heat stable. Others aim to create vaccine "delivery systems" that can be eaten, inhaled, or sprayed into the nose. Several projects relate to the development of a malaria vaccine. Others concern efforts to develop strategies for genetically engineering mosquitoes so that they will be unable to spread the dengue virus.[13]

Several of the projects that were funded will try to use genetic engineering to biofortify plants, such as making bananas contain more usable vitamin A, vitamin E, and iron in Uganda, where bananas are a staple food. Similar work would be done on rice with vitamins A and E, iron, zinc, and improved protein quality. Additional projects would focus on the science relating to the development of drugs for addressing latent TB and vaccines for the human papillomavirus.[13]

CONSTRAINTS TO APPLYING SCIENCE AND TECHNOLOGY TO GLOBAL HEALTH PROBLEMS

Given the strengths of existing scientific knowledge, why is it that some of the products that could make an important difference to the health of the poor globally have not been developed? Beyond the inherent scientific difficulties in some of these efforts, such as the development of HIV and malaria vaccines, there are several common constraints to the development of desired products. First, much of the research and development on new diagnostics, vaccines, drugs, and delivery devices is carried out in the for-profit sector and that sector has historically believed that it could not make a sufficient return from products oriented toward the developing world. These firms see the market for their goods in the developing world as a small one. They also doubt the ability of low-income individuals to pay prices for their products that would give them a sufficient return on their capital. In addition, they doubt that governments in low-income countries could afford their products. As evidence of this, for example, they point to the slow uptake in developing countries of the vaccines against *Haemophilus influenzae* type b (Hib) and hepatitis B.

Moreover, the costs of research and development on new products can be very high, some suggesting as high as $800 million, to bring a new drug from research to market.

Given these costs, profit-making firms will invariably want to use their capital to develop, for example, a potential "blockbuster" drug against high cholesterol, that can be sold in the developed countries, rather than develop a drug for low-income countries on which the firm believes it will not be able to recoup its investment.[14]

In addition, vaccine markets have some particular constraints to entry. Vaccine development requires a considerable amount of upstream investment, the costs of developing vaccine candidates is very high, and governmental regulations may also reduce the prospects that firms can make sufficient profit from vaccines to attract them to this market. In addition, the number of firms engaged in vaccine production worldwide is small and production capacity is limited. Developing vaccines for low- and middle-income countries is also complicated by the fact that there is an increasing divergence between the vaccines used in the immunization programs of low- and middle-income countries and the vaccines used in developed countries. This relates primarily to the relatively expensive combination vaccines that are increasingly used in developed countries. Moreover, pharmaceutical companies can generally earn a higher return on money invested in the development of drugs than money invested in developing vaccines.[15]

Another constraint to greater focus on the health conditions of the developing world until recently has been insufficient attention to them by some of the major national research institutions. The basic research that is conducted at places like the U.S. National Institutes of Health often sets a foundation for product development later by the for-profit manufacturers. The greater the attention that national research institutes in developed countries pay to high-burden problems of developing countries, the greater the likelihood that new products for them will eventually be developed.

Some of the above constraints are reflected in the extent to which drugs have been developed to address diseases that most affect poor people in developing countries. A study of drugs that were approved for marketing showed that between 1975 and 1999, for example, there were 1393 new chemicals approved but only about 3% were relevant to infectious and parasitic diseases that are the most significant burdens of disease in low-income countries. The same study looked at the number of new drugs approved for every million DALYs lost and found that two to three times more drugs were produced for every million DALYs lost to diseases of the developed world, rather than diseases of the developing world.[16] Over the same period, only about 1% of the drugs approved concerned the "neglected tropical diseases" and only about 0.2% concerned TB.[16]

A study of 20 major pharmaceutical manufacturers found that several of the firms spent less than 1% of their research and development budget the previous fiscal year on TB, malaria, African trypanosomiasis, Chagas' disease, and leishmaniasis. Only malaria appears to be an area of infectious diseases which is attracting any substantial investment from pharmaceutical manufacturers. Yet, the amount of investment by drug companies in asthma drugs was about 20 times the amount they invested in malaria drugs.

Moreover, about 90% of expenditure on research and development on health is oriented toward the diseases of the developed world and only about 10% toward the diseases of the developing world. The Global Forum for Health Research called this the "10/90 gap."[17,18]

ENHANCING NEW PRODUCT DEVELOPMENT

We have seen that gaps in the development of diagnostics, drugs, vaccines, and medical devices that can serve the needs of the developing world reflect failures of the market. In general, the public sector tries to reduce its risks by waiting for such products to be developed by the private sector. However, the private sector generally believes that it is too risky to produce products that are expensive to develop and for which an adequate return on investment can not be assured. Is it possible to change the market for these products? Can one reduce the cost of product research and development to the point where the private for-profit sector might be interested in such products? What other steps can be taken to speed product development?

Push Mechanisms

There are a number of steps that could encourage a larger share of research and development to focus on the needs of the developing world. Some of these are shown in Figure 16-1, which depicts push and pull mechanisms and where in the product development cycle they have the most impact.

One type of effort is called "push mechanisms." These refer to mechanisms meant to encourage product development by helping to "reduce the risks and costs of investments."[15] Push mechanisms could include:

- Direct financing—government financing or carrying out of research activities needed to develop a product
- Performing or facilitating clinical trials—this could include government measures to make it easier to carry out clinical trials for the product and to help with the ethical issues involved in such trials
- Tax credits for research and development—governments can lower the cost to firms of research and

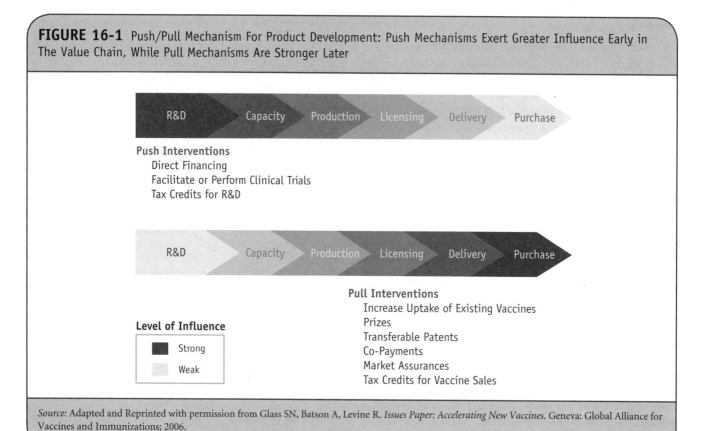

FIGURE 16-1 Push/Pull Mechanism For Product Development: Push Mechanisms Exert Greater Influence Early in The Value Chain, While Pull Mechanisms Are Stronger Later

Source: Adapted and Reprinted with permission from Glass SN, Batson A, Levine R. *Issues Paper: Accelerating New Vaccines.* Geneva: Global Alliance for Vaccines and Immunizations; 2006.

development by giving them credits against their taxes for certain investments[15]

These push mechanisms operate on the early stages of product development. Such mechanisms have been used successfully before. In addition, they can reduce risk and, thereby, encourage investment in product development. The disadvantage of push mechanisms, however, is that there is no guarantee that they will produce a product. Even if a product is developed, it may not be the best one and product developers will then not produce what might have been better candidates. Furthermore, when the money is spent on push mechanisms it is gone whether or not a product has been developed.[15]

Some of the direct financing and facilitation of clinical trials could be done through programs like the U.S. National Institutes of Health or similar institutes in other countries. Additional money could also be channeled, for example, to the Special Program for Research and Training in Tropical Diseases that is sponsored by WHO, the United Nations Development Program, and the World Bank.[19] Some of the financing of the Bill & Melinda Gates Foundation, like that for the Grand Challenges, is meant to push new product development.

In conjunction with these efforts, it is important to strengthen the links between researchers in developed and developing counties. The links can also be enhanced between researchers in developing countries. The aim of these efforts would be to attract more research money to institutions within the developing countries that are engaged in research and development on the most important burdens of disease in low- and middle-income countries. A number of developing countries, especially India, China, Brazil, South Africa, Mexico, Indonesia, and Cuba, have the ability to carry out basic research and to develop products that emanate from that research.[20]

It is also important to comment on some aspects of governmental regulation of pharmaceutical and vaccine development. Regulation is necessary but it is also an important part of the costs of research and development. By arranging to speed drug approvals and harmonize approval processes across countries, the costs of research and development can be reduced to provide some incentives to manufacturers. Granting fast track approval for generic AIDS drugs, for example, *has* encouraged the development of such drugs.[16]

Pull Mechanisms

There are a number of mechanisms that are intended to help "assure a future return in the event that a product is produced." These are called pull mechanisms.[15,19] Some of the most important pull mechanisms include:

- Increasing the uptake of existing vaccines—using public funds to increase the use of vaccines that have not been taken up sufficiently, such as the vaccines for Hib and hepatitis B
- Prizes—offering monetary rewards to those firms that develop desired products
- Transferable patents—in exchange for the development of the desired product, providing the manufacturer with the right to extend a patent on another of their products or patents in developed world markets on the new product
- Co-payments—governments can provide the manufacturer with a payment for every product sold
- Market assurances—the public sector can promise to buy the products if they are produced
- Tax credits for vaccine sales—governments can offer tax credits for products that are sold[15]

From the point of view of the public sector, pull mechanisms have the advantage of providing funding only when desired products have been developed. However, there is little experience with such mechanisms to date. Governments and the private sector have to agree early on what such arrangements would be for any product, and neither party might be satisfied with these arrangements when products do emerge.[15]

Related to the pull mechanisms noted above, we should note that the government of the United Kingdom has developed a proposal for an "International Finance Facility." In this case, bonds would be sold to raise money for health and development projects and the flows from development assistance from developed countries would help to retire the bond debt. This would help to raise funds that could be available over a multi-year period, which is often a problem for development assistance, much of which can only be committed on a 1 year at a time basis. Such a fund is meant to signal to the private sector that financing is available to pay for needed products and, thereby, help to encourage product development.[21]

A mechanism that has been used for vaccines for some time and more recently for AIDS drugs is called "tiered pricing." This is a mechanism by which a firm charges different prices in different markets. The idea behind tiered pricing is that a firm can charge enough to make a profit in developed country markets to offset the fact that the products will not make a profit in developing country markets. The profits from one market could cross-subsidize the sales at reduced prices in other markets. This is being practiced now for some drugs for which there is a global market. However, tiered pricing is not likely to work effectively for products that are needed exclusively in the developing world because the basis for cross-subsidizing will not exist.[16] Efforts are now being proposed to develop tiered pricing mechanisms for products as soon as they are available, rather than wait until many years after their development, as has been the case until now.[22]

In addition, as discussed in Chapter 15, considerable hope is being put into the role that public-private partnerships can play in encouraging the development of the diagnostics, drugs, vaccines, and medical devices that could have a significant impact on the health of the poor in low- and middle-income countries. As indicated earlier, many of these efforts are organized around the search for new products for particular diseases, such as HIV, TB, and malaria. These public-private partnerships are also referred to as product development partnerships (PDP) and are organized on a not-for-profit basis. They aim to attract private, public, and philanthropic funds to invest in needed research and development, tapping the strengths of the private sector in product development as they do so. There are now PDPs for a large number of vaccines and drugs, including, for example, TB and malaria.

Meeting product development goals will probably require a combination of the above efforts. First, they can start with a greater focus by developed country research institutions on the problems of the developing world and greater networking of research institutions in the developing world. This can help encourage product development, with other push mechanisms. At the same time, it will be important to change the market and perceptions of the market for needed products through "pull" mechanisms that can ensure that money will be available for products it they are developed. Third, the public and private sectors can collaborate with each other, bringing complementary skills and financing to the partnership. Over the next several years, evidence should emerge which will allow one to evaluate the effectiveness of PDPs and the push and pull mechanisms that are discussed above.

CASE STUDIES

Three case studies follow. The first concerns the effort to develop a vaccine for hookworm. It centers on a public-private product development partnership that is being funded by the Bill & Melinda Gates Foundation. This is especially significant, given the burden of disease from hookworm, the fact that treatment has to be repeated every 6 months, and the fact there is no vaccine at the moment for any of the neglected tropical diseases. The second case concerns efforts to ensure that a relatively new vaccine against pneumonia is used as widely as possible and as soon as possible in developing countries. This is especially important given the extent of pneumonia deaths and the long time it has taken historically to expand the use of vaccines from the developed to the developing world. The last case concerns efforts to spread the use of relatively new vaccines for Hib and hepatitis B in Chile and The Gambia. This case also highlights the measures that can be taken to speed the uptake of both existing and new vaccines.

The Human Hookworm Vaccine Initiative

Background

The neglected tropical diseases are a group of chronic disabling and poverty-promoting conditions that affect the world's poorest people in rural areas of low-income countries. They include, among other diseases, a group of helminth infections, of which some of the most important are ascariasis, hookworm, trichuriasis, dracunculiasis (guinea worm), lymphatic filariasis (elephantiasis), and onchocerciasis (river blindness). The neglected tropical diseases cause human suffering and impede economic development either because of their disfiguring consequences or through their impact on child health and development, maternal health and pregnancy outcome, and worker productivity. The combined disease burden of the neglected tropical diseases is equivalent to HIV/AIDS, malaria, or tuberculosis, and their economic impact results in losses of tens of billions of dollars annually.

Despite their enormous health and economic importance, there has been little interest in developing new drugs or vaccines for the neglected tropical diseases. A major reason for this situation is the absence of any commercial market for products related to these diseases because they affect almost exclusively the world's three billion people who live on less than $2 per day. As a result, many of the drugs in use for the neglected tropical diseases were first developed during the early or middle parts of the 20th century and are highly toxic or difficult to administer in resource poor settings.

Similarly, there are no licensed vaccines available for the neglected tropical diseases, even though there have been significant basic research efforts related to their development over the last 20 years.

Human hookworm infection is an example of a neglected tropical disease that would benefit from the development of a vaccine. Hookworm affects an estimated 600 million people, almost all of them impoverished individuals living in rural areas of Sub-Saharan Africa, Southeast Asia, and tropical regions of the Americas. The infection is caused by nematode parasites that attach to the inside of the intestine and ingest host blood. When individuals are infected with large numbers of hookworms, blood loss is sufficient to cause iron deficiency, iron-deficiency anemia, and protein deficiency. This is especially a problem for young children and pregnant women.

There are inexpensive drugs available to treat human hookworm infection. The two major drugs for hookworm are albendazole and mebendazole, which are typically administered to school-aged children in mass treatment programs, sometimes referred to as "de-worming" programs. However, de-worming does not prevent hookworm reinfection, which can occur within 4–12 months following treatment in areas of high transmission. Moreover, there is evidence that the efficacy of drugs against hookworm diminishes with increasing use and there is concern that the hookworm parasites are becoming resistant to them. These concerns have prompted interest in controlling the infection through vaccination.

The Intervention

The Human Hookworm Vaccine Initiative (HHVI) was established at the Sabin Vaccine Institute in Washington, DC, USA, in 2000 with major funding from the Bill & Melinda Gates Foundation. The HHVI is comprised of a network of laboratories and clinical trial sites, with program management, quality assurance, and regulatory affairs units based at the Sabin Vaccine Institute. Two different vaccines are under development—each building on well-established academic research and development efforts based at The George Washington University (Washington, DC) and the Queensland Institute of Medical Research (QIMR, Brisbane, Australia), respectively. Eventually, the two vaccines will be reformulated and combined into a single human hookworm vaccine.

Critical to the success of the HHVI is the concept that it is possible to develop and test vaccines in non-profit and academic settings. This required the purchase and operation of special equipment and the recruitment of scientists with industrial manufacturing experience, as well as experts in quality control, quality assurance, and documentation. The process development and quality control facilities for the HHVI are located at The George Washington University, near the Sabin Vaccine Institute.

In 2005, the HHVI sponsored the development of its first vaccine. In 2006, the vaccine completed the first phase of trials meant to test safety and whether or not the vaccine produces an immune response. Efforts will follow to conduct a series of trials to test safety and immune response in hookworm-infected individuals living in Brazil. This will be done in collaboration with the Oswaldo Cruz Foundation (FIOCRUZ), a Brazilian governmental organization that combines research and public health activities. Process development and manufacture of a second hookworm vaccine is scheduled to begin in 2007.

Impact

To ensure that any safe and effective vaccine that might be developed will be distributed to the people who need it, the HHVI is working with public sector vaccine manufacturers in countries where hookworm infection is endemic. Initially, the HHVI is working with the non-profit and state-owned Instituto Butantan in Sao Paulo, Brazil, to ultimately ensure a supply of locally made and affordable hookworm vaccine.

Another component of the HHVI's global access plan is to work out strategies for administering the vaccine in settings where de-worming is currently practiced. For most of the developing world, de-worming is conducted in schools because school children on average harbor the greatest numbers of intestinal worms. A human hookworm vaccine will likely be administered following de-worming in a strategy of vaccine-linked chemotherapy. Additional efforts are underway to conduct cost-effectiveness analyses in order to compare hookworm vaccination with de-worming.

Lessons Learned

Several important and useful lessons have been learned so far from the HHVI experience, including:

- It is feasible to produce and test vaccines in the non-profit sector through a Product Development Partnership
- Achieving these goals, however, requires very tight program management for maintaining timelines and achieving milestones
- There are important advantages to cooperating with scientifically capable developing countries for both manufacture and clinical testing of new products and looking to these countries as a means to initiate global access for neglected tropical disease vaccines
- There is a need to consider novel healthcare delivery systems, such as schools, to ensure that products will be accessible to the populations who need them the most

PneumoADIP

Background

The Pneumococcal Vaccines Accelerated Development and Introduction Plan (PneumoADIP) was launched in June 2003 by the Global Alliance for Vaccines and Immunization. PneumoADIP represents an innovative approach to accelerating access to pneumococcal vaccines in developing countries. The initiative is based at the Johns Hopkins Bloomberg School of Public Health in Baltimore, Maryland. It is supported by a $30 million grant from the GAVI Alliance. Through a combination of translational research, partnership with the private sector, and efforts to secure financing for the vaccine, this initiative aims to save hundreds of thousands of children's lives annually by reducing the time it would normally take to introduce life-saving pneumococcal vaccines.

According to the estimates of the World Health Organization, pneumococcal infections kill up to one million children who are younger than five years every year. This is more than any other vaccine-preventable infection, including measles.[23] Pneumococcal bacteria are also the most severe cause of bacterial meningitis worldwide, a disease that disables survivors, creating long-term education and economic consequences for people of all ages.[24,25] More than 90 strains (serotypes) of pneumococcus bacteria exist, of which 7 to 11 serotypes are most common and cause most disease in children.[4] Children with HIV/AIDS are 20 to 40 times more likely to get pneumococcal disease than children without HIV/AIDS.[26,27] Antibiotic resistance[28–30] and HIV increase the urgency of expanding the uptake of pneumococcal vaccine.

Unlike HIV and malaria, effective vaccines for the prevention of pneumococcal infections are currently available.[31] However, historically the use of new vaccines in developing countries takes 15 to 20 years after the actual introduction of the vaccine in the developed world. The long delays in using "new" vaccines in the developing world is partly a result of a vicious cycle of uncertain demand for the new vaccine from developing countries, leading to limited supply by the manufacturers, which keeps prices high and, in turn keeps these vaccines away from the people who need them.

The Intervention

In light of these constraints to satisfactory supply of vaccines at affordable prices, PneumoADIP is designed to:

- Engage in research that can help to determine the importance of pneumococcal infections in different settings
- Help countries to understand the importance of vaccines for the health of their own people

- Assist countries in financing the use of pneumo-coccus vaccines as they become more interested in adopting them

PneumoADIP refers to these measures as steps to establish the value, communicate the value, and deliver the value of pneumococcal vaccines.

To establish the value of the vaccine, PneumoADIP is supporting research and surveillance to help provide decision makers in developing countries with data on the burden of penumococcal disease and efficacy of the pneumococcal vaccine at a local and regional level. This evidence-based approach will help facilitate informed decision-making and provide leaders with the information necessary to justify dedicating resources to combating pneumococcal disease with vaccines.

Coordinated and proactive communications efforts are already succeeding in raising the profile of pneumococcal disease and increasing the awareness of the associated burden and existence of life-saving vaccines in a number of developing countries. PneumoADIP continues its efforts to communicate the value of pneumococcal vaccines by working with its partners to make information about pneumococcal disease accessible to all audiences and to further highlight the economic benefits of investing in prevention of this disease through immunization.

Delivering the value of the vaccine requires that the financing and delivery system and the vaccine itself are available to translate demand into actual vaccination. To this end, PneumoADIP has worked with a variety of stakeholders to develop and test an innovative demand forecasting model. The aim of this strategy is to work with industry willing to supply vaccine, countries willing to introduce it, and donors/countries willing to finance these vaccination programs to find agreed solutions to ensuring access to sufficient supplies of affordable vaccines.

Impact

In collaboration with the World Health Organization, PnuemoADIP has helped to establish rigorous, systemic methods for estimating the global, regional, and local burden of pneumococcal disease. The pneumococcal surveillance networks are collecting standardized pneumococcal disease data and communicating their local data to regional network partners that include surveillance sites, ministries of health, multilateral organizations, and donors supporting vaccination. New networks continue to be established and expand pneumococcal disease surveillance around the world. Additionally, 20 small grants were awarded to support local

researchers in 17 developing countries to establish and communicate the burden of pneumococcal disease and the value of vaccination.

Since PneumoADIP has been in operation, pneumococcal disease has moved up the media agenda. PneumoADIP documented a seven-fold increase in media coverage of pneumococcal disease and vaccine issues, driven in large part by their media outreach efforts. 45% of these articles were in the developing world and PneumoADIP was responsible for generating 36% of these. Additionally, 13% of the coverage was related to a pneumococcal conjugate vaccine trial in The Gambia, further demonstrating the effectiveness of the PneumoADIP campaign to communicate effectively about scientific matters. The global information campaign on pneumococcal vaccines was successful in achieving its aim to raise awareness of pneumococcal disease as a leading cause of death in children and the need for an effective pneumococcal vaccine in the developing world.

Lessons Learned

The PneumoADIP strategy is a departure from previous public-sector efforts to accelerate the introduction of vaccines in developing countries. It focuses on reducing the uncertainty of demand for vaccines by engaging and communicating with national and international decision makers even before the research to establish the potential benefit of these vaccines is complete. This strategy recognizes that accelerated accessibility to vaccines requires that stakeholders must be willing to assume some risks that industry typically assumes in high-income countries so that time is not lost in the event that the research supports the widespread use of these vaccines. The strategic demand forecasting model helps each stakeholder to understand the size and timing of their potential commitments. By bringing together multiple stakeholders and communicating as early in the vaccine development process as possible, this strategy has the potential to successfully influence planning of the production capacity for the vaccine, availability of the vaccine, affordable pricing of the product, and therefore, increased use of the vaccine in developing countries.

Preventing Hib Disease in Chile and The Gambia

Background

Although the microbe *Haemophilus influenzae* type b (Hib) causes 450,000 deaths worldwide each year, it has avoided the notoriety of other major killers. Hib disease occurs in many invasive forms such as meningitis, pneumonia, and bacteremia. Hib meningitis is particularly lethal, killing 20–40%

of the children who get it, and leaving many survivors with lasting impairments such as deafness or mental retardation.[32] Children under the age of 5 are most susceptible to Hib disease—particularly when they are between 6 to 11 months—and 23 per 100,000 develop Hib meningitis every year. Infection and fatality rates are highest in Sub-Saharan Africa.

Many low- and middle-income countries have not been able to afford Hib vaccines, available since the late 1980s, unlike industrialized nations where Hib has been dramatically reduced. However, the successful experience of two very different countries—Chile and The Gambia—has persuaded other developing countries to introduce the vaccine. In Chile, a study in the late 1980s revealed the extent of Hib meningitis in Santiago: 32 per 100,000 among infants up to 5 months and 63 per 100,000 among infants aged 6 to 11 months.[33,34] The disease was fatal for 16% of Hib cases. In The Gambia, surveillance of hospitals in the western region in the 1990s showed that more than 200 children per 100,000 had Hib meningitis each year.[35]

The Intervention

Chile is a middle-income country with largely modern infrastructure, where 95% of infants receive routine vaccines. Nonetheless, Hib vaccines were not previously included because of their cost. Research done in the 1980s, however, showing the prevalence of Hib disease, persuaded the government to launch a program to further explore the efficacy of the vaccine. Hib immunization was provided at 36 health centers and their results compared with other centers where no Hib inoculations were provided. The vaccine, donated by Aventis Pasteur, was injected along with the usual DTP antigens in the same syringe. The dramatic results of this study convinced the government to include Hib in the routine immunization program, starting in 1996.

The Gambia is among the world's poorest countries, with a far less developed infrastructure than Chile. Although immunization coverage of 85% is higher than in many parts of Africa,[32] infant mortality in The Gambia remains high. However, once the government recognized the severity of the Hib problem through the 1990s survey, it began a large, controlled trial of the Hib vaccine in 1993. Here too, Aventis Pasteur donated the vaccine, and WHO, UNICEF, USAID, and other organizations supported the program. The government improved its vaccine cold chain with the use of solar power, decentralizing vaccine storage and healthcare management to improve supply. As in Chile, the results were impressive, and in 1997, a 5-year program of immunization and surveillance was launched in the western region.

The Impact

Among children at Chile's health centers who received the vaccine, Hib meningitis was reduced by 91%, and pneumonia and other forms of Hib disease by 80%, compared to the children in the DTP-only centers.[36] In The Gambia, the 5-year program yielded equally remarkable results. Within the first year, the number of children developing Hib meningitis dropped almost tenfold, from 200 per 100,000 to 21 per 100,000. In the last 2 years of the study, there were only 2 cases.

Costs and Benefits

The government of Chile paid $3.39 million for the combined DTP-Hib vaccine, which is 23% of the total immunization budget. The price per Hib dose has declined from $15 in 1996 to $3 today,[37] and the government saves an estimated $78 for every case of Hib prevented. In The Gambia, the 5-year program was made possible by Aventis Pasteur's donation of Hib vaccines. Financial support from the Vaccine Fund and the Global Alliance for Vaccines and Immunization (GAVI) has helped sustain the program through 2008.

Lessons Learned

The governments of Chile and The Gambia both found ways of overcoming the obstacle of cost, which remains the main impediment to adoption of the vaccine by other countries. The success of the program in The Gambia demonstrated the effectiveness of the vaccine in a country where the health system is severely underfunded at every level. Other developing countries have since adopted the Hib vaccine, often with the help of GAVI or PAHO.

However, it is not yet known whether some other developing countries, where Hib is a major problem, will introduce the vaccine. The answer depends in part on how and whether financing is made available, and on how expensive the vaccine will be over the medium term. The effects on regions without the vaccine is still undocumented, and it remains to be seen whether the positive experiences now being consolidated in Latin America and the Caribbean, and parts of Africa, will be shared elsewhere. Another unknown element lies in the spread of antibiotic-resistant strains of the Hib microbe, complicating treatment of the disease in the future.

MAIN MESSAGES

Science and technology have the potential to make major contributions to the development of diagnostics, vaccines, drugs, and medical devices that can help address the highest burdens of disease in low- and middle-income countries. Progress in scientific areas like the sequencing of genes, information technology, chemistry, robotics, and biotechnology can help, for example, to engineer mosquitoes that will not carry disease, discover new drugs much more rapidly than before, and develop less expensive and more effective vaccines.

In a more "ideal" world, diagnostics, vaccines, drugs, and medical devices would be appropriate to the needs of the health conditions that cause the largest burden of disease in low- and middle-income countries. They would also be appropriate to the ability of countries to manage their health systems. If these were the case, they would be affordable by low-income patients and countries that are unable to spend much on health. They would also be heat stable, not require refrigeration, and be easy to store and transport. The number of pills needed to cure a disease would be few and require a short course of therapy. Ideal vaccines would be a combination of many of the vaccines that exist today, so that children would need fewer vaccinations to be "fully covered." Given the risks of injections being unsafe, the "delivery devices" for vaccines would increasingly rely on non-invasive means, such as nasal sprays, skin patches, or perhaps, vaccines that are edible.

Unfortunately, the needed advances are unlikely to come about on their own. This is largely a reflection of the fact that the for-profit sector has historically been a major developer of diagnostics, vaccines, and drugs but does not believe that the market for these products in the developing world is sufficient to give it an adequate return on its investment. In addition, the public sector is risk averse and would prefer to purchase a product developed by the private sector rather than to try to develop these products itself. The failure of the market is reflected, as an example, in the very small number of drugs that have been developed over the last 20 years to address the main burdens of disease among the poor in low- and middle-income countries. Moreover, vaccine development is constrained by the need for substantial investments, limited capacity in an industry with a very small number of producers, and an increasing divergence between the vaccines used in developed countries and those used in developing countries.

Overcoming these market failures and encouraging the development of the desired products will probably require a series of measures. Some of these can be "push mechanisms" that are meant to lower the cost of research and development for the private sector. These could include, for example, direct financing by government of research; the facilitation by government of clinical trials; or, government's offering tax credits for research and development. Push mechanisms do lower the cost of research and development but they provide no certainty that the desired product will be produced.

Another set of efforts could focus on "pull mechanisms," which are intended to help assure a satisfactory return to investors in the event that a product is produced. These mechanisms could include increasing the uptake of existing vaccines; prizes; transferable patents; co-payments; market assurances; and, tax credits for vaccine sales. Pull mechanisms have the advantage of providing funding only when the desired product is available. However, they have the disadvantage of having to be negotiated far in advance of product availability and parties may not be satisfied with the terms of their agreement at the time in the future when the products are available.

A mechanism already in use for vaccines and for AIDS drugs is tiered pricing. This is an arrangement in which products are sold at different prices in different markets, with the principle being that the price of sales in developed country markets will help defray the low cost of the products in developing country markets. However, these arrangements have generally been put in place only when products were established and efforts are now underway to try to put them in place at the early stages of a product's life.

Considerable hope for new product development is being placed in public-private product development partnerships, such as the International AIDS Vaccine Initiative, the Global Alliance for TB Drug Development, and the Medicines for Malaria Venture. The aim of these ventures is to bring the strengths of the public and private sector together in complementary ways that can spur the development of new products. The chapter suggests in its case studies on hookworm vaccine, pneumococcal vaccines, and the dissemination of Hib and hepatitis B vaccines in Chile and The Gambia, some steps that can be taken both to develop products that are needed and to see that they are widely used once they are developed.

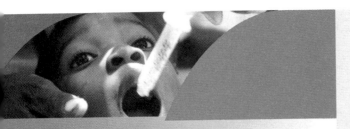

Study Questions

1. What are some of the "ideal" properties that diagnostics, vaccines, and drugs should have to be most appropriate to the health and health system needs of low- and middle-income countries?

2. What is the extent to which some of the available vaccines for the six basic antigens and the vaccination schedule for them meet the "ideal"?

3. What are the health conditions and risk factors that deserve additional attention from science and technology? Why have you chosen those conditions and risk factors?

4. What are some of the specific gaps in diagnostics, drugs, vaccines, and other medical equipment that could most improve global health if filled?

5. What have been some of the major constraints to the development of drugs and vaccines that could better meet health needs in low- and middle-income countries?

6. Why does only 10% of all research expenditure worldwide focus on the diseases that most affect the poor in the developing world? What is the 10/90 research gap?

7. What steps can be taken to overcome those constraints? What are the roles in this of publicly supported research? What are the roles of public-private partnerships for health?

8. What "push" and "pull" mechanisms could most help to encourage the development of new diagnostics, drugs, and vaccines?

9. What lessons do the case studies on hookworm and pneumococcal vaccine suggest for the discovery of other drugs and vaccines?

10. If you were the Bill & Melinda Gates Foundation, how would you spend money on research and development of new products for global health? Why?

REFERENCES

1. UNAIDS. Botswana Country Profile. Available at: http://www.unaids.org/en/Regions_Countries/Countries/botswana.asp. Accessed March 9, 2007.

2. Birn AE. Gates's grandest challenge: transcending technology as public health ideology. *Lancet*. 2005;366(9484):514–519.

3. UNICEF. Facts for Life. Available at: http://www.unicef.org/ffl/pdf/factsforlife-en-part7.pdf. Accessed October 27, 2006.

4. Centers for Disease Control and Prevention. BCG Vaccine. Available at: http://www.cdc.gov/nchstp/tb/pubs/tbfactsheets/250120.htm. Accessed October 27, 2006.

5. Global Alliance for TB Drug Development. New TB Drugs Urgently Needed to Replace Treatment from the 1960s. Second Gates Grant to TB Alliance Quadruples Initial Support. Available at: http://www.tballiance.org/gates.asp. Accessed October 27, 2006.

6. Roll Back Malaria. Facts on ACTs (Artemisinin-based Combination Therapies): January 2006 update. Available at: http://www.rbm.who.int/malariacmc_upload/0/000/015/364/RBMInfosheet_9.htm. Accessed April 13, 2007.

7. Fauci AS. Infectious diseases: considerations for the 21st century. *Clin Infect Dis*. 2001;32(5):675–685.

8. World Health Organization. Genomics and World Health: A Report of the Advisory Committee on Health Research. Available at: http://whqlibdoc.who.int/hq/2002/a74580.pdf. Accessed October 27, 2006.

9. Weatherall D, Greenwood B, Chee HL, Wasi P. Science and technology for disease control: past, present, and future. In: Jamison DT, Breman JG, Measham AR, et al., eds. *Disease Control Priorities in Developing Countries*. 2nd ed. New York: Oxford University Press; 2006:127.

10. Weatherall D, Greenwood B, Chee HL, Wasi P. Science and technology for disease control: past, present, and future. In: Jamison DT, Breman JG, Measham AR, et al., eds. *Disease Control Priorities in Developing Countries*. 2nd ed. New York: Oxford University Press; 2006:132.

11. Daar AS, Thorsteinsdottir H, Martin DK, Smith AC, Nast S, Singer PA. Top ten biotechnologies for improving health in developing countries. *Nat Genet*. 2002;32(2):229–232.

12. The Bill & Melinda Gates Foundation. Fourteen Grand Challenges in Global Health Announced in $200 Million Initiative. Available at: http://www.gatesfoundation.org/GlobalHealth/BreakthroughScience/GrandChallenges/Announcements/Announce-031016.htm. Accessed October 4, 2006.

13. The Bill & Melinda Gates Foundation. Grand Challenges in Global Health Initiative Selects 43 Groundbreaking Research Projects for More Than $436 Million in Funding. Available at: http://www.gatesfoundation.org/GlobalHealth/BreakthroughScience/GrandChallenges/Announcements/Announce-031016.htm. Accessed October 14, 2006.

14. Mahmoud A, Danzon PM, Barton JH, Mugerwa RD. Product development priorities. In: Jamison DT, Breman JG, Measham AR, et al., eds. *Disease Control Priorities in Developing Countries*. 2nd ed. New York: Oxford University Press; 2006:141.

15. Glass SN, Batson A, Levine R. *Issues Paper: Accelerating New Vaccines*. Geneva: Global Alliance for Vaccines and Immunizations; 2006.

16. Trouiller P, Torreele E, Olliaro P, et al. Drugs for neglected diseases: a failure of the market and a public health failure? *Trop Med Int Health*. 2001;6(11):945–951.

17. Bloom BR, Michaud CM, LaMontagne JR, Simonsen L. Priorities for global research and development interventions. In: Jamison DT, Breman JG, Measham AR, et al., eds. *Disease Control Priorities in Developing Countries*. 2nd ed. New York: Oxford University Press; 2006:106.

18. Global Forum for Health Research. Available at: http://www.globalforumhealth.org/Site/000__Home.php. Accessed October 27, 2006.

19. Reich MR. The global drug gap. *Science*. 2000;287(5460):1979–1981.

20. Morel CM, Acharya T, Broun D, et al. Health innovation networks to help developing countries address neglected diseases. *Science*. 2005;309(5733):401–404.

21. HM Treasury. International Issues. Available at: http://www.hm-treasury.gov.uk/documents/international_issues/int_gnd_intfinance.cfm. Accessed October 27, 2006.

22. Batson A, Glass SN, Levine R. *Differential Pricing of Vaccines, Draft Report*. Geneva: Global Alliance for Vaccines and Immunization; 2006.

23. World Health Organization. Pneumococcal vaccines. *Weekly Epidemiol Record*. 2003;14:110–119.

24. Goetghebuer T, West TE, Wermenbol V, et al. Outcome of meningitis caused by Streptococcus pneumoniae and *Haemophilus influenzae* type b in children in The Gambia. *Trop Med Int Health*. 2000;5(3):207–213.

25. Madhi SA, Petersen K, Madhi A, Wasas A, Klugman KP. Impact of human immunodeficiency virus type 1 on the disease spectrum of Streptococcus pneumoniae in South African children. *Pediatr Infect Dis J*. 2000;19(12):1141–1147.

26. Mao C, Harper M, McIntosh K, et al. Invasive pneumococcal infections in human immunodeficiency virus-infected children. *J Infect Dis*. 1996;173(4):870–876.

27. Klugman KP, Madhi SA, Huebner RE, Kohberger R, Mbelle N, Pierce N. A trial of a 9-valent pneumococcal conjugate vaccine in children with and those without HIV infection. *N Engl J Med*. 2003;349(14):1341–1348.

28. Baraff LJ, Lee SI, Schriger DL. Outcomes of bacterial meningitis in children: a meta-analysis. *Pediatr Infect Dis J*. 1993;12(5):389–394.

29. Klugman KP. Bacteriological evidence of antibiotic failure in pneumococcal lower respiratory tract infections. *Eur Respir J Suppl*. 2002;36:3s–8s.

30. Dagan R. Clinical significance of resistant organisms in otitis media. *Pediatr Infect Dis J*. 2000;19(4):378–382.

31. Whitney CG, Pickering LK. The potential of pneumococcal conjugate vaccines for children. *Pediatr Infect Dis J*. 2002;21(10):961–970.

32. Adegbola R, Usen SO, Weber MW, et al. *Haemophilus influenzae* type b meningitis in the gambia after the introduction of a conjugate vaccine. *Lancet*. 1999;354(9184):1091–1092.

33. Ferreccio C, Ortiz E, Astriza L, Rivera C, Clemens J, Levine MM. A population based retrospective assessment of the disease burden resulting from invasive *Haemophilis influenzae* in infants and young children in santiago, chile. *Ped Infect Dis J*. 1990;9(7):488–494.

34. Lagos R, Levine OS, Avendano A, Horwitz I, Levine MM. The introduction of routine *Haemophilus influenzae* type b conjugate vaccine in Chile: a framework for evauating new vaccines in newly industrializing countries. *Ped Infect Dis J*. 1998;(Supplement 17):S139–S148.

35. Mulholland K, Hilton S, Adegbola R, et al. Randomised trial of *Haemophilus influenzae* type b tetanus protein conjugate for prevention of penumonia and meningitis in gambian infants. *Lancet*. 1997;349:1191–1197.

36. Lagos R, Horwitz I, Toro J, Martin O, Bustamante P. Large scale post-licensure, selective vaccination of Chilean infants with PRP-T conjugate vaccine: practicality and effectiveness in preventing *Haemophilus influenzae* type b infections. *Ped Infect Dis J*. 1996;15:216–222.

37. Dr. Fernando Muniz of the Chilean Ministry of Health. In: *Development CfG*, ed; 2003.

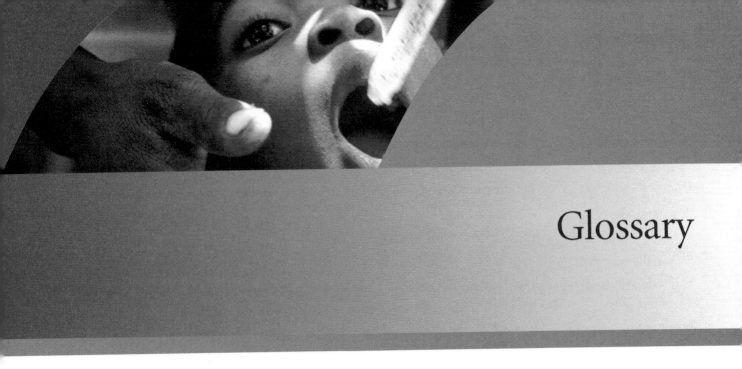

Glossary

Abortion	Premature expulsion or loss of embryo, which may be induced or spontaneous
Anemia	Low level of hemoglobin in the blood
Asphyxsia	A condition of severely deficient supply of oxygen to the body
Body Mass Index	Body weight in kilograms divided by height in meters squared
Cardiovascular Disease	A disease of the heart or blood vessels
Cataract	A clouding of the lens of the eye
Case Fatality Rate	The proportion of cases of a specified condition which is fatal within a specified period of time
Cesarean Delivery (Section)	The delivery of a fetus by surgical incision through the abdominal wall and uterus
Communicable Disease	Illnesses that are caused by a particular infectious agent and that spread directly or indirectly from people to people, from animals to animals, from animals to people, or from people to animals
Control	Reduction of disease incidence, prevalence, morbidity, or mortality to a locally acceptable level
Cost-effectiveness Analysis	In health, a tool for comparing the relative cost of two or more investments with the amount of health that can be purchased with those investments
Culture	A set of rules or standards shared by members of a society, which when acted upon by the members, produce behavior that falls within a range of variation that members consider proper and acceptable
Demographic Transition	The shift from high fertility and high mortality to low fertility and low mortality
Diabetes	Medical illness caused by too little insulin or poor response to insulin
Diarrhea	A condition in which the sufferer has frequent and watery or loose bowel movements

Disability	The temporary or long-term reduction in a person's capacity to function
Disability Adjusted Life Year	A composite measure of premature deaths and losses due to illnesses and disabilities in a population
Drug Resistance	The extent to which infectious and parasitic agents develop an ability to resist drug treatment
Eclampsia	A serious, life-threatening condition in late pregnancy in which very high blood pressure can cause a woman to have seizures
Elimination	Reduction of case transmission to a predetermined very low level
Epidemiologic Transition	A shift in the pattern of disease from largely communicable diseases to non-communicable diseases
Eradication	Termination of all transmission of infection by extermination of the infectious agent through surveillance or containment
Family Planning	The conscious effort of couples to regulate the number and spacing of births through artificial and natural methods of contraception. Family planning connotes conception control to avoid pregnancy and abortion, but it also includes efforts of couples to induce pregnancy
Female Genital Cutting (also called female circumcision and female genital mutilation)	A collective term for various traditional practices which are all related to the cutting of the female genital organs. Four different forms and grades of female genital cutting are usually distinguished
Gestational Diabetes	Diabetes that develops during pregnancy because of improper regulation of blood sugar. It usually goes away after delivery, but can increase the woman's risk of developing type II diabetes later
Global Health	Health problems, issues, and concerns that transcend national boundaries and may best be addressed by cooperative actions
Gross Domestic Product	The total market value of all the goods and services produced within a country during a specified period of time
Gross National Product	A measure of the incomes of residents of a country, including income they receive from abroad but subtracting similar payments made to those abroad
Health-adjusted Life Expectancy	A composite health indicator that measures the equivalent number of years in full health that a newborn can expect to live, based on current rates of ill health and mortality
Health System	The combination of resources, organization, and management that culminate in the delivery of health services to the population
Hemorrhage (related to pregnancy)	Significant and uncontrolled loss of blood, either internally or externally from the body. Antepartum (prenatal) hemorrhage occurs after the 20th week of gestation but before delivery of the baby. Postpartum hemorrhage is the loss of 500 ml or more of blood from the genital tract after delivery of the baby. Primary postpartum hemorrhage occurs in the first 24 hours after delivery
Hookworm	A parasite that lives in the small intestine of its host, which may be a mammal such as a dog, cat, or human
Hypertension	High blood pressure

Incidence Rate	The rate at which new cases of a disease occur in a population
Infant Mortality Rate	The number of deaths of infants under age 1 per 1000 live births in a given year
Injury	The result of an act that damages, harms, or hurts; unintentional or intentional damage to the body resulting from acute exposure to thermal, mechanical, electrical, or chemical energy or from the absence of such essentials as heat or oxygen
Life Expectancy at Birth	The average number of years a newborn baby could expect to live if current mortality trends were to continue for the rest of the newborn's life
Low birthweight	Birthweight less than 2500 grams
Malaria	A disease of humans caused by blood parasites of the species *Plasmodium falciparum*, vivax, ovale, or malariae and transmitted by anopheline mosquitoes
Maternal Death	The death of a woman while pregnant, during delivery, or within 42 days of delivery, irrespective of the duration and the site of pregnancy. The cause of death is always related to or aggravated by the pregnancy or its management; it does not include accidental or incidental causes.
Maternal Mortality Ratio	The number of women who die as a result of pregnancy and childbirth complications per 100,000 live births in a given year
Measles	A highly communicable disease characterized by fever, general malaise, sneezing, nasal congestion, a brassy cough, conjunctivitis, and an eruption over the entire body, caused by the rubeola virus
Morbidity	Illness
Mortality	Death
Neonatal Mortality Rate	Number of deaths to infants under 28 days of age in a given year per 1000 live births in that year
Neonatal Tetanus	A bacterial infection usually contracted by a puncture wound with a dirty object
Non-communicable Disease	Illnesses that are not spread by any infectious agent
Non-governmental Organization	A non-profit group or association organized outside of institutionalized political structures to realize particular social objectives, such as environmental protection, or serve particular constituencies, such as indigenous peoples
Obesity	Excessive body fat content
Obstetric Fistula	An injury in the birth canal that allows leakage from the bladder or rectum into the vagina, leaving a woman permanently incontinent, often leading to isolation and exclusion from the family and community
Overweight	Excess weight relative to height
Parasite	An animal or vegetable organism that lives on or in another and derives its nourishment therefrom
Pneumonia	An inflammation, usually caused by infection, involving the alveoli of the lungs
Poliomyelitis (Polio)	Infantile paralysis, a viral paralytic disease

Preeclampsia (previously called toxemia)	A hypertensive disorder of pregnancy. It is said to exist when a pregnant woman with gestational hypertension develops proteinuria. Originally, edema was considered part of the syndrome of preeclampsia, but presently the former two symptoms are sufficient for a diagnosis of preeclampsia
Prevalence	The number of people suffering from a certain condition over a specific time period. The "prevalence rate" is the share of the population, which is being measured, who have the condition
Public Health	The science and art of preventing disease; prolonging life; and promoting physical health and mental health and efficiency through organized community efforts toward a sanitary environment, control of community infections, education in hygiene, and the development of social machinery to ensure capacity in the community to maintain health
Pull Mechanism	Interventions that reduce the risks and costs of investments
Push Mechanism	Interventions that assure a future return in the event that a product is produced
Risk Factor	An aspect or personal behavior or lifestyle, an environmental exposure, or an inborn or inherited characteristic that, on the basis of epidemiologic evidence, is known to be associated with health related conditions
Sepsis	Infection in the blood
Sex Selective Abortion	The practice of aborting a fetus after a determination, usually by ultrasound but also rarely by amniocentesis or another procedure, that the fetus is an undesired sex, typically female
Sexually Transmitted Infections (STIs)	Diseases, also known as sexually-transmitted diseases (STDs), that are commonly transmitted between partners through some form of sexual activity, most commonly vaginal intercourse, oral sex, or anal sex
Society	A group of people who occupy a specific locality and share the same cultural traditions
Stroke	Temporary or permanent loss of the blood supply to the brain
Stunting	Failure to reach linear growth potential because of inadequate nutrition or poor health; two z-scores below the international reference
Under-five Child Mortality Rate	The annual number of deaths in children under five years, expressed as a rate per thousand live births, averaged over the previous 5 years
Undernutrition	Low weight-for-age; two z-scores below the international reference for weight-for-age
Unintentional Injury	That subset of injuries for which there is no evidence of predetermined intent
Uterine Prolapse	A condition in which the uterus protrudes into, and sometimes out of, the vagina
Wasting	Weight, measured in kilograms, divided by height in meters squared that is two z-scores below the international reference

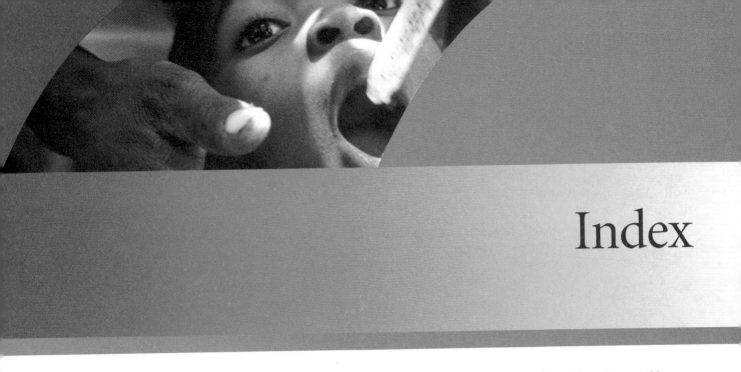

Index

Page numbers in italic denote figures; those followed by *n* denote footnotes, and those followed by *t* denote tables

total deaths by region, low- and middle-income
countries, 236, 237*t*
total deaths from road traffic accidents, by region,
low- and middle-income countries, 236, 237*t*
case studies
motorcycle helmet use in Taiwan, 240
rumble strips and speed bumps in Ghana, 240
childhood injuries, 236
costs and consequences of, 237–238
definition of, 300
emergency medical services, 239
future challenges, 240–241
importance of, 233–234
incidence of in mature young persons, 236–237
main messages, 241
risk factors for, 236–237
vignettes, 233
United Kingdom (UK), healthcare system, 76, 77
United Nations Agencies, 274
United Nations Development Program (UNDP), 157, 278,
288
United Nations Millennium Summit, 10
United Nations Population Fund (UNFPA), 158
United States
healthcare system, 77–78
lack of health insurance in, 73
Universal Declaration of Human Rights (UDHR), 60, 61
U.S. Commission for the Protection of Human Subjects of
Biomedical and Behavioral Research (1974), 65
U.S. National Institutes of Health, 286, 287
U.S. National Research Act, 65
USAID (United States Agency for International
Development), 157, 268–269, 268*t*, 274, 275
funding of ORT, 175
Uterine prolapse, definition of, 149*t*, 300

V

Vaccine
BCG, for TB, 200
constraints to development of, 287
design and manufacture of new and improved vaccines,
285–286
DTP-Hib vaccine, 292–293
Haemophilus influenza type b (Hib) vaccine, 180, 286
hepatitis B, 180, 223, 286
ideal characteristics of, 284*t*, 285
measles, 42, 43*f*
polio, 3, 263
rate of coverage in the poorest countries, 263

vignette:lack of malaria vaccine in Kenya, 283
Vaccine Fund, 270, 293
Vaccine-preventable diseases, 4, 182–183, 188
Vector control, 188
Venezuela, human rights issues in, 62
Vertical programs, 87–88
Veterans Administration, healthcare, 77, 78
Violence, against women, 152
Viral pathogens, 119*t*
H5N1 strain of the influenza virus, 206
Vitamin A deficiency, 133, 137, 138*t*
case study:reducing child mortality in Nepal through
vitamin A
background, 175–176
costs and benefits, 176–177
impact, 176
interventions, 176
lessons learned, 177
definition of, 130*t*
Vitamin A-Ivermectin integrated treatment approach
costs and benefits, 91
impact, 90–91
interventions, 90
introduction, 89–90
lessons learned, 91
Vitamin and mineral supplementation, 142
Volatile organic compounds (VOCs), 116*t*
Volcanoes, 251
Voluntary Health Services-India, 76*t*

W

Wars and conflicts, impact on child health, 174
Wasting
definition of, 130*t*, 300
rates of, 136
Water supply
improving, 188
integrating investment choices about water, sanitation,
and hygiene, 122–123, 123*t*
methods for improving water sources, 121–122
potential morbidity reduction from excellent water
supply, 122*t*
unsafe, 117, 118
Waterborne diseases, 117, 117*t*
Waterborne pathogens, 119*t*
Welcome Trust, 286
West, Keith, 176
West Nile virus
origination of, 3